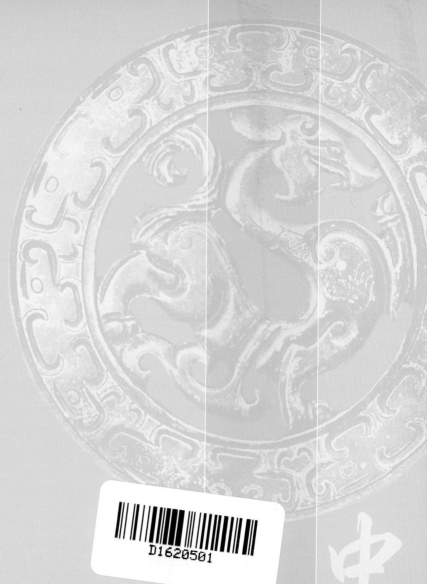

*The plant shown on the cover is Prunnus armeniaca L., whose dried mature, bitter seed is known as kǔ xìng rén*苦杏仁 *(Semen Armeniacae Amarum) in Chinese medicine, commonly known as bitter apricot seed. Kǔ xìng rén (Semen Armeniacae Amarum) can suppress cough, calm panting, and moisten the intestines to unblock the stool. In Chinese medicine, it is widely used in the treatment of respiratory diseases such as asthma and chronic obstructive pulmonary diseases (COPD).*

Project Editor: Liu Shui, Jiang Qian & Zeng Chun
Book Designer: Li Xi
Cover Designer: Li Xi
Typesetter: Wei Hong-bo

The Clinical Practice of Chinese Medicine

COPD & Asthma

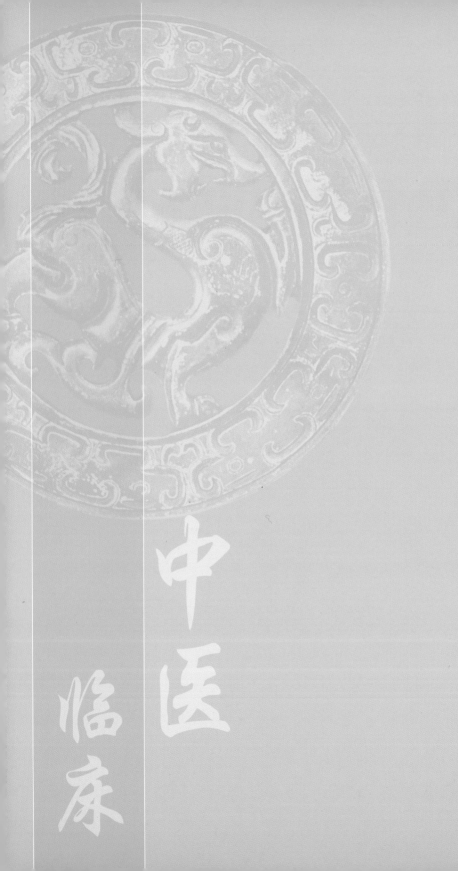

The Clinical Practice of Chinese Medicine

COPD & Asthma

Liu Wei-sheng
Master of the National Master and Apprentice Education Program, Professor of Chinese Internal Medicine, Division of Respiratory & Oncology, the Second Teaching Hospital of Guangzhou University of CM

Lin Lin
Professor of Chinese Internal Medicine, Director of Department of Respiratory, the Second Teaching Hospital of Guangzhou University of CM

Contributors

He De-ping
Associate Chief Physician, M.S. TCM

Huang Dong-hui
Associate Chief Physician, M.S. TCM

Lin Yan-zhao
Associate Chief Physician, M.S. TCM

Xu Yin-ji
Associate Chief Physician, M.S. TCM

Han Yun
Chief Physician, M.S. TCM

Wu Lei
Resident, M.S. TCM

Feng Wei-bin
Professor of Chinese Internal Medicine, Chief Physician

Translator-in-Chief
Zhang Qing-rong, Professor of Chinese Medicine, Chief Physician

Translators
Hui Shi-yang, M.S. TCM **Ma Jin**, M.S. TCM **Lu Jian**, M.S. TCM
Yi Qiu-xia, M.S. TCM **Zhu Hui**, Ph.D. TCM

Edited by **Andrea Kurts**, L.Ac.

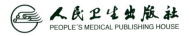
PEOPLE'S MEDICAL PUBLISHING HOUSE

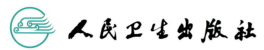

PMPH PEOPLE'S MEDICAL PUBLISHING HOUSE

Website: http://www.pmph.com

Book Title: The Clinical Practice of Chinese Medicine: **COPD & Asthma**
中医临床实用系列：慢性阻塞性肺疾病与哮喘

Copyright © 2007 by People's Medical Publishing House. All rights reserved. No part of this publication may be reproduced, stored in a database or retrieval system, or transmitted in any form or by any electronic, mechanical, photocopy, or other recording means, without the prior written permission of the publisher.

Contact address: Bldg 3, 3 Qu, Fang Qun Yuan, Fang Zhuang, Beijing 100078, P. R. China, phone/fax: 86 10 6761 7315, E-mail: pmph@pmph.com

---

Disclaimer

This book is for educational and reference purposes only. In view of the possibility of human error or changes in medical science, neither the author, editor nor the publisher nor any other party who has been involved in the preparation or publication of this work guarantees that the information contained herein is in every respect accurate or complete. The medicinal therapy and treatment techniques presented in this book are provided for the purpose of reference only. If readers wish to attempt any of the techniques or utilize any of the medicinal therapies contained in this book, the publisher assumes no responsibility for any such actions.

It is the responsibility of the readers to understand and adhere to local laws and regulations concerning the practice of these techniques and methods. The authors, editors and publishers disclaim all responsibility for any liability, loss, injury, or damage incurred as a consequence, directly or indirectly, of the use and application of any of the contents of this book.

First published: 2007
ISBN: 978-7-117-09112-1/R·9113

Cataloguing in Publication Data:
A catalog record for this book is available from the CIP-Database China.

Printed in P.R. China

About the Authors

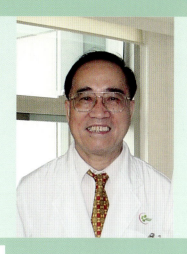

刘伟胜　教授

    Professor **Liu Wei-sheng** is a chief physician, professor, state-approved Doctoral Supervisor, and academic leader of the Tumor Department at the Second Teaching Hospital of the Guangzhou University of Chinese Medicine (also known as Guangdong Provincial Hospital of TCM). He is also a standing member of the following associations: the Committee of Chinese Medicine Oncology Association, the Anticancer Society of the Oncology Traditional Medicine Board of China, and the Committee of National Chinese Medicine. Professor Liu is also a lifelong member of the Guangdong Provincial Chinese Medicine and Pharmacological Society, the honorary director of the Respiratory Specialty Board of the Guangdong Provincial Chinese Medicine Association, the vice-director of the Oncology Specialty Board of the Guangdong Provincial Chinese Medicine Association, an expert on the Council for Drug Examination and Appraisal under the State Food and Drug Administration, and an expert on the Council for Drug Examination and Appraisal of the board of the Guangdong Provincial Food and Drug Administration. Professor Liu is one of the famous doctors in Guangdong province, and one of the national veteran Chinese medical experts in the second group appointed by the State Ministry of Personnel, Ministry of Public Health and the State Administration of Traditional Chinese Medicine. And he is also a member of the Appraisal Committee for Medical Events in Guangdong Province and Guangzhou City.

He has long been engaged in clinical practice, teaching, and scientific research, with expertise in the treatment of respiratory and oncological diseases by using an approach that integrates Chinese and Western medical treatments. He has fostered over 10 Master's and Doctoral level students.

Professor Liu authored *"The Diagnosis and Treatment of Chronic Bronchitis by Pattern Differentiation with an Integration of Chinese and Western Medical Approaches"* which won the first prize at a national scientific conference in 1978 (collective prize). He also wrote *"Tongue Diagnosis of COPD"* which won the third prize from the Guangdong Provincial Higher Education Bureau. In 1985, his "Qi-Lowering and Panting-Calming Granule 降气定喘颗粒" for the treatment of chronic bronchitis, won the fourth prize given by the Guangzhou City Scientific & Technical Committee for scientific and technological achievements. This formula and the empirical formula "Phlegm-Dispelling and Cough-Arresting Granule 祛痰止咳冲剂" passed provincial level appraisal, and was transferred to factory production, with a good effect in terms of both benefiting society and economy. He has participated in 10 scientific research projects through the national "Eighth, Ninth and Tenth Five Year" Key Programs, at the provincial level. He has published over 40 research papers, and been the chief editor or editor of 10 books.

In 2003, Professor Liu won a prize from the China Scientific & Technological Society honoring his excellent work in the national anti-SARS campaign. In 2004, he also won a second prize from the State Education Ministry for his clinical study on treating SARS through an integration of Chinese and Western medical approaches. In 2005 Professor Liu won a second prize from the State Education Ministry for his clinical study on treatment of SARS using an integration of Chinese and Western medical approaches.

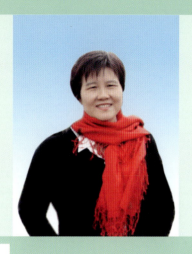

林琳 教授

Professor **Lin Lin** is a chief physician, professor, and state-approved Master's level Supervisor at the Chinese Medicine Hospital of Guangdong Province. She is also the director of the Respiratory Department of the hospital. In addition, she serves as the vice-president of the Specialty Committee of Respiratory Disease of World Federation of Chinese Medical Societies (WFCMS), the director of the Respiratory Specialty Board of the Guangdong Provincial Chinese Medicine Association, the vice-director of the Respiratory Specialty Board of the Guangdong Provincial Integrated Chinese and Western Medicine Association, and as a Chinese Medicinal Specialist of the "Guangdong Provincial Expert Group for First Aid" and the "Guangdong Provincial Expert Group for Emergency Treatment of Respiratory and Infectious Diseases". She is also a part time editor of the *China Journal of Chinese Medicine and Pharmacology*. For over 20 years, in addition to clinical practice, she has taught, done scientific research, hosted 2 projects of scientific research on the national level and 4 projects on the provincial and bureau levels, participated in 20 or more projects on various levels, and published more than 30 research papers. She is the chief editor of 3 monographs. Professor Lin has long specialized in the prevention and treatment of respiratory diseases through the use of integrated Chinese and Western medicine. She has persevered seeking truth and fact with a scientific and researching attitude that includes careful observation, strict analysis, and an objective, scientific, tenacious and hard struggling principle in academic pursuits. She has rich clinical experiences in the prevention and treatment of COPD, asthma, and pulmonary infections by using TCM. She pays attention to the holistic treatment of phlegm, stasis, heat and deficiency, and she has had successive breakthroughs in clinical studies. Professor Lin has won many awards, including one for young female Chinese scientists, a national "May 1st" labor medal, a Guangdong provincial "May 1st" labor medal, and a first grade of achievement in anti-SARS work in the Guangdong province.

Foreword

Chinese medicine is a broad and profound art of healing. It is a well-established and comprehensive system of medicine with an ancient origin and a long rich history. Throughout the ages, it has made a significant contribution to the prosperity of the Chinese civilization. The system of pattern differentiation and treatment fully reflects the Chinese medical view of health and disease as a holistic concept, the emphasis on the body's ability to regulate itself and adapt to the environment, and the need for individualized treatment. The integration of diseases and syndromes is the consummation of treatment based on pattern differentiation; it fully displays the superior characteristic of this discipline, and has an extensive influence on the development of the art of Chinese medicine.

The intention of this series of books is to introduce accurate Chinese medical diagnosis and treatment of various diseases to overseas readers.

The Chinese edition of *The Clinical Practice of Chinese Medicine* was edited by the Second Teaching Hospital of Guangzhou University of CM (also known as Guangdong Provincial Hospital of TCM), and published by People's Medical Publishing House. When the series was published in 2000, it was widely accepted in clinical practice due to its originality, distinguishing features, richness in content, completeness, accuracy, and outstanding emphases. This series has become a trademark of standard in the eyes of Chinese and integrative medical practitioners. During the second printing of this series of books, Professor Deng Tie-tao praised, "For a series to be printed a multiple number of times, shows that it is highly regarded and has received excellent reviews." In order to keep up with the constant development of medical science, this series was revised and re-published in 2004 by People's Medical Publishing House. Due to its popularity, it has been reprinted numerous times since.

The English edition of this series of books includes 20 volumes:

- *COPD & Asthma*
- *Coronary Artery Disease & Hyperlipidemia*
- *Stroke & Parkinson's Disease*
- *Chronic Gastritis & Irritable Bowel Syndrome*
- *Diabetes & Obesity*
- *Gout & Rheumatoid Arthritis*
- *Menstrual Disorders I: Dysfunctional Uterine Bleeding & Amenorrhea*
- *Menstrual Disorders II: Premenstrual Syndrome, Dysmenorrhea & Perimenopause*
- *Endometriosis & Uterine Fibroids*
- *Pelvic Inflammatory Disease & Miscarriage*
- *Postpartum Hypogalactia & Breast Hyperplasia*
- *Male & Female Infertility*
- *Urticaria*
- *Eczema & Atopic Dermatitis*
- *Lupus Erythematosus*
- *Scleroderma & Dermatomyositis*
- *Diseases of the Accessory Organs of the Skin*
- *Psoriasis & Cutaneous Pruritis*
- *Herpes Zoster & Fungal Skin Infections*
- *Chloasma & Vitiligo*

Clinical application varies by individual and by location; when this is combined with the rapid development of medical science, the treatment methods and medicinal dosages may also vary accordingly. When using these books as a reference guide, overseas readers should confirm the formulas and dosages of medicinals according to the individual health condition of the patient, as well as take into account the origin of the Chinese medicinals.

The quotes in these books were taken from various medical literature during the compilation process. We have deleted some of the contents of the original texts for the purpose of uniformity and ease in readability. We ask for the reader's forgiveness and express our respect and gratitude toward the original authors.

Due to the complicated nature of the diagnoses and treatments covered in these books, and the wide range of topics they touch upon, it is inevitable that one may encounter errors while reading through them. We respectively welcome constructive criticism and corrections from our readers.

The clinical practice of medicine changes with the constant development of medical science. The books in this series will be revised regularly to continuously adapt to the development of traditional Chinese medicine.

Editorial Board for the English edition of
The Clinical Practice of Chinese Medicine series
September, 2006

Editorial Board

for the English edition of

The Clinical Practice of Chinese Medicine Series

Academic Consultants

Deng Tie-tao

Master of the National Master and Apprentice Education Program, Tenured Professor of Guangzhou University of CM, Former vice President of Guangzhou University of CM

Yan De-xin

Professor of Chinese Medicine, Medical College, Shanghai Railway University, Specialized in the theory & clinical practice of Chinese medicine

Lu Zhi-zheng

Master of the National Master and Apprentice Education Program, Professor of Chinese Medicine, China Academy of Chinese Medical Science

Ren Ji-xue

Master of the National Master and Apprentice Education Program, Professor of Changchun University of CM, Visiting Professor of Guangzhou University of CM

Jiao Shu-de

Master of the National Master and Apprentice Education Program, Professor of Chinese Medicine, China-Japan Hospital, Ministry of Health

Gan Zu-wang

Master of the National Master and Apprentice Education Program, Professor of Chinese Medicine, Nanjing University of TCM, A founder of otolaryngology of Chinese medicine

Wu Xian-zhong

Specialist of Integrative Medicine, Academician of Chinese Academy of Engineering, Professor, Tianjin Medical University, Chairman of Tianjin Institute of Acute Abdomen Research on Integrative Medicine

Wang Yong-yan

Specialist of Chinese Internal Medicine, Academician of Chinese Academy of Engineering, Professor and former President of Beijing University of CM, and Honorary President of China Academy of Chinese Medical Science

Chen Ke-ji

Specialist of Cardiovascular & Aging Diseases, Academician of Chinese Academy of Science, Professor of Medicine, Xiyuan Hospital, and Institute of Aging Medicine, China Academy of Chinese Medical Science, Consultant on Traditional Medicine, WHO

General Coordinator

Lü Yu-bo
Professor & Vice President, Guangzhou University of CM,
President, the Second Teaching Hospital of Guangzhou University of CM

Editors-in-Chief

Luo Yun-jian

Guangdong Province Entitled Famous Chinese Medicine Physician, Professor of Chinese Internal Medicine & former Vice President of the Second Teaching Hospital of Guangzhou University of CM

Liu Mao-cai

Guangdong Province Entitled Famous Chinese Medicine Physician, Professor of Chinese Internal Medicine & former Vice President of the Second Teaching Hospital of Guangzhou University of CM, Former Chairman of Institute for Aging Cerebral Diseases, Guangzhou University of CM

Associate Editors-in-Chief

Xuan Guo-wei

Guangdong Province Entitled Famous Chinese Medicine Physician, Director & Professor, Department of Chinese External Medicine, Guangzhou University of CM, Former Vice President of the Second Teaching Hospital of Guangzhou University of CM

Huang Chun-lin

Professor of Chinese Internal Medicine, & former Associate-Director of the Second Institute for Clinical Research, Guangzhou University of CM

Chen Da-can

Professor of Chinese External Medicine, Vice President of the Second Teaching Hospital of Guangzhou University of CM

Chen Zhi-qiang

Professor of Chinese External Medicine, Director of the Department of Surgery, Vice President of the Second Teaching Hospital of Guangzhou University of CM

Feng Wei-bin

Professor of Chinese Internal Medicine, the Second Teaching Hospital of Guangzhou University of CM

Yang Zhi-min

Professor of Chinese Internal Medicine, Vice President of the Second Teaching Hospital of Guangzhou University of CM

Lu Chuan-jian

Professor of Chinese External Medicine, Vice President of the Second Teaching Hospital of Guangzhou University of CM

Zou Xu

Professor of Chinese Internal Medicine, Vice President of the Second Teaching Hospital of Guangzhou University of CM

Members (Listed alphabetically by name)

Deng Zhao-zhi
Professor of Chinese Internal Medicine, Guangzhou University of CM

Fan Guan-jie
Professor of Chinese Internal Medicine, Director of Department of Education, the Second Teaching Hospital of Guangzhou University of CM

Fan Rui-qiang
Professor of Chinese External Medicine, Director of Department of Dermatology, the Second Teaching Hospital of Guangzhou University of CM

Huang Jian-ling
Professor of Chinese Medicine Gynecology, Director of the First Department of Gynecology, the Second Teaching Hospital of Guangzhou University of CM

Huang Pei-xin
Professor of Chinese Internal Medicine, the Second Teaching Hospital of Guangzhou University of CM, Head of the Research Project of Cerebral Disease Treatment on Chinese Internal Medicine, Sponsored by SATCM China

Huang Sui-ping
Professor of Chinese Internal Medicine, Director of Department of Digestion, the Second Teaching Hospital of Guangzhou University of CM

Li Li-yun
Guangdong Province Entitled Famous Chinese Medicine Physician, Professor of Chinese Medicine Gynecology, the Second Teaching Hospital of Guangzhou University of CM

Liang Xue-fang
Professor of Chinese Medicine Gynecology, Director of the Third Department of Gynecology, the Second Teaching Hospital of Guangzhou University of CM

Lin Lin

Professor of Chinese Internal Medicine, Director of Department of Respiratory, the Second Teaching Hospital of Guangzhou University of CM

Liu Wei-sheng

Master of the National Master and Apprentice Education Program, Professor of Chinese Internal Medicine, the Second Teaching Hospital of Guangzhou University of CM

Wang Xiao-yun

Professor of Chinese Medicine Gynecology, Director of Department of Gynecology, Head of Teaching Division of Gynecology, the Second Teaching Hospital of Guangzhou University of CM

Lin Yi

Professor of Mastopathy in Chinese Medicine, the Second Teaching Hospital of Guangzhou University of CM, Head of the National Key Subject – Mastopathy in Chinese Medicine

Si-tu Yi

Professor of Chinese Medicine Gynecology, the Second Teaching Hospital of Guangzhou University of CM, Head of the National Key Subject – Chinese Medicine Gynecology

Sponsored by

The Second Teaching Hospital of Guangzhou University of CM, also known as **Guangdong Provincial Hospital of TCM**

Preface

Since its publication in 2000, the Chinese edition of *Clinical Diagnoses and Treatment of Respiratory Diseases in Chinese Medicine*, has been widely accepted because of its rich content and outstanding clinical characteristics. The second edition was published in 2004. This book has actively influenced the establishment of a respiratory specialty within Chinese medicine. Now a part of the book - Chronic Obstructive Pulmonary Disease (COPD) & Asthma - has been combined and translated into English edition. As such, we hope to extend the influence of Chinese medicine to overseas areas and to increase the theoretical accumulation and clinical knowledge of this specialty area.

The authors of this book are both Chinese medical experts who have engaged in clinical practice and scientific research on respiratory diseases; thus they have accumulated rich clinical experiences, and work at a high academic level. In the compilation process, the authors consulted a large number of reference literatures, summarized famous Chinese medical physicians' academic thinking and clinical experiences, and blended their own knowledge into the book. At the same time, the authors deeply and comprehensively summarized the clinical achievements of research into these specific diseases, so as to reflect new and more effective diagnostic and therapeutic techniques that are now used to treat these illnesses. They also discuss the simple, convenient, proven, and cheap techniques of traditional Chinese medicine in treating these special diseases. On the whole, the book summarizes clinical practice experiences in treating COPD and asthma by Chinese medicine in China. It also reflects our deep thoughts on key and difficult points of diagnosing and treating these diseases.

In the book, the most commonly encountered diseases of the respiratory system - COPD and asthma - are discussed in detail. COPD is a disease characterized by airflow limitation, with progressive decreases of pulmonary function, finally developing into respiratory failure. At the present time, there are no drugs that can reverse its course. Chinese medicine has better effects to stop cough and resolve sputum, reduce the number of acute episodes, and relieve respiratory muscle fatigue. Asthma is a chronic airway inflammation associated with several cells. Its pathogenic mechanism is linked to allergic reactions, airway inflammation, airway hyperactivity, and nervous factors. So far it cannot be radically cured. The anti-asthmatic actions of Chinese medicine are slower than those of biomedical drugs; however they do have a certain effects on mild asthma attacks, and is especially advantageous for treatment during the remission stage. Primary clinical investigations have suggested that Chinese medicine can reduce the number of acute asthma episodes, and can, to a given extent, reduce the dosages of glucocorticoids and bronchodilators.

In this book, the following sections are included for each disease: a brief overview, etiology and pathomechanisms in terms of Chinese medicine, Chinese medical treatment using various modalities, prognosis, preventive healthcare practices, comments from famous physicians, integrative treatment approaches, quotes from classical texts, and summaries of modern research. In the brief **overview**, the recognition of the disease by biomedicine is briefly introduced. In the chapters on **etiology and pathomechanisms** in terms of Chinese medicine, and **Chinese medical treatment** using various modalities, the occurrence, diagnosis and treatment based on pattern differentiation are expounded upon in detail from the angle of Chinese medicine. These sections summarize the traditional thinking and methods of treatment based on pattern differentiation in Chinese medicine so that readers can understand the systemic knowledge of diagnosis and treatment of the disease in Chinese medicine. In the section of **comments from famous physicians**, a great number of proven cases and experiences by renown doctors are included. These experiences are definitely effective and proven through clinical practice, and are chosen so as to help the readers understand how modern Chinese physicians treat diseases based on traditional diagnostic and treating methods. In the chapter on **integrative treatment approaches**, the advantages of Chinese medical treatment and the opportune time for biomedical intervention are introduced, so as to provide foreign readers with a clear method of thinking about integrative diagnosis and treatment. In section of **quotes from classical texts**, penetrating discussions on these diseases by Chinese physicians throughout the ages are selected and translated. In the chapter on **modern research**, the readers will find the newest advances in both clinical and basic research. The book, being rich in content, caters to readers with its comprehensive diagnostic and treatment experiences of various distinguished schools and experts in both modern and contemporary times. The recent status of research on these diseases and the academic results that have been achieved are also discussed.

This book may serve as a text and reference book for teachers and students in Chinese medical colleges, medical practitioners in Chinese medicine, as well as biomedical physicians who are interested in the clinical application of Chinese medicine. It is also suitable for general readers who want to understand the characteristics and advantages of Chinese medicine. The diagnostic and therapeutic methods introduced in the book should be carried out only under the guidance of professional Chinese medical physicians, and no unauthorized application should be performed by non-professionals. If these methods are utilized by professionals, they should have a solid foundation in the theories of Traditional Chinese Medicine, and should fully take into consideration the patient's individuality, region and ethnicity in treating according to pattern differentiation so as to reasonably prescribe a formula with the proper medicinals. At the same time, practitioners should also pay attention to the dosages of medicinals and their place of origin. It is very important in countries without Chinese medicinals, that practitioners have a deep understanding of the functions and incompatibilities of the herbs. On the basis of these understandings, they can choose similar medicinals, or medicinals with the same functions, for substitution in a prescription.

In the compilation of this book, the authors wish to acknowledge the leaders of Guangdong Provincial Hospital of TCM, many medical experts and professors, as well as the Publishing House for their great support. Because of the limitation of the authors' ability and experience, and the quick and constant development of medical science, we apologize for any errors or shortcomings that may appear in the book. We hope that the experts and readers will not hesitate to point them out to us for further improvement.

Liu Wei-sheng & Lin Lin
Guangzhou China
April 2007

Contents

Chronic Obstructive Pulmonary Disease ··· 001

OVERVIEW ··· 009
CHINESE MEDICAL ETIOLOGY AND PATHOMECHANISM ··· 013
    Etiology of COPD in Chinese Medicine ··· 013
    Pathomechanism of COPD in Chinese Medicine ··· 014
CHINESE MEDICAL TREATMENT ··· 016
    Pattern Differentiation and Treatment ··· 016
    Additional treatment modalities ··· 033
PROGNOSIS ··· 040
PREVENTIVE HEALTHCARE ··· 040
    Lifestyle Modification ··· 041
    Dietary Recommendation ··· 043
    Regulation of Emotional and Mental Health ··· 047
CLINICAL EXPERIENCE OF RENOWNED PHYSICIANS ··· 048
    Empirical Formulas ··· 048
    Selected Case Studies ··· 069
    Discussions ··· 096
PERSPECTIVES OF INTEGRATIVE MEDICINE ··· 156
    Challenges and Solutions ··· 157
    Insight from Empirical Wisdom ··· 168
    Summary ··· 175
SELECTED QUOTES FROM CLASSICAL TEXTS ··· 176
MODERN RESEARCH ··· 185

Clinical Research	185
Experimental Studies	200
REFERENCES	204

Bronchial Asthma 211

OVERVIEW	217
CHINESE MEDICAL ETIOLOGY AND PATHOMECHANISM	219
CHINESE MEDICAL TREATMENT	220
Pattern Differentiation and Treatment	220
Additional Treatment Modalities	233
PROGNOSIS	247
PREVENTIVE HEALTHCARE	248
Lifestyle Modification	248
Dietary Recommendation	249
Regulation of Emotional and Mental Health	253
CLINICAL EXPERIENCE OF RENOWNED PHYSICIANS	254
Empirical Formulas	254
Selected Case Studies	265
Discussions	283
PERSPECTIVES OF INTEGRATIVE MEDICINE	316
Challenges and Solutions	316
Insight from Empirical Wisdom	323
Summary	332
SELECTED QUOTES FROM CLASSICAL TEXTS	335
MODERN RESEARCH	339
Clinical Research	339
Experimental Studies	363

REFERENCES 369
Index by Disease Names and Symptoms 375
Index by Chinese Medicinals and Formulas 384
General Index 401

Chronic Obstructive Pulmonary Disease

by **Lin Lin**, Professor of Chinese Internal Medicine
He De-ping, M.S. TCM
Xu Yin-ji, M.S. TCM
Wu Lei, M.S. TCM
Huang Dong-hui, M.S. TCM

OVERVIEW 009
CHINESE MEDICAL ETIOLOGY AND PATHOMECHANISM 013
  Etiology of COPD in Chinese Medicine 013
  Pathomechanism of COPD in Chinese Medicine 014
CHINESE MEDICAL TREATMENT 016
  Pattern Differentiation and Treatment 016
    1. During the Acute Attack Stage 017
    2. During the Remission Stage 028
  Additional treatment modalities 033
    1. Chinese Patent Medicine 033
    2. Acupuncture and Moxibustion 034
    3. Simple Prescriptions and Empirical Formulas 038
PROGNOSIS 040
PREVENTIVE HEALTHCARE 040
  Lifestyle Modification 041
    1. Engage in Cold-Resistance Exercises such as Rubbing the Body Down with Cold Water 041
    2. Persist in Doing Abdominal Breathing and Pursed-lip Respiration in order to Improve Pulmonary Ventilation 041
    3. Do Exercises to Restore Health, like *Taiji*, Walking, and Jogging 041
    4. Rubbing the Nose 042
    5. Expanding the Chest 042
    6. Pressing the Abdomen 042
    7. Clenching the Fists 042
    8. Massage 043
    9. Keep the Indoor Air Circulating, and Maintain Appropriate Temperature and Humidity 043
  Dietary Recommendation 043
    1. *Gǒu Qǐ Zǐ* (Fructus Lycii) Stewed Pig Heart (枸杞子炖猪心) 044

2. Crucian Carp, Xìng Rén (Armeniacae Semen Amarum) and Brown Sugar Soup (鲫鱼杏仁红糖汤) ·· 044

3. Xìng Rén (Armeniacae Semen Amarum) and Pig Lung Decoction (杏仁猪肺汤) ·· 045

4. Hé Táo (Semen Juglandis) Stewed Xìng Rén (Armeniacae Semen Amarum) (核桃炖杏仁) ·· 045

5. Radish and Sugar Liquid (萝卜糖水) ·································· 045

6. Bǔ Fèi Yì Shèn Gāo (补肾益肺糕) ·· 046

7. Dān Shēn (Radix et Rhizoma Salviae Miltiorrhizae) and Huáng Qí (Radix Astragali) Porridge (参芪粥) ··· 046

8. Pí Pá Yè (Folium Eriobotryae) Decoction (枇杷叶煎汤) ············· 047

9. Rén Shēn (Radix Ginseng) and Hé Táo (Semen Juglandis) Decoction (人参核桃煎) ··· 047

Regulation of Emotional and Mental Health ·················· 047
CLINICAL EXPERIENCE OF RENOWNED PHYSICIANS ··············· 048
Empirical Formulas ·· 048

1. The Treatment of Cough due to Deficiency of both the Lung and Spleen with Qì Zhǒng Fāng (气肿方) (Deng Tie-tao) ·· 048

2. The Treatment of Cough due to Accumulation of Cold Phlegm in the Lung with Jié Chuǎn Tāng (截喘汤) (Jiang Chun-hua) ··························· 049

3. The Treatment of Cough and Panting with Copious Sputum due to Invasion of Wind-Cold with Zhǐ Ké Dìng Chuǎn Tāng (止咳定喘汤) (Yu Shen-chu) ··· 050

4. The Treatment of Cough due to Yang Deficiency of the Lung and Kidney with Fèi Qì Zhǒng Yàn Fāng (肺气肿验方) (Li Ke-shao) ······················ 051

5. The Treatment of Chronic Bronchitis with Chú Yún Zhǐ Ké Tāng (锄云止咳汤) (Yue Mei-zhong) ·· 052

6. The Treatment of Cough and Panting due to Deficiency Cold of the Kidney and Du Vessel, Coagulation and Stagnation of Phlegm and Stasis with Yáng Hé Píng Chuǎn Tāng (阳和平喘汤) (Hu Qiao-wu) ···················· 054

7. The Treatment of Cough and Panting due to Dual Deficiency of the Lung and Kidney with *Jiā Wèi Mài Wèi Dì Huáng Tāng* (加味麦味地黄汤) (Dong Jian-hua) ⋯⋯⋯⋯⋯⋯057

8. The Treatment of Cough due to Deficiency of Both Qi and Yin with *Dài Mài Yǎng Fèi Zhǐ Ké Tāng* (黛麦养肺止咳汤) (Li Bing-nan) ⋯⋯⋯⋯⋯058

9. The Treatment of Cough and Panting due to Kidney Deficiency Failing to Receive Qi, with Phlegm and Fluids Lodged in the Lung with *Sì Zǐ Píng Chuǎn Tāng* (四子平喘汤) (Lu Zhi-qing) ⋯⋯⋯⋯⋯⋯⋯⋯⋯⋯⋯061

10. The Treatment of Dry Cough due to Lung-Heat with *Qīng Fèi Dìng Chuǎn Tāng* (清肺定咳汤) (Zhu Liang-chun) ⋯⋯⋯⋯⋯⋯⋯⋯⋯063

11. The Treatment of Acute and Chronic Bronchitis, and Bronchiectasis, with *Jiā Jiǎn Zé Qī Tāng* (加减泽漆汤) (Huang Ji-geng) ⋯⋯⋯065

12. The Treatment of Dual Deficiency of Lung and Kidney of Chronic Bronchitis with *Pí Gōng Fāng* (脾功方) (Huang Ji-geng) ⋯⋯⋯⋯⋯⋯066

13. The Treatment of Phlegm-Damp Cough with *Qū Tán Zhǐ Ké Chōng Jì* (祛痰止咳冲剂) (Liu Wei-sheng) ⋯⋯⋯⋯⋯⋯⋯⋯⋯068

14. The Treatment of Cough due to Accumulation of Phlegm-Heat with *Yín Huáng Hé Jì* (银黄合剂) (Liu Wei-sheng) ⋯⋯⋯⋯⋯⋯⋯069

Selected Case Studies ⋯⋯⋯⋯⋯⋯⋯⋯⋯⋯⋯⋯⋯⋯⋯⋯069

1. Professor Liu Du-zhou's Case Study: Cold Fluid-Retention in the Lung ⋯⋯069

2. Professor Gao Hui-yuan's Case Study: Dual Deficiency of Qi and Yin, With Phlegm-Heat Obstructing the Lung ⋯⋯⋯⋯⋯⋯⋯⋯074

3. He Yan-shen's Case Study: Warm Evil Transforming into Heat, Contending With Cold Fluids ⋯⋯⋯⋯⋯⋯⋯⋯⋯⋯⋯⋯⋯⋯076

4. Yan Zheng-hua's Case Study: Phlegm-Heat Internally Accumulating, Failure of the Lung to Clear and Depurate ⋯⋯⋯⋯⋯⋯⋯⋯080

5. Shi Jin-mo's Case Study: Phlegm-Damp Obstructing the Middle Jiao, with Dual Deficiency of the Lung and Spleen ⋯⋯⋯⋯⋯⋯⋯⋯084

6. Liu Wei-sheng's Case Study: Lung Deficiency and Phlegm-Damp, Compounded

  by a Contraction of Wind-Heat ···086

 7. Yang Ji-shun's Case Study: Accumulation of Phlegm-Heat Mixed with

  Stasis ··089

 8. Jiao Shu-de's Case Study: Yang Deficiency with Water Flooding, Upwardly

  Insulting the Heart and Lung ···092

 9. Li Kong-ding's Case Study: Dual Deficiency of the Spleen ···············094

 10. Wang Zhi-zhong's Song Dynasty Case Study ······························096

Discussions ·· 096

 1. Professor Jiao Shu-de Believes that the Concept of Two Classes, Six Patterns

  and Three Principles must be Grasped in Order to Treat Panting ···············096

 2. Professor Shao Chang-rong Believes that in the Treatment of Chronic

  Bronchitis, Importance should be Attached to Cold, Heat, Phlegm, Dampness,

  and Deficiency ··104

 3. Professor Xie Chang-ren Believes that in the Treatment of Cough and Panting

  Three Stages Need to be Differentiated ···105

 4. Professor Wang Zheng-gong's Opinion on the Methods to Reverse Chronic

  Obstructive Pulmonary Disease ···109

 5. Professor Wu Sheng-nong Believes that in the Treatment of Chronic Bronchitis,

  Diffusing Lung Qi and Transforming Turbid Phlegm should be Used during

  the Attack Stage, and Consolidating the Defensive (Wei) Qi and Warming the

  Original Yang in the Remission Stage ···113

 6. Professor Huo Jing-tang's Discussion of His Experience in Treating Panting and

  Cough due to Internal Damage ···116

 7. Professor Pu Fu-zhou's Discussion on Panting and Cough ···············120

 8. Professor Hong Guang-xiang Believes that the Warming Method is Indispensable

  for Treating the Lung ···125

 9. Professor Yue Mei-zhong Emphasizes that the Treatment of Cough Requires

  Combining General Aspects with Specific Aspects ·····························128

 10. Professor Jiang Chun-hua's Discussion on the Treatment of Cough ······134

11. Professor Li Ji-ren's Discussion of Clearing Phlegm and Disinhibiting Qi as the Primary Method to Treat Cough ... 142

12. Professor Chao En-xiang's Discussion on the Failure of the Kidney to Receive Qi, and the Internal Obstruction of Turbid Phlegm ... 144

13. Professor Zhang Zhen-ru: Determine the Treatment of Lung Distention (Emphysema) According to the Deficiency and Damage of the Five *Zang* Organs from Phlegm Turbidity, Water Fluids, and Blood Stasis ... 144

14. Professor Yu Shen-chu's Discussion of His Experience Treating Cough and Panting ... 148

15. Professor Li Shi-qing: Treatment of Cough in Bronchitis ... 154

PERSPECTIVES OF INTEGRATIVE MEDICINE ... 156

Challenges and Solutions ... 157

Challenge #1: Treatment of Respiratory Failure ... 157

Challenge #2: Treatment of Respiratory Tract Infection is the Key Point to Relieving Acute Exacerbation ... 160

Challenge #3: Preventing the Acute Exacerbation of COPD as an Important Key in Delaying the Progression of COPD ... 163

Challenge #4: Treatment of Pulmonary Artery Hypertension ... 165

Insight from Empirical Wisdom ... 168

1. When Encountering Any of the Below, Quickly Treat with Combined Western and Chinese Medicine ... 168

2. Treatment of Respiratory Muscle Fatigue ... 168

3. The Pathogenesis and Treatment of Blood Stasis in COPD ... 172

4. Pay attention to opening the *Fu* Organs, Draining Heat, and Downbearing the Lung to Calm Panting ... 174

Summary ... 175

SELECTED QUOTES FROM CLASSICAL TEXTS ... 176

MODERN RESEARCH ... 185

Clinical Research ... 185

1. Pattern Differentiation and Corresponding Treatment ·····························185
2. Specific Formulas ···191
3. Acupuncture and Moxibustion ···195

Experimental Studies ·· 200
1. Research on the Efficacy of Single Chinese Medicinals ························200
2. Research on the Efficacy of Herbal Prescriptions ·······························200
3. Studies on Forms of Chinese Medicinals ··202

REFERENCES ··· 204

008 COPD & Asthma

OVERVIEW

Chronic obstructive pulmonary disease (COPD) is characterized by airflow limitation, which is partially reversible, and progressive in nature. It is associated with abnormal inflammatory reactions to harmful gases or particles. The course of COPD can be divided into the acute exacerbation phase and the stable phase. The acute exacerbation phase is defined as having cough, expectoration, shortness of breath and/or aggravated gasping all occurring within a short duration of time, as well as an increased volume of purulent or mucopurulent sputum. This phase may be accompanied by symptoms of an apparent worsening of inflammation, such as fever. The stable phase refers to the fact that the cough, expectoration, shortness of breath and other symptoms are stable or mild. The clinical manifestations of COPD include cough, expectoration, shortness of breath or dyspnea, wheezing, and chest oppression. In the advanced stage, there is often weight loss, poor appetite and, if the disease is complicated by infection, expectoration of bloody sputum (hemoptysis). In the early stage of COPD, the physical signs are not obvious. As the disease progresses, emerging signs usually include abnormal changes of the thorax or over inflation of the chest with an enlarged anteroposterior diameter, widened epigastric angle, and abdominal prominence. There are often signs such as tachypnea, and respiratory movements involving the accessory respiratory muscles such as scalene muscles and sternocleidomastoid muscles. In severe cases there can be paradoxical thoraco-abdominal movements. If there is hypoxemia, cyanosis of the mucosa and skin can occur. If there is right-sided heart failure, there will be and edema of the lower limbs and hepatomegaly. Upon percussion the following signs can be found: a decreased border of cardiac dullness, a lowered pulmonohepatic border, and a hyper resonance of the lung. Upon auscultation, the following signs may be audible: diminished respiratory sounds over the two lungs with a prolonged expiratory phase, dry rales with normal respiration, and moist rales over the two lung bases or over other lung fields. The cardiac sounds are distant, with clear and loud heart sounds over the xiphoid area.

In recent years, it is thought that these pathogenic factors of COPD are two-fold and interactive with each other: individual susceptibility and environmental factors. So far, the more definite factor in individual susceptibility is a shortage of α-antitrypsin; while the most important environmental factors are smoking and exposure to occupational dust or chemicals (such as smog, allergic antigens, waste fumes, and indoor air pollution). Pulmonary function tests play the most important role in the diagnosis, assessment of severity, progression, prognosis, and treatment of COPD. After the administration of an inhaled bronchodilator, if the forced expiratory volume (FEV_1) in 1 second drops to less than 80% of the predicted value, and the ratio of the FEV_1 to the forced vital capacity (FVC) drops to less than 70%, then a partially reversible airflow limitation can be confirmed. The major X-ray changes include lung over-inflation: enlarged lung volume, a lengthened thoracic cavity (in the anteroposterior diameter), flattened ribs, a decreased density of lung fields, a low and flattened diaphragm, a elongated pendulous heart, residual root-like vascular markings of the pulmonary hila, tenuous markings of peripheral lung fields, and occasionally, the development of bullae. In cases complicated by pulmonary hypertension and cor pulmonale, in addition to right cardiomegaly, there may also be bulging of the pulmonary conus, enlargement of hilar vascular shadows, and a widened right lower pulmonary artery. A blood gas analysis during the early stage shows only slight or moderate hypoxemia. As the disease develops, hypoxemia gradually becomes more severe, often leading to hypercapnia. When complicated by infection, a large amount of neutrophilic leukocytes can be detected in the sputum smear. A bacterial culture of the sputum will reveal various pathogenic bacteria, including Streptococcus Pneumoniae, Haemophilus influenzae, Moraxella Catarrhalis, and Klebsiella Pneumoniae. The diagnosis of COPD should be based on comprehensive analysis of the case history, history of relevant risk factors, signs, and the results of laboratory examinations. Partially reversible airflow limitation is a necessary condition, and a pulmonary function test is the golden standard for diagnosis.

The treatment principles during the acute exacerbation phase of COPD are as follows. First, evaluate the severity of the disease according to the symptoms, blood gas analyses and chest X-ray results. Use controlled oxygen therapy. Oxygen therapy is the basic treatment for hospitalized patients with exacerbated COPD. Antibiotics should be chosen according to the local common pathogenic bacteria and drug sensitivity for patients with deteriorated dyspnea and cough with increased volume of sputum and/or purulent sputum. The long-term application of broad-spectrum antibiotics and glucocorticoids is likely to result in a secondary fungal infection, so antifungal drugs are needed for either prevention or treatment. Bronchodilators are the main approach of controlling COPD symptoms; they can relax the bronchial smooth muscle, dilate the bronchi and reduce airflow limitation. Short-acting β_2-receptor excitants are suitable for the acute exacerbation phase of COPD. If this is ineffective, anticholinergics can also be added. An intravenous drip of theophylline is necessary in cases of severely deteriorated COPD. COPD in-patients should be given a glucocorticoid orally or by intravenous injection based on the premise of bronchodilator application. For COPD patients in the acute exacerbation stage, non-invasive positive pressure ventilation can reduce $PaCO_2$ and relieve dyspnea, so as to reduce the use of endotracheal intubation and invasive mechanical ventilation, shorten the duration of hospitalization, and reduce case fatality rate. Under conditions of active medication, if respiratory failure is still getting progressively worse, with life-threatening acid-base imbalances and/or unconsciousness, invasive mechanical ventilation is necessary. During the whole course of treatment, attention should be paid to the water-electrolyte balance and the nutritional state, recognizing and treating potential complications (such as heart failure and cardiac arrhythmia).

The treatment principles during the stable phase of COPD are as follows. Through education, increase the ability of COPD patients (and everyone involved in their care) to recognize and treat the disease in order to provide better management, prevention and treatment as well as stabilize pathogenetic conditions. The control of occupational and environmental pollution is also necessary. In terms of medication, drugs are necessary for preventing and controlling symptoms, raising exercise tolerance and improving quality of life. The commonly used drugs are bronchodilators such as β_2-receptor excitants, anticholinergics and methylxanthines. They should be chosen according to drug effectiveness and the individual response of the patient. Glucocorticoids may be applied via inhalation for the patients whose FEV_1 is less than 50% of the predicted value, and who need antibiotics or glucocorticoids orally because of repeated exacerbation. COPD patients are not advised to take glucocorticoids orally over a long period of time, and glucocorticoid inhalation in the stable phase cannot check the falling of FEV_1. Other drugs include apophlegmatics (mucolytics), antioxidants, immunomodulators, and vaccines. $LTDO_2$ (long-term domiciliary oxygen therapy) can increase the survival rate for COPD patients with chronic respiratory failure. Rehabilitative care can increase the exercise capacity and improve the quality of life in patients who have seldom exercised because of progressive airflow limitation and severe dyspnea.

COPD belongs to the category of *fèi zhàng* (肺胀 , Lung distention) or *chuǎn zhèng* (喘证 , panting pattern) in Chinese medicine.

CHINESE MEDICAL ETIOLOGY AND PATHOMECHANISM

In Chinese medicine there is no disease named COPD. As far as the clinical features of COPD (such as repeated cough with white and sticky or yellow sputum, panting, dyspnea, gasping with the shoulder shrugged, cyanosis of the lips and fingers) are concerned, they are quite similar to the characteristics of *fèi zhàng* (Lung distention) or *chuǎn zhèng* (panting pattern) in Chinese medicine. There are detailed descriptions of the symptoms, signs, and prognoses of these diseases in ancient medical literature.

Etiology of COPD in Chinese Medicine

(1) Six Climatic Evils

Six climatic evils invade the body either through the skin or through the mouth and nose. The skin and fine hair corresponds to the Lung, and the Lung has its opening in the nose. Exogenous evils invade and block the defense (*wei*) phase, thus the Lung fails to diffuse, qi congests in the Lung, the movement cannot be depurative and downbearing, but counterflows upward, causing cough and panting.

(2) Phlegm-Fluid Retention in the Lung

Unregulated diet harms the Spleen and Stomach, or inhibited emotions cause the Liver to assail the Spleen. All these changes result in dysfunction of the Spleen in transportation and transformation, thus turbid phlegm will generate internally and accumulate in the Lung. The phlegm-fluid retention block the airway to make it narrow, then the Lung will fail to diffuse and depurate, leading to cough, expectoration, and dyspnea.

(3) Deficiency of the Spleen and Stomach

The deficient and weak Spleen and Stomach cannot transport and transform food and drink, thus causing the ingested material to turn into turbid phlegm. The phlegm may then accumulate in the Lung and affect the diffusion and depuration of the Lung qi, leading to cough with profuse sputum, and panting.

(4) Deficiency of the Lung and Kidney

Prolonged illness results in physical weakness and deficiency of the Lung and Kidney. Protracted Lung disease affects the Kidney (in the five phase doctrine, "the disorder of the mother involves the child"), thus resulting in deficiency of both the Lung and Kidney. The deficient Lung will fail to govern qi, and the deficient Kidney will fail to receive qi, which leads to shortness of breath aggravated by exertion. Failure of the Kidney to govern the water will cause impairment of fluid metabolism, leading to edema.

Pathomechanism of COPD in Chinese Medicine

COPD is a chronic disease. Its clinical progression can go through a long course, consisting of early, middle and late stages. The pathological presentation varies at the different stages.

(1) During the Early Stage, the Focus is the Lung, with Invasion of the Six Climatic Evils, and Blockage of the Lung by Phlegm

In the early stage of COPD, six climatic evils (wind, cold, summer-heat, dampness, dryness and fire) repeatedly invade the body, or endogenous turbid phlegm blocks the Lung, causing the Lung to fail to diffuse and depurate, hence there is panting and cough. The causes are exogenous evils and turbid phlegm, and the focus is mainly the Lung. The major manifestations are cough, expectoration, and mild shortness of breath. The exogenous evils, invading the body through the mouth and nose or the skin and fine hair, first injure the Lung. This may impair the Lung's function of diffusion and descent, giving rise to cough. This may also cause the Lung to fail in diffusing fluids, leading to a disturbance in fluid distribution, which leads to the formation of phlegm. As the phlegm blocks the Lung, the airway will be obstructed, thus resulting in expectoration and panting. There are also cases in which unregulated diet harms the Spleen and Stomach, or inhibited emotions cause the Liver to assail the Spleen. All these changes may result in a dysfunction of the Spleen in transportation and transformation, thus turbid phlegm will generate internally. "The Spleen is the source of the generation of phlegm, and the Lung is the container for the storage of phlegm." As the phlegm blocks the Lung, it leads to cough, panting and expectoration.

(2) During the Middle Stage, the Illness Affects the Spleen and Kidney. Over the Protracted Course of the Disease, there is a Deficiency of the Lung, Spleen and Kidney, and Retention of Turbid Phlegm

A prolonged cough will damage the Lung, and in turn, affect the Spleen (in the five phase doctrine, "the child consumes the qi of the mother"), thus deficiency of both the Lung and Spleen develops. The Lung, when deficient, will fail to govern qi, giving rise to shortness of breath upon exertion. The Spleen, when deficient, will cause turbid phlegm to generate internally, leading to cough and expectoration. The turbid phlegm can exacerbate the shortness of breath. Lung deficiency may affect the Kidney (in the five phase doctrine "metal fails to promote water"). When both the Lung and Kidney are deficient, qi will lose its ability to govern and receive, then the panting will worsen day by day, and the dyspnea will be aggravated by exertion.

(3) During the Late Stage, the Illness Involves the Heart (Brain), Qi and Yang are Deficient and Weak, Phlegm and Stasis Internally Obstruct, Water and Fluids Flow Outside Normal Boundaries, So the Clear Orifices Will be Clouded

The Lung communicates with the Heart-vessels. The Lung qi assists the Heart in circulating blood. When the Lung qi becomes insufficient, it will fail to govern and regulate the qi of the whole body. After a while, it may involve the Heart, leading to stagnation of the Heart-vessels. Heart yang stems from the primordial fire of the life gate (Kidney yang). When Kidney yang declines, it will subsequently result in the deficiency of Heart yang. If the qi and yang of the Lung, Spleen, Heart and Kidney decline, the transportation and transformation of water will be disrupted. Water may then turn into the phlegm-fluid retention. The latter can go upward and cloud the clear orifices, resulting in unconsciousness, lethargy, and coma. It can also accumulate in the Lung, leading to exacerbation of panting, and cough with profuse sputum, or it can attack the Heart and injure the Lung to give rise to palpitations and dyspnea. These fluids can also exudate subcutaneously, leading to *yì yǐn* (溢饮, anasarca); or stagnate in the hypochondria or abdomen to cause *xuán yǐn* (悬饮, fluid retention in the hypochondria) or *shuǐ gǔ* (水臌, ascites); or go into the gastrointestinal tract leading to *tán yǐn* (痰饮, fluid retention in the gastrointestinal tract). The phlegm-fluid retention may combine with the stagnated blood to block qi movement, impairing the Lung's function of diffusion and depuration, and leading to aggravated panting. As it is said in *Teachings of Zhu Dan-xi* (丹溪心法, *Dān Xī Xīn Fǎ*): "The Lung distends to cause panting; the patient cannot sleep on either the left or right lateral positions. This is a disorder of qi due to obstruction by phlegm mixed with static blood." Briefly, as COPD develops into the advanced stage, the pathomechanism consists of deficiency of the right qi and an excess of evil qi. The former is the decline in yang qi of the Lung, Spleen, Kidney and Heart; and the latter is turbid phlegm mixed with static blood and stagnant qi.

CHINESE MEDICAL TREATMENT

Pattern Differentiation and Treatment

In the treatment of COPD one should clearly differentiate between the branch and root, deficiency and excess. Generally speaking, the pathogenic excess is the contraction of external evils, but during normal times there is a root deficiency. For cases of excess, there needs to be differentiation of whether the case is wind-cold, wind-heat, turbid phlegm (fluid retention), phlegm-heat, or stagnated blood. For cases of deficiency, differentiation between the nature of qi (yang) and yin, should be made. In addition, the disorders of the Lung, Heart, Spleen, and Kidney need to be ranked in terms of treatment priority. Both cases [excess and deficiency] often appear simultaneously, therefore the patterns are complex and various. Nevertheless, the different aspects of treating both the branch and the root should be understood from a clinical perspective.

1. During the Acute Attack Stage

(1) Cold in the Exterior and Fluid Retention in the Interior

【Syndrome Characteristics】

Cough, panting, dyspnea, a large amount of thin and frothy sputum, a dry mouth with no desire to drink, accompanied by severe aversion to cold, fever, soreness of the limbs, general pain with no sweating. In severe cases there can also be a puffy complexion and cyanosis of the lips and tongue. There is a pale tongue with a white and glossy coating, and a floating and tight pulse.

【Treatment Principle】

Diffuse the Lung and scatter cold; warm and move the water-fluids.

【Commonly Used Medicinals】

Use *má huáng* (Herba Ephedrae), *fáng fēng* (Radix Saposhnikoviae) and *sū yè* (Folium Perillae) to diffuse the Lung and dispel the cold. Use *xì xīn* (Radix et Rhizoma Asari), *gān jiāng* (Rhizoma Zingiberis), *guì zhī* (Ramulus Cinnamomi), *fǎ xià* (Rhizoma Pinelliae Ternatae Praeparata), *chén pí* (Pericarpium Citri Reticulatae) and *bái zhú* (Rhizoma Atractylodis Macrocephalae) to warm and transform the water-fluids.

【Representative Formula】
Modified *Xiǎo Qīng Lóng Tāng* (小青龙汤)

【Ingredients】

麻黄	má huáng	5g	Herba Ephedrae
桂枝	guì zhī	10g	Ramulus Cinnamomi
白芍	bái sháo	10g	Radix Paeoniae Alba
细辛	xì xīn	3g	Radix et Rhizoma Asari
干姜	gān jiāng	5g	Rhizoma Zingiberis
法夏	fǎ xià	10g	Rhizoma Pinelliae Praeparatum
五味子	wǔ wèi zǐ	5g	Fructus Schisandrae Chinensis
茯苓	fú líng	15g	Poria
陈皮	chén pí	5g	Pericarpium Citri Reticulatae
葶苈子	tíng lì zǐ	15g	Semen Lepidii seu Descurainiae
大枣	dà zǎo	10 pcs	Fructus Jujubae
炙甘草	zhì gān cǎo	5g	Radix et Rhizoma Glycyrrhizae Praeparata

Decoct in 500ml of water until 200ml of the decoction is left. Divide into two portions and take warm, 1 dose a day.

【Formula Analysis】
Within this formula, *má huáng* (Herba Ephedrae) and *guì zhī* (Ramulus Cinnamomi) diffuse the Lung, dispel cold and resolve the exterior. *Bái sháo* (Radix Paeoniae Alba), in combination with *guì zhī* (Ramulus Cinnamomi) regulates the nutrient (*ying*) and defense (*wei*) phases. *Tíng lì zǐ* (Semen Lepidii seu Descurainiae) drains the Lung, transforms fluids and calms panting. *Gān jiāng* (Rhizoma Zingiberis), *xì xīn* (Radix et Rhizoma Asari) and *fǎ xià* (Rhizoma Pinelliae Praeparata) warm the Lung and transform fluids. The astringency of *wǔ wèi zǐ* (Fructus Schisandrae Chinensis) prevents over-consumption of Lung qi. *Chén pí* (Pericarpium Citri Reticulatae) and *fú líng* (Poria) strengthen the Spleen, regulate qi and resolve phlegm. *Gān cǎo* (Radix et Rhizoma Glycyrrhizae) and *dà zǎo* (Fructus Jujubae) regulate the Spleen and Stomach. Together

they affect a cure by diffusing the Lung, scattering cold, warming the Lung and transforming fluids.

(2) Accumulation of Phlegm-Heat in the Lung

【Syndrome Characteristics】

Cough, panting, vexation and agitation, dyspnea, fullness of the chest, thick and yellow sputum, a dry and bitter taste in the mouth, and halitosis. This can be accompanied by fever and sweating. There is a red tongue with a yellow and greasy coating, and a wiry and slippery or slippery and rapid pulse.

【Treatment Principle】

Clear heat and transform phlegm; eliminate phlegm and calm panting.

【Commonly Used Medicinals】

Use *huáng qín* (Radix Scutellariae), *shēng shí gāo* (Gypsum Fibrosum), *wěi jīng* (Coulis Phragmitis), *yú xīng cǎo* (Herba Houttuyniae) and *jīn qiáo mài gēn* (Rhizoma Fagopyri Dibotryis) to clear heat and transform phlegm. Use *zhì má huáng* (Herba Ephedrae Praeparata), *xìng rén* (Armenicae Semen Amarum), *tiān zhú huáng* (Concretio Silicea Bambusae), *zhè bèi mǔ* (Bulbus Fritillariae Thunbergii), *quán guā lóu* (Fructus Trichosanthis), and *zhú lì* (Succus Bambusae) to eliminate phlegm and calm panting.

【Representative Formula】

Modified *Má Xìng Shí Gān Tāng* (麻杏石甘汤) plus *Wěi Jīng Tāng* (苇茎汤) with modifications, or Modified *Qīng Qì Huà Tán Tāng* (清气化痰汤)

【Ingredients】

炙麻黄	zhì má huáng	5g	Herba Ephedrae Praeparata
生石膏	shēng shí gāo	30g (decocted first)	Gypsum Fibrosum
杏仁	xìng rén	10g	Armenicae Semen Amarum
薏苡仁	yì yǐ rén	30g	Semen Coicis
苇茎	wěi jīng	30g	Coulis Phragmitis
桃仁	táo rén	10g	Semen Persicae

鱼腥草	yú xīng cǎo	30g	Herba Houttuyniae
黄芩	huáng qín	15g	Radix Scutellariae
天竺黄	tiān zhú huáng	10g	Concretio Silicea Bambusae
全瓜蒌	quán guā lóu	15g	Fructus Trichosanthis
生甘草	shēng gān cǎo	5g	Radix et Rhizoma Glycyrrhizae Recens
冬瓜仁	dōng guā rén	20g	Semen Benincasae

Decoct in 1000ml of water until 200ml of the decoction is left. Divide into two portions and take warm for one day.

【Formula Analysis】

Zhì má huáng (Herba Ephedrae Praeparata) diffuses the Lung and checks panting. *Shēng shí gāo* (Gypsum Fibrosum), *wěi jīng* (Coulis Phragmitis), *huáng qín* (Radix Scutellariae) and *yú xīng cǎo* (Herba Houttuyniae) clear heat and produce liquids to reduce vexation. *Xìng rén* (Armeniacae Semen Amarum), *dōng guā rén* (Semen Benincasae), *tiān zhú huáng* (Concretio Silicea Bambusae), *quán guā lóu* (Fructus Trichosanthis) and *yì yǐ rén* (Semen Coicis) clear heat and resolve phlegm. *Táo rén* (Semen Persicae) invigorates blood and eliminates phlegm. *Shēng gān cǎo* (Radix et Rhizoma Glycyrrhizae Recens) clears heat, harmonizes the middle jiao, and regulates all of the medicinals.

【Modifications】

➢ For difficulty in expectoration because of sticky sputum, add *tiān huā fěn* (Radix Trichosanthis) 30g, or *hǎi gé ké* (Concha Meretricis seu Cyclinae) 15g to clear the Lung, produce liquids and resolve phlegm.

➢ For throat pain, add *shè gān* (Rhizoma Belamcandae) 10g, or *niú bàng zǐ* (Fructus Arctii) 10g, *xuán shēn* (Radix Scrophulariae) 15g to clear heat so as to relieve throat pain.

➢ For a dry mouth and polydipsia, add *tiān huā fěn* (Radix Trichosanthis) 30g, and *zhī mǔ* (Rhizoma Anemarrhenae) 10g so as to clear heat and produce liquids.

➢ For gurgling sounds of phlegm in the throat, and constipation, add *shēng dà huáng* (Radix et Rhizoma Rhei) 10g or *hǔ zhàng* (Radix et Rhizoma Polygoni Cuspidati) 15g to purge the bowels and reduce heat.

(3) Accumulation of Phlegm-Stasis in the Lung

【Syndrome Characteristics】

Cough with copious white and frothy sputum, stridor in the throat, panting and inability to lie flat, hyperinflation and oppression of the chest, a gray and dark complexion, cyanosis of the lips and nails, a dark tongue with a greasy or turbid greasy coating, and a wiry and slippery pulse.

【Treatment Principle】

Flush phlegm and dispel stasis, drain the Lung and calm panting.

【Commonly Used Medicinals】

Use *bái jiè zǐ* (Semen Sinapis Albae), *sū zǐ* (Fructus Perillae), *lái fú zǐ* (Semen Raphani), *táo rén* (Semen Persicae), *dān shēn* (Radix et Rhizoma Salviae Miltiorrhizae), and *yù jīn* (Radix Curcumae) to clear phlegm and remove stasis. Use *tíng lì zǐ* (Semen Lepidii seu Descurainiae), *sāng bái pí* (Cortex Mori), *xìng rén* (Armenicae Semen Amarum), *fǎ bàn xià* (Rhizoma Pinelliae Praeparatum), and *fú líng* (Poria) to flush phlegm and dispel stasis.

【Representative Formula】

Modified *Tíng Lì Dà Zǎo Xiè Fèi Tāng* (葶苈大枣泻肺汤) plus *Sān Zǐ Yǎng Qīn Tāng* (三子养亲汤) and *Guì Zhī Fú Líng Wán* (桂枝茯苓丸).

【Ingredients】

葶苈子	tíng lì zǐ	15g	Semen Lepidii seu Descurainiae
白芥子	bái jiè zǐ	10g	Semen Sinapis Albae
苏子	sū zǐ	15g	Fructus Perillae
莱菔子	lái fú zǐ	15g	Semen Raphani
桃仁	táo rén	10g	Semen Persicae
丹皮	dān pí	15g	Cortex Moutan

桑白皮	sāng bái pí	15g	Cortex Mori
杏仁	xìng rén	10g	Armeniacae Semen Amarum
法半夏	fǎ bàn xià	10g	Rhizoma Pinelliae Praeparatum
茯苓	fú líng	15g	Poria
桂枝	guì zhī	10g	Ramulus Cinnamomi

Decoct in 800ml of water until 200ml of the decoction is left. Divide into 2 portions, take warm for one day.

【Formula Analysis】

Tíng lì zǐ (Semen Lepidii seu Descurainiae) and *sāng bái pí* (Cortex Mori) drain the Lung and calm panting. *Bái jiè zǐ* (Semen Sinapis Albae), *sū zǐ* (Fructus Perillae), and *lái fú zǐ* (Semen Raphani) dispel phlegm and disinhibit qi. *Fǎ bàn xià* (Rhizoma Pinelliae Praeparatum), *xìng rén* (Armeniacae Semen Amarum), and *fú líng* (Poria) fortify the Spleen and transform phlegm. *Dān pí* (Cortex Moutan), *táo rén* (Semen Persicae), and *guì zhī* (Ramulus Cinnamomi) invigorate blood and eliminate stasis.

【Modifications】

➤ For distention and fullness of the chest and abdomen, with a thick and greasy tongue coating, add *cāng zhú* (Rhizoma Atractylodis) 10g and *hòu pò* (Cortex Magnoliae Officinalis) 10g so as to dry dampness and fortify the Spleen.

➤ For white, sticky and frothy sputum, add *gān jiāng* (Rhizoma Zingiberis) 5g and *xì xīn* (Radix et Rhizoma Asari) 3g so as to warm and transform phlegm fluids.

➤ For cases with qi deficiency of both the Lung and Spleen marked by susceptibility to sweating, shortness of breath, and weakness in expectoration, add *dǎng shēn* (Radix Codonopsis) 15g, *huáng qí* (Radix Astragali) 15g, and *bái zhú* (Rhizoma Atractylodis Macrocephalae) 15g so as to tonify and boost the Lung and Spleen.

(4) Phlegm Clouding the Spirit-orifice

【Syndrome Characteristics】

Blurred consciousness or restlessness, a red complexion, delirium, a stiff tongue with slurred speech, gasping with gurgling sounds, difficulty in expectoration, a dark red tongue with a yellow and turbid coating, and a slippery or rapid-irregular pulse.

【Treatment Principle】

Transform phlegm and open the orifice; purge the bowels and promote resuscitation.

【Commonly Used Medicinals】

Use *shí chāng pú* (Rhizoma Acori Tatarinowii), *yù jīn* (Radix Curcumae), *zhú lì shuǐ* (Bambusae Succus), *dǎn nán xīng* (Arisaema cum Bile), *zhǐ shí* (Fructus Aurantii Immaturus), *fǎ bàn xià* (Rhizoma Pinelliae Praeparatum), *tiān zhú huáng* (Concretio Silicea Bambusae), and *tíng lì zǐ* (Semen Lepidii seu Descurainiae) to transform phlegm and open the orifice. Use *quán guā lóu* (Fructus Trichosanthis), *dà huáng* (Radix et Rhizoma Rhei), and *hǔ zhàng* (Radix et Rhizoma Polygoni Cuspidati) to purge the bowels and promote resuscitation.

【Representative Formula】

Modified *Chāng Pú Yù Jīn Tāng* (菖蒲郁金汤)

【Ingredients】

石菖蒲	shí chāng pú	10g	Rhizoma Acori Tatarinowii
郁金	yù jīn	15g	Radix Curcumae
竹沥水	zhú lì shuǐ	100ml	Bambusae Succus
胆南星	dǎn nán xīng	10g	Arisaema cum Bile
枳实	zhǐ shí	10g	Fructus Aurantii Immaturus
葶苈子	tíng lì zǐ	15g	Semen Lepidii seu Descurainiae
大黄	dà huáng	6g	Radix et Rhizoma Rhei

Decoct in 500ml of water until 200ml of the decoction is left. Divide into two portions.

【Formula Analysis】

Shí chāng pú (Rhizoma Acori Tatarinowii), *yù jīn* (Radix Curcumae), *zhú lì* (Bambusae Succus), *dǎn xīng* (Arisaema cum Bile), *zhǐ shí* (Fructus Aurantii Immaturus) and *tíng lì zǐ* (Semen Lepidii seu Descurainiae) disinhibit qi, clear and transform turbid phlegm. *Dà huáng* (Radix et Rhizoma Rhei) purges the bowels to promote resuscitation.

【Modifications】

➢ For tetany with Liver-wind internally stirring, add *gōu téng* (Ramulus Uncariae cum Uncis) 30g, *bái sháo* (Radix Paeoniae Alba) 15g, and *tiān má* (Rhizoma Gastrodiae) 10g (dissolved in hot water before taking).

➢ For cyanosis of the lips and nails, add *táo rén* (Semen Persicae) 10g, *dān shēn* (Radix et Rhizoma Salviae Miltiorrhizae) 15g, and *hóng huā* (Flos Carthami) 5g so as to invigorate blood and resolve stasis.

(5) Retention of Water due to Yang Deficiency

【Syndrome Characteristics】

Palpitations, cough and dyspnea, expectoration of clear and thin sputum, panting aggravated by exertion, inability to lie flat, edema that is more severe in the lower limbs, scanty or profuse urine, a dark and gloomy complexion, cyanosis of the lips, cold body and limbs, soreness and weakness of the waist and knees, occasional cold sweats, a pale and swollen or dark purple tongue with a white and glossy coating, and a deep and slippery or knotted or intermittent pulse.

【Treatment Principle】

Warm yang and disinhibit water; invigorate blood and transform stasis.

【Commonly Used Medicinals】

Use *shú fù zǐ* (Radix Aconiti Lateralis Praeparata), *gān jiāng* (Rhizoma Zingiberis), *ròu guì* (Cortex Cinnamomi), *bái zhú* (Rhizoma

Atractylodis Macrocephalae), *fú líng* (Poria), *tíng lì zǐ* (Semen Lepidii seu Descurainiae), *chē qián zǐ* (Semen Plantaginis), and *sāng bái pí* (Cortex Mori) to warm yang and disinhibit water. Use *chì sháo* (Radix Paeoniae Rubra), *dān shēn* (Radix et Rhizoma Salviae Miltiorrhizae), *yì mǔ cǎo* (Herba Leonuri), and *zé lán* (Herba Lycopi) to invigorate blood and transform stasis.

【Representative Formula】

Zhēn Wǔ Tāng (真武汤) with modifications

【Ingredients】

熟附子	shú fù zǐ	10g (decocted first)	Radix Aconiti Lateralis Praeparata
干姜	gān jiāng	6g	Rhizoma Zingiberis
肉桂	ròu guì	1.5g	Cortex Cinnamomi
白术	bái zhú	15g	Rhizoma Atractylodis Macrocephalae
茯苓	fú líng	30g	Poria
葶苈子	tíng lì zǐ	15g	Semen Lepidii seu Descurainiae
桑白皮	sāng bái pí	15g	Cortex Mori
白芍	bái sháo	15g	Radix Paeoniae Alba
丹参	dān shēn	15g	Radix et Rhizoma Salviae Miltiorrhizae
益母草	yì mǔ cǎo	20g	Herba Leonuri

Decoct in 800ml of water until 200ml of the decoction is left. Divide into two portions and take warm for one day.

【Formula Analysis】

Within this formula, *shú fù zǐ* (Radix Aconiti Lateralis Praeparata), *gān jiāng* (Rhizoma Zingiberis), and *ròu guì* (Cortex Cinnamomi) warm yang of the Heart and Kidney to invigorate the yang qi. *Bái zhú* (Rhizoma Atractylodis Macrocephalae) fortifies the Spleen to eliminate dampness; a larger quantity of *fú líng* (Poria) fortifies the Spleen to disinhibit water. *Tíng lì zǐ* (Semen Lepidii seu Descurainiae) and *sāng bái pí* (Cortex Mori) drain the Lung and disinhibit water. *Bái sháo* (Radix Paeoniae Alba), *dān shēn* (Radix et Rhizoma Salviae Miltiorrhizae) and *yì mǔ cǎo* (Herba leonuri) invigorate blood, transform stasis and disinhibit water.

【Modifications】

➢ For edema, add *chē qián zǐ* (Semen Plantaginis) 30g and *zé xiè* (Rhizoma Alismatis) 20g so as to dsinhibit water to relieve swelling.

➢ For severe blood stasis, add *zé lán* (Herba Lycopi) 15g and *wǔ jiā pí* (Cortex Acanthopanacis) 15g.

➢ For potential collapse due to qi deficiency, add *hóng shēn* (Radix et Rhizoma Ginseng Rubra) 10g (simmered separately).

(6) Original Yang about to Expire

【Syndrome Characteristics】

Unconsciousness, dyspnea with over-inflation of the chest, rhonchi in the throat, forehead sweats or spontaneous cold sweats, intense coldness of the limbs, cold nasal tip and head, and a faint pulse that is hard to detect.

【Treatment Principle】

Restore yang and consolidate yin so as to rescue the patient from collapse.

【Commonly Used Medicinals】

Use *hóng shēn* (Radix et Rhizoma Ginseng Rubra), *shú fù zǐ* (Radix Aconiti Lateralis Praeparata), *gān jiāng* (Rhizoma Zingiberis), *wǔ wèi zǐ* (Fructus Schisandrae Chinensis), *shān zhū yú* (Fructus Corni), *duàn lóng gǔ* (Os Draconis Calcinatun), *duàn mǔ lì* (Concha Ostreae Calcinatun), and *bái sháo* (Radix Paeoniae Alba) to restore yang and consolidate yin to rescue the patient from collapse.

【Representative Formula】

Shēn Fù Lóng Mǔ Tāng (参附龙牡汤) plus *Shēn Mài Sǎn* (参麦散) with modifications

【Ingredients】

红参	hóng shēn	10g (simmered separately)	Radix et Rhizoma Ginseng Rubra
熟附子	shú fù zǐ	10g (decocted first)	Radix Aconiti Lateralis Praeparata
干姜	gān jiāng	6g	Rhizoma Zingiberis
五味子	wǔ wèi zǐ	9g	Fructus Schisandrae Chinensis
山茱萸	shān zhū yú	10g	Fructus Corni
煅龙骨	duàn lóng gǔ	30g	Os Draconis Calcinatun
煅牡蛎	duàn mǔ lì	30g	Concha Ostreae Calcinatun
麦冬	mài dōng	15g	Radix Ophiopogonis
炙甘草	zhì gān cǎo	10g	Radix et Rhizoma Glycyrrhizae Praeparata

Decoct in 800ml of water until 200ml of the decoction is left. Take in small portions at short intervals.

【Formula Analysis】

Shú fù zǐ (Radix Aconiti Lateralis Praeparata), *gān jiāng* (Rhizoma Zingiberis) and *zhì gān cǎo* (Radix et Rhizoma Glycyrrhizae Praeparata) restore yang and rescue the patient from collapse. *Hóng shēn* (Radix et Rhizoma Ginseng Rubra) greatly supplements the yang qi to supplement the exhausted qi. *Mài dōng* (Radix Ophiopogonis), *wǔ wèi zǐ* (Fructus Schisandrae Chinensis) and *shān zhū yú* (Fructus Corni) nourish and astringe. *Duàn lóng gǔ* (Os Draconis Calcinatun) and *duàn mǔ lì* (Concha Ostreae Calcinatun) astringe in order to stop perspiration and consolidate yin.

【Modifications】

➢ For cyanosis of the lips with a dark purple tongue, add *dān shēn* (Radix et Rhizoma Salviae Miltiorrhizae) 15g, *táo rén* (Semen Persicae) 10g, and *hóng huā* (Flos Carthami) 10g in order to invigorate blood and resolve stasis.

➢ For patients that have accompanying vexation due to internal heat, dry mouth, flushed cheeks, and viscous sweats, this indicates the exhaustion of both qi and yin. Therefore subtract *fù zǐ* (Radix Aconiti Lateralis Praeparata), and add *xī yáng shēn* (Radix Panacis Quinquefolii) 10g (simmered separately).

2. During the Remission Stage

(1) Deficiency of Lung Qi

【Syndrome Characteristics】

Mild cough with little sputum, breathlessness induced by exertion, a complexion with little luster, a low voice and a reluctance to speak, spontaneous sweating, susceptibility to catch colds, a pale tongue with a thin white coating, and a thready and weak pulse.

【Treatment Principle】

Supplement the Lung, nourish qi and consolidate the exterior.

【Commonly Used Medicinals】

Use *huáng qí* (Radix Astragali), *bái zhú* (Rhizoma Atractylodis Macrocephalae), *fáng fēng* (Radix Saposhnikoviae), *dǎng shēn* (Radix Codonopsitis) and *zhì gān cǎo* (Radix et Rhizoma Glycyrrhizae Praeparata) to supplement qi and consolidate the exterior.

【Representative Formula】

Yù Píng Fēng Sǎn (玉屏风散) with additions

【Ingredients】

黄芪	huáng qí	30g	Radix Astragali
白术	bái zhú	15g	Rhizoma Atractylodis Macrocephalae
防风	fáng fēng	10g	Radix Saposhnikoviae
党参	dǎng shēn	20g	Radix Codonopsitis
炙甘草	zhì gān cǎo	5g	Radix et Rhizoma Glycyrrhizae Praeparata
炙紫菀	zhì zǐ wǎn	10g	Radix et Rhizoma Asteris Praeparata
炙冬花	zhì dōng huā	10g	Flos Farfarae Praeparata

Decoct in 500ml of water until 200ml of the decoction is left. Take warm, 1 dose a day.

【Formula Analysis】

Huáng qí (Radix Astragali) nourishes qi and consolidates the exterior. As the auxiliary herbs, *bái zhú* (Rhizoma Atractylodis Macrocephalae) fortifies the Spleen, and *fáng fēng* (Radix Saposhnikoviae) dispels wind. The three medicinals in combination nourish qi and consolidate the exterior. Without retaining the evil, they eliminate the evil and do not injure the right qi. *Dǎng shēn* (Radix Codonopsis) and *zhì gān cǎo* (Radix et Rhizoma Glycyrrhizae Praeparata) assist *huáng qí* (Radix Astragali) to nourish qi. *Zhì zǐ wǎn* (Radix et Rhizoma Asteris Praeparata) and *zhì dōng huā* (Flos Farfarae Praeparata) stop cough and eliminate phlegm.

【Modifications】

➤ For copious sputum, add *bàn xià* (Rhizoma Pinelliae) 10g, *chén pí* (Pericarpium Citri Reticulatae) 5g, and *sū zǐ* (Fructus Perillae) 15g in order to eliminate phlegm.

➤ For excessive sweating, add *fú xiǎo mài* (Fructus Tritici Levis) 30g and *duàn mǔ lì* (Concha Ostreae Calcinatun) 30g in order to astringe sweat.

(2) Dual Deficiency of the Lung and Spleen

【Syndrome Characteristics】

Panting and cough, shortness of breath, much phlegm, fatigued spirit, lack of strength, spontaneous sweating, aversion to wind, poor appetite, loose stools, a pale and enlarged tongue with a white coating, and a thready and weak pulse.

【Treatment Principle】

Fortify the Spleen and nourish the Lung; transform phlegm and stop panting.

【Commonly Used Medicinals】

Use *huáng qí* (Radix Astragali), *bái zhú* (Rhizoma Atractylodis

Macrocephalae), *dǎng shēn* (Radix Codonopsis), *fú líng* (Poria), *zhì gān cǎo* (Radix et Rhizoma Glycyrrhizae Praeparata), and *shān yào* (Rhizoma Dioscoreae) to fortify the Spleen and boost the Lung. Use *xìng rén* (Armenicae Semen Amarum), *chén pí* (Pericarpium Citri Reticulatae), *fǎ bàn xià* (Rhizoma Pinelliae Praeparatum), and *sū zǐ* (Fructus Perillae) to transform phlegm and stop panting.

【Representative Formula】

Yù Píng Fēng Sǎn (玉屏风散) plus *Liù Jūn Zǐ Tāng* (六君子汤) with modifications

【Ingredients】

黄芪	huáng qí	30g	Radix Astragali
白术	bái zhú	15g	Rhizoma Atractylodis Macrocephalae
党参	dǎng shēn	20g	Radix Codonopsitis
茯苓	fú líng	15g	Poria
炙甘草	zhì gān cǎo	5g	Radix et Rhizoma Glycyrrhizae Praeparata
杏仁	xìng rén	10g	Armeniacae Semen Amarum
陈皮	chén pí	5g	Pericarpium Citri Reticulatae
法半夏	fǎ bàn xià	10g	Rhizoma Pinelliae Praeparatum
防风	fáng fēng	10g	Radix Saposhnikoviae

Decoct in 800ml of water until 200ml of the decoction is left. Take warm, 1 dose a day.

【Formula Analysis】

Huáng qí (Radix Astragali), *bái zhú* (Rhizoma Atractylodis Macrocephalae), and *fáng fēng* (Radix Saposhnikoviae) nourish qi and consolidate the exterior. *Dǎng shēn* (Radix Codonopsitis), *fú líng* (Poria), and *zhì gān cǎo* (Radix et Rhizoma Glycyrrhizae Praeparata) fortify the Spleen and boost qi. *Fǎ xià* (Rhizoma Pinelliae Praeparatum), *chén pí* (Pericarpium Citri Reticulatae), and *xìng rén* (Armeniacae Semen Amarum) transform phlegm and stop cough.

【Modifications】

➢ For severe panting, add *zhì má huáng* (Herba Ephedrae Praeparata) 5g and *sū zǐ* (Fructus Perillae) 15g in order to stop panting.

➢ For cases with copious and tenacious yellow sputum, add *sāng bái pí* (Cortex Mori) 15g, *huáng qín* (Radix Scutellariae) 15g, and *wěi jīng* (Coulis Phragmitis) 15g to clear heat and transform phlegm.

(3) Dual Deficiency of the Lung and Kidney

【Syndrome Characteristics】

Breathlessness, panting aggravated by exertion, or shallow, short and incontinuous breaths, a low voice and weak speech, cough with little sputum, a dark complexion, a pale tongue with a white coating, and a deep and weak pulse.

【Treatment Principle】

Tonify the Lung and boost qi; warm the Kidney to receive qi.

【Commonly Used Medicinals】

Use *rén shēn* (Radix Ginseng), *huáng qí* (Radix Astragali), *bái zhú* (Rhizoma Atractylodis Macrocephalae), *shān yào* (Rhizoma Dioscoreae) and *huáng jīng* (Rhizoma Polygonati) to tonify the Lung and boost qi. Use *gé jiè* (Gecko), *dōng chóng xià cǎo* (Cordyceps Sinensis), *hú táo ròu* (Semen Juglandis Regiae), *cí shí* (Magnetitum), and *chén xiāng* (Lignum Aquilariae Resinatum) to warm the Kidney so as to receive qi.

【Representative Formula】

Píng Chuǎn Gù Běn Tāng (平喘固本汤) with modifications

【Ingredients】

红参	hóng shēn	10g (simmered separately)	Radix et Rhizoma Ginseng Rubra
黄芪	huáng qí	30g	Radix Astragali
白术	bái zhú	15g	Rhizoma Atractylodis Macrocephalae
蛤蚧粉	gé jiè fěn	5g (dissolved in hot water before taking)	Gecko
胡桃肉	hú táo ròu	15g	Semen Juglandis Regiae

茯苓	fú líng	15g	Poria
杏仁	xìng rén	10g	Armeniacae Semen Amarum
川贝母粉	chuān bèi mǔ fěn	3g (dissolved in hot water before taking)	Bulbus Fritillariae Cirrhosae
磁石	cí shí	30g	Magnetitum
炙紫菀	zhì zǐ wǎn	10g	Radix et Rhizoma Asteris Praeparata
炙甘草	zhì gān cǎo	5g	Radix et Rhizoma Glycyrrhizae Praeparata
陈皮	chén pí	5g	Pericarpium Citri Reticulatae

Decoct in 800ml of water until 200ml of the decoction is left. Divide into two portions and take warm, 1 dose a day.

【Formula Analysis】

Hóng shēn (Radix et Rhizoma Ginseng Rubra) and *huáng qí* (Radix Astragali) tonify the Lung and boost qi. *Bái zhú* (Rhizoma Atractylodis Macrocephalae), *fú líng* (Poria), and *zhì gān cǎo* (Radix et Rhizoma Glycyrrhizae Praeparata) fortify the Spleen and boost qi. *Gé jiè* (Gecko), *hú táo ròu* (Semen Juglandis Regiae), and *cí shí* (Magnetitum) warm the Kidney to receive qi. *Chuān bèi* (Bulbus Fritillariae Cirrhosae), *xìng rén* (Armeniacae Semen Amarum), *zǐ wǎn* (Radix et Rhizoma Asteris) and *chén pí* (Pericarpium Citri Reticulatae) transform phlegm, stop cough and rectify qi.

【Modifications】

➢ For cases with obvious blood stasis like dark purplish lips and nails, add *dāng guī* (Radix Angelicae Sinensis) 10g and *chì sháo* (Radix Paeoniae Rubra) 15g to nourish and invigorate blood.

➢ For cases with intolerance of cold and cold limbs, white and thin or frothy sputum due to depletion of Kidney yang and a blockage of cold phlegm, add *lù jiǎo jiāo* (Colla Cornus Cervi) 15g (melted before used), *ròu guì* (Cortex Cinnamomi) 1.5g, *bái jiè zǐ* (Semen Sinapis Albae) 10g, and *gān jiāng* (Rhizoma Zingiberis Officinalis) 6g in order to warm yang and transform phlegm.

Additional treatment modalities

1. Chinese Patent Medicine

(1) *Qū Tán Zhǐ Ké Chōng Jì* (祛痰止咳冲剂)

Fortifies the Spleen and dries dampness, eliminates phlegm and stops cough. Taken orally, one bag three times a day.

(2) *Ān Dá Píng Kǒu Fú Yè* (安达平口服液)

Nourishes yin and astringes the Lung, stops cough and eliminates phlegm. Taken orally, 15ml, 3 times a day.

(3) *Zhū Bèi Dìng Chuǎn Wán* (珠贝定喘丸)

Rectifies qi and transforms phlegm, stops cough and calms panting, supplements qi and warms the Kidney. Taken by holding it in the mouth, or orally with warm boiled water, 6 pills, 3 times a day.

(4) *Xiān Zhú Lì Kǒu Fú Yè* (鲜竹沥口服液)

Clears heat and transforms phlegm. Taken orally, 10ml, 3 times a day.

(5) *Xuán Mài Gān Jú Jiāo Náng* (玄麦柑橘胶囊)

Clears heat and nourishes yin, eliminates phlegm and benefits the throat. Taken orally, 3 to 4 pills, three times a day.

(6) *Jú Hóng Tán Ké Gāo* (橘红痰咳膏)

Rectifies qi and eliminates phlegm, moistens the Lung and stops cough. Taken orally, 15ml, 3 times a day.

(7) *Bǎi Lìng Jiāo Náng* (百令胶囊)

Tonifies the deficient and damaged, nourishes the *jing* qi (essential qi), protects the Lungs and boosts the Kidneys, stops cough and transforms phlegm, astringes, settles and tranquilizes. Taken orally, 5 pills, 3 times a day.

(8) *Jīn Shuǐ Bǎo* (金水宝)

Tonifies and boosts the Lung and Kidney, contains the *jing* (essence), and boosts qi. Taken orally, 3 pills, 3 times a day.

(9) *Shēng Mài Jiāo Náng* (生脉胶囊)

Boosts qi and restores the pulse, nourishes yin and engenders fluids. Taken orally, 3 pills, 3 times a day.

(10) *Hóu Zǎo Sǎn* (猴枣散)

This is suitable for patients with an accumulation of phlegm-heat in the Lung. Taken orally, 1 vial, 3 times a day.

(11) *Shé Dǎn Chuān Bèi Yè* (蛇胆川贝液)

This is suitable for patients with phlegm-heat accumulating in the Lung. Taken orally, 1 vial, 3 times a day.

2. Acupuncture and Moxibustion

(1) Body Acupuncture

【Point Selection】

BL 13	fèi shù	肺俞
RN 17	dàn zhōng	膻中
EX-B1	dìng chuǎn	定喘

【Point Modifications】

➢ For cases of exterior cold and interior heat, add LU 5 (*chǐ zé*), LI 4 (*hé gǔ*), and DU 14 (*dà zhuī*).

➢ For cases with accumulation of phlegm-heat in the Lung, add LU 5 (*chǐ zé*), LI 4 (*hé gǔ*), and ST 40 (*fēng lóng*).

➢ For cases with a blockage of damp-phlegm in the Lung, add RN 12 (*zhōng wǎn*), ST 40 (*fēng lóng*), BL 20 (*pí shù*), and ST 36 (*zú sān lǐ*).

➢ For deficiency panting, add BL 43 (*gāo huāng*), ST 36 (*zú sān lǐ*), BL 20 (*pí shù*), BL 23 (*shèn shù*), RN 4 (*guān yuán*) and RN 6 (*qì hǎi*).

【Manipulation】

Use even supplementation and drainage, and retain the needles for 30 minutes. Do once a day.

(2) Electro-Acupuncture

【Point Selection】

BL 13	fèi shù	肺俞
EX-B1	dìng chuǎn	定喘
RN 17	dàn zhōng	膻中
RN 22	tiān tū	天突
ST 36	zú sān lǐ	足三里
ST 40	fēng lóng	丰隆

【Manipulation】

Use sparse-dense waves for 30 minutes of electro-acupuncture therapy, once daily or every other day. Ten times makes up a course of treatment.

(3) Ear Acupuncture

【Point Selection】

apex of tragus	TG1p	píng jiān	屏尖
Anti-asthma		píng chuǎn	平喘
brain		nǎo	脑
Xiajiaoduan		xià jiǎo duān	下脚端
Intertragal notch		píng jiān	屏间

【Manipulation】

Use filiform needles, with perpendicular insertion, and moderate stimulation. Retain the needles for 20 minutes, once a day. This is suitable for every pattern of this disease.

(4) External Application

Take equal portions of *má huáng* (Herba Ephedrae), *gān cǎo* (Radix et

Rhizoma Glycyrrhizae), *wǔ wèi zǐ* (Fructus Schisandrae Chinensis), and *zhū shā* (Cinnabaris). Dry them in an oven and grind them together into a fine powder. Then the sieved powder is prepared by mixing it with wine into a paste. This paste is then plastered on at EX-B1 (*dìng chuǎn*), BL 13 (*fèi shù*), and RN 22 (*tiān tū*). The paste is covered with moxa piece and gauze, and fixed with adhesive tape. The dressing should be changed every 24 hours. Ten times makes up a course of treatment, with a week interval between two courses. This is suitable for patients with productive cough, panting, fever and insomnia.

Use 3g each of *dǎng shēn* (Radix Codonopsis), *zhì gān cǎo* (Radix et Rhizoma Glycyrrhizae Praeparata), and *gān jiāng* (Rhizoma Zingiberis), and 6g of *bái zhú* (Rhizoma Atractylodis Macrocephalae). Grind them together into a powder, and then add 20g of *Huà Shān Shēn Jìn Gāo* (华山参浸膏, the extract of *huà shān shēn* [Radix Physochlainae]). Mix them until uniform and then grind them into a fine powder. Make this into a paste with wine, and apply topically at RN 8 (*shén quē*). Cover the paste with gauze and fix with a plaster. The dressing should be changed every three days, successively 4－5 times. This is used for deficiency panting.

(5) Suture Embedding at Points
【Point Selection】

1) Clinical attack stage：

DU 14	dà zhuī	大椎
EX-B1	dìng chuǎn	定喘
BL 12	fēng mén	风门
RN 17	dàn zhōng	膻中
ST 40	fēng lóng	丰隆
ST 36	zú sān lǐ	足三里
BL 13	fèi shù	肺俞

2) Clinical remission stage:

BL 23	shèn shù	肾俞
BL 20	pí shù	脾俞
BL 13	fèi shù	肺俞
ST 36	zú sān lǐ	足三里
RN 4	guān yuán	关元
RN 17	dàn zhōng	膻中
ST 40	fēng lóng	丰隆
KI 13	tài xī	太溪

【Point Modification】

➢ For cases mainly with cough, add LU 6 (kǒng zuì).
➢ For cases mainly with panting, add LU 10 (yú jì).
➢ For cases with obvious blood stasis, add BL 17 (gé shù).
➢ Except for DU 14 (dà zhuī), RN 17 (dàn zhōng), and RN 4 (guān yuán), all other points may be used bilaterally.

【Manipulation】

Disinfect the points using conventional methods, and anesthetize locally. Forceps are used in the left hand to pick up the prepared suture. It is placed onto the local anesthetized point. With the right hand, the embedding needle is held, and pressed downward on the suture with the tip of the needle. It is placed in the point with an angle of 15°—45°. The depth is the same as for acupuncture. There should be no deeper insertion in the trunk points. No bleeding should occur from stimulation. After the withdrawal of the needle, place an alcohol-soaked cotton-ball on the hole, and fix it in place with a plaster for 1 to 3 days. This is done once every 1½ months as a course of treatment. Six courses later the effect was statistically analyzed. During the period of treatment, no raw, cold, greasy or irritating foods should be eaten, and there should be no overeating. Heavy physical labor should be avoided within a week of the procedure.

3. Simple Prescriptions and Empirical Formulas

(1) *Xìng Rén Hú Táo Sǎn* (杏仁胡桃散)

杏仁	xìng rén	Armeniacae Semen Amarum
胡桃仁	hú táo rén	Semen Juglandis Regiae

The two herbs are used in equal portions and are ground into a fine powder. This is taken orally, 3g, three times a day. It can be mixed with a little bit of honey before taken. As it can tonify the Kidney and boost the Lung, it is suitable for cases with qi deficiency of the Lung and Kidney.

(2)

紫花杜鹃	zǐ huā dù juān	75g	Rhododendron Mariae Hance
矮地茶	ǎi dì chá	50g	Herba Ardisiae Japonicae

Decoct them twice, and divide into two portions. Take orally, one dosage per day. This prescription is for cases of deficiency of both the Lung and Spleen.

(3)

人参	rén shēn	15g	Radix Ginseng
胡桃	hú táo	9g	Semen Juglandis Regiae
生姜	shēng jiāng	3 slices	Rhizoma Zingiberis Recens

This is suitable for patients with general weakness.

(4)

千年矮 (紫金牛)	qiān nián ǎi (zǐ jīn niú)	25g	Herba Ardisiae Japonicae
干枝	gān zhī	25g	Radix Campylotropis Harmsii
石膏	shí gāo	15g	Gypsum Fibrosum
桔梗	jié gěng	12g	Radix Platycodonis
干地龙	gān dì lóng	9g	Lumbricus
蜂蜜	fēng mì	30g	Mel

| 猪苦胆 | zhū kǔ dǎn | 1 piece | Pig Gallbladder |
| 甘草 | gān cǎo | 5g | Radix et Rhizoma Glycyrrhizae |

Decoct with water. This prescription is suitable for excess or heat-type panting.

(5)

| 生梨 | shēng lí | 1 piece | Raw Pear |
| 柿饼 | shì bǐng | 2 pieces | Preserved Persimmon |

Decoct with water. The indication is *fèi zhàng* (Lung distention) caused by yin deficiency of both the Lung and Kidney.

(6) *Fèi Fù Kāng Hé Jì* (肺复康合剂)

桃仁	táo rén	50g	Semen Persicae
红花	hóng huā	50g	Flos Carthami
川芎	chuān xiōng	50g	Rhizoma Chuanxiong
杏仁	xìng rén	50g	Armeniacae Semen Amarum
当归	dāng guī	75g	Radix Angelicae Sinensis
赤芍	chì sháo	75g	Radix Paeoniae Rubra
麻黄	má huáng	75g	Herba Ephedrae
车前子	chē qián zǐ	75g	Semen Plantaginis
百部	bǎi bù	60g	Radix Stemonae

All of the medicinals are decocted together twice with water, then condensed to 500ml. Take 100ml daily, in 3 portions. One course of treatment is 2 successive months. Its indication is *fèi zhàng* (Lung distention) due to qi deficiency and blood stasis, and accumulation of turbid phlegm in the Lung.

(7) *Ké Chuǎn Hé Jì* (咳喘合剂)

| 蔓荆子 | màn jīng zǐ | 15g | Fructus Viticis |
| 金荞麦 | jīn qiáo mài | 15g | Rhizoma Fagopyri Dibotryis |

佛耳草	fó ěr cǎo	10g	Herba Gnaphalii
天竺子	tiān zhú zǐ	10g	Fructus Nandinae Domesticae

Decoct with water. This is suitable for cases with excess or heat-type panting during the acute exacerbated stage of COPD.

PROGNOSIS

Once COPD has developed, the destruction of the lung tissues is irreversible, and recovery is difficult. In addition, due to decreased immunity of the body, there can be repeated respiratory tract infections. These occur especially during the winter and spring seasons, or during times of markedly changing weather. Each infection can lead to further decreases in lung function, finally resulting in a gradual aggravation of the cardiopulmonary function. Hence there can be respiratory failure or right-sided heart failure. Thus there can be an unfavorable prognosis. Nevertheless, if appropriate treatment is conducted during the progression of COPD, the cardiopulmonary function can be, to a certain degree, restored. Therefore it is extremely important to give to COPD and high-risk patients rehabilitative treatments and preventative education. Based on differing patient circumstances, also give lifestyle, dietary, and mental-emotional recommendations.

PREVENTIVE HEALTHCARE

The prevention strategies for COPD include avoiding high risk factors like pathogens and other agents that can induce acute aggravations of the disease, as well as enhancing the body's immunity. Giving up smoking is essential, and also the most simple and practical measure — it is good at any time during COPD in order to prevent the onset and development of the disease. Controlling vocational and environmental pollution, so as to lessen the inhalation of harmful gases or particles, can reduce abnormal inflammatory reactions of the airway and lung. Actively preventing and treating respiratory tract infections in infanthood and childhood may be helpful in reducing the chance of the disease occurring later in life. The influenza virus vaccine and Streptococcus pneumoniae vaccine may be useful in stopping repeated infections. Increasing physical exercise in order to improve the constitution and raise the body's immunity can improve the general condition of the body. In addition, monitoring of lung function should be performed regularly in high-risk COPD patients so as to recognize the illness and to give prompt intervention.

Lifestyle Modification

The COPD patient should pay attention to protecting against cold, keeping warm, and increasing strength.

1. Engage in Cold-Resistance Exercises such as Rubbing the Body Down with Cold Water

This strengthens the constitution and protects against catching colds.

2. Persist in Doing Abdominal Breathing and Pursed-lip Respiration in order to Improve Pulmonary Ventilation

3. Do Exercises to Restore Health, like *Taiji*, Walking, and Jogging

These strengthen resistance to cold and enhance the constitution. Exercises should be chosen according to the individual condition of the patient's physique and disease state, or the amount of exercise should depend on the results of cardiopulmonary exercise testing under ECG and respiratory function monitoring, so that their exercises for pulmonary rehabilitation can be beneficial. Generally the amount of exercise should increase from less to more, and the duration should increase from shorter to longer. Strenuous exercise should be avoided.

4. Rubbing the Nose

Use the two index fingers to rub on LI 20 (*yíng xiāng*) and along the sides of the bridge of the nose for 10–20 times. Massage DU 25 (*sù liáo*) from right to left, then in the opposite direction, for 10–20 times each way.

5. Expanding the Chest

Move the left foot a half-step to the left, and stand with the feet shoulder-width apart. Raise the arms upward while inhaling forcefully; draw the arms back to the front of the chest while exhaling forcefully, and move the left foot back, standing at attention. Repeat the movement, reversing sides. The movements are done alternately reversing the left and the right, for 4 times.

6. Pressing the Abdomen

Move the left foot to the left a half-step, raise the arms to the sides and upward with the palms turned up. Turn the head slightly backward while inhaling forcefully; quickly draw back the arms to press the abdomen (with the right hand on the top of the left hand), with the torso slightly bent foreword while exhaling forcefully. Draw back the left foot and stand still with both hands down. Repeat the above movement, reversing sides. The movements are done alternating left and right, 4 times each.

7. Clenching the Fists

Clench both fists at the front of the chest with the palms facing inward. With the elbows bent, swing both the arms upward and backward for 3 successive times while inhaling. Repeat the movement, in the opposite direction, for 3 successive times while exhaling. Draw the arms back to the starting position. Repeat the above movements 3 times.

8. Massage

The patient can massage the points on his Lung channel, as well as RN 22 (*tiān tū*) and RN 17 (*dàn zhōng*). He can also use his hands to lightly tap the points alongside the spine, from the top to the bottom, several times in a row. This is helpful to expel sputum. In addition, the patient can also do training or relaxing of the respiratory muscles: take a sitting position, with the torso slightly bent forward, elbows bent at an angle of 90°, and the shoulders relaxed. Circle the arms and shoulder joints from the front to the back for 10－20 cycles. This action should be done gently and slowly.

9. Keep the Indoor Air Circulating, and Maintain Appropriate Temperature and Humidity

The patients should not go to places where the air is unclean, or where large crowds of people gather.

Dietary Recommendation

The COPD patient should carry out active dietary regulations, such as eating medicinal foods that can cooperate with pharmacotherapies so as to enhance their effect. The food should be light, nutritive-rich, and easy to digest. This includes soft rice, well cooked rice, porridge, noodles, breads, and fresh milk. These dietary changes should be done in an orderly and gradual way, with regular intake of frequent small meals, avoiding immoderate drinking and eating and overeating. The patient should also avoid raw, cold, overly sweet, greasy, pungent, dry, and hot foods. Dietary therapy assists to greatly fortify the Spleen, Lung and Kidney, supplementing the right qi and strengthening the constitution, and raising the resistance of the body against the illness.

The medicinals that can be used for dietary therapy include *bǎi hé* (Bulbus Lilii), *bái guǒ* (Semen Ginkgo), *xìng rén* (Armeniacae Semen

Amarum), *luó hàn guǒ* (Fructus Momordicae), *chuān bèi mǔ* (Bulbus Fritillariae Cirrhosae), *hé táo* (Semen Juglandis), *chén pí* (Pericarpium Citri Reticulatae), *fó shǒu* (Fructus Citri Sarcodactylis), *dīng xiāng* (Flos Caryophylli), *rén shēn* (Radix Ginseng), *fú líng* (Poria), *shān yào* (Rhizoma Dioscoreae), *qiàn shí* (Semen Euryales), *dāng guī* (Radix Angelicae Sinensis), *huáng qí* (Radix Astragali), *gé jiè* (Gecko), *mài dōng* (Radix Ophiopogonis), *shā shēn* (Radix Glehniae seu Adenophorae), *lián zǐ* (Stamen Nelumbinis), *xuě ěr* (Tremela), *dōng chóng xià cǎo* (Cordyceps Sinensis) and foods like lean pork meal, chicken, tortoise and turtle, fish air bladder and bird's (swallow's) nest.

1. *Gǒu Qǐ Zǐ* (Fructus Lycii) Stewed Pig Heart (枸杞子炖猪心)

枸杞子	gǒu qǐ zǐ	10g	Fructus Lycii
鲜猪心	xiān zhū xīn	1 piece	Fresh Pig Heart

Wash the pig heart until clean and dry, then stew it together with *gǒu qǐ zǐ* (Fructus Lycii) on a slow fire for about 1 hour, season the soup with a little bit of salt. It is suitable for deficiency of Kidney qi.

2. Crucian Carp, *Xìng Rén* (Armeniacae Semen Amarum) and Brown Sugar Soup (鲫鱼杏仁红糖汤)

鲫鱼	jì yú	1 piece	Crucian Carp
甜杏仁	tián xìng rén	9g	Armeniacae Semen Amarum

Remove the scales, gills and internal organs of the carp, and clean it, then put it into a pot together with *tián xìng rén* (Armeniacae Semen Amarum) and appropriate amount of water to cook. Then add a reasonable amount of brown sugar and cook continuously for a few moments. This remedy is suitable for cases of internal blockage by turbid phlegm with symptoms of cough, excessive sputum, dyspnea, and emaciation.

3. *Xìng Rén* (Armeniacae Semen Amarum) and Pig Lung Decoction (杏仁猪肺汤)

猪肺	zhū fèi	250g	Pig Lung
杏仁	xìng rén	10g	Armeniacae Semen Amarum

Cut the pig lung into pieces; clean and put them in water together with *xìng rén* (Armeniacae Semen Amarum) in enough water. Decoct, and just before well cooked, add 1－2 spoons of ginger liquid. Season the soup with table salt. Drink the soup and eat the lung, twice a day. The quantity may be dependent upon individual conditions. It is suitable for a pattern of Lung qi deficiency.

4. *Hé Táo* (Semen Juglandis) Stewed *Xìng Rén* (Armeniacae Semen Amarum) (核桃炖杏仁)

生姜	shēng jiāng	30g	Rhizoma Zingiberis Recens
苦杏仁	kǔ xìng rén	15g	Armeniacae Semen Amarum
核桃仁	hé táo rén	30g	Semen Juglandis
蜂蜜	fēng mì	15g	Mel (honey)

Pound the *shēng jiāng* (Rhizoma Zingiberis Recens) 30g into a pulp and squeeze out its juice. Take off the skin and tips of *kǔ xìng rén* (Armeniacae Semen Amarum). Put the ginger juice, prepared *kǔ xìng rén* (Armeniacae Semen Amarum) 15g and *hé táo rén* (Semen Juglandis) 30g together, then pound them into a pulp and add 15g of honey. Cook well, then divide into 2 portions for one day's use. This is suitable for patients with cold panting. No honey should be added for patients with a thick greasy tongue coating and copious sputum.

5. Radish and Sugar Liquid (萝卜糖水)

红皮辣萝卜	hóng pí là luó bo	200g	Crimson Radish
白糖	bái táng	5g	Sugar

Clean the crimson radish and cut it into thin slices, then put the slices into a bowl and put the sugar on them. Let it rest overnight. On the next day, drink small portions of the liquid at short intervals. This is suitable for patients with cough and copious sputum due to heat.

6. *Bǔ Fèi Yì Shèn Gāo* (补肺益肾糕)

核桃仁	hé táo rén	30g	Semen Juglandis
莲米	lián mǐ	20g	Stamen Nelumbinis
柏子仁	bǎi zǐ rén	20g	Semen Platycladi
白果	bái guǒ	30g	Semen Ginkgo
陈皮	chén pí	10g	Pericarpium Citri Reticulatae
玉米粉	yù mǐ fěn	200g	Maize powder
淮山药	huái shān yào	200g	Rhizoma Dioscoreae

Grind *hé táo rén* (Semen Juglandis), *lián mǐ* (Stamen Nelumbini), *bǎi zǐ rén* (Semen Platycladi), *bái guǒ* (Semen Ginkgo), and *chén pí* (Pericarpium Citri Reticulatae) into a powder and mix them. Add a little bit of brown sugar, then add the maize powder and the powder of *huái shān yào* (Rhizoma Dioscoreae) to make cakes. The cake can be taken long-term. The indication is COPD in the remission stage, manifesting as soreness and weakness of the waist and legs, shortness of breath, panting, and cough, which are aggravated upon exertion.

7. *Dān Shēn* (Radix et Rhizoma Salviae Miltiorrhizae) and *Huáng Qí* (Radix Astragali) Porridge (参芪粥)

丹参	dān shēn	20g	Radix et Rhizoma Salviae Miltiorrhizae
黄芪	huáng qí	20g	Radix Astragali
粳米	jīng mǐ	100g	Oryza Sativa

Decoct *dān shēn* (Radix et Rhizoma Salviae Miltiorrhizae) and *huáng qí* (Radix Astragali) twice with water. Add *jīng mǐ* (Oryza Sativa) into the prepared decoction and boil it into a porridge. This remedy can nourish the Lung and invigorate blood.

8. Pí Pá Yè (Folium Eriobotryae) Decoction (枇杷叶煎汤)

| 枇杷叶 | pí pá yè | 15g | Folium Eriobotryae |

Remove the hair of the herb, decoct it, and melt a little rock sugar in the decoction before taking. Divide into 2 portions for one day.

9. Rén Shēn (Radix Ginseng) and Hé Táo (Semen Juglandis) Decoction (人参核桃煎)

人参	rén shēn	6g	Radix Ginseng
核桃仁	hé táo rén	6 – 12 pieces	Semen Juglandis
生姜	shēng jiāng	3 slices	Rhizoma Zingiberis Recens

Put the *rén shēn* (Radix Ginseng), *hé táo* (Semen Juglandis) and *shēng jiāng* (Rhizoma Zingiberis Recens) into an earthen pot, and decoct the medicinals with an appropriate amount of water for about 1 hour. Drink the decoction and eat the *rén shēn* (Radix Ginseng) and *hé táo ròu* (Semen Juglandis), once a day. This remedy can supplement the Lung and Kidney, receive qi and calm panting. The contraindication is panting due to heat-phlegm.

Regulation of Emotional and Mental Health

Because of many years of illness without cure, COPD patients often need hospitalization for treatment during repeated acute aggravations of the disease. In addition, they ordinarily have cough, expectoration of sputum, dyspnea upon exertion, a poor quality of life, and heavy mental stress. Some patients may suffer from different degrees of anxiety and melancholy. Therefore pay attention to lifestyle and dietary regulation as the basis for self care. Even more so, the patient must have mental emotional healthcare, in order to aid them in establishing confidence in a victory over the disease. Encourage the patient to have a steady state of mind, and optimistic and positive ways of thinking. The patient should have dynamic cooperation with doctors, nurses and staff, in the treatment and restoration of his health. Lectures on COPD should be regularly held with wardmates, in order to help the patient understand the disease, strengthen communication, and increase confidence. If there emerges a serious mental-emotional disturbance, psychological counseling should be carried out in a timely manner.

CLINICAL EXPERIENCE OF RENOWNED PHYSICIANS

Empirical Formulas

1. The Treatment of Cough due to Deficiency of both the Lung and Spleen with Qì Zhǒng Fāng (气肿方) (Deng Tie-tao)

【Ingredients】

五爪龙	wǔ zhuǎ lóng	30g	Herba Tetrastigmatis Hypoglauci
太子参	tài zǐ shēn	30g	Radix Pseudostellariae
白术	bái zhú	15g	Rhizoma Atractylodis Macrocephalae
茯苓	fú líng	15g	Poria
甘草	gān cǎo	5g	Radix et Rhizoma Glycyrrhizae
苏子	sū zǐ	10g	Fructus Perillae
莱菔子	lái fú zǐ	10g	Semen Raphani
白芥子	bái jiè zǐ	10g	Semen Sinapis Albae
鹅管石	é guǎn shí	30g	Balanophyllia

【Indications】

Cough and panting in chronic bronchitis and emphysema during the remission stage.

【Modifications】

➢ For cases with severe cough, add *bǎi bù* (Radix Stemonae) 10g, *zǐ wǎn* (Radix et Rhizoma Asteris) 10g, and *jú luò* (Retinervs Citri Reticulatae Fructus) 10g.

➢ For cases with severe panting, add *má huáng* (Herba Ephedrae) 6g and *dì lóng* (Lumbricus) 10g.

➢ For cases accompanied by a stagnant complexion, add *máng guǒ hé* (Mangifera indicae) 10g and *bù zhā yè* (Folium Microcotis) 15g.

(Deng Tie-tao. *Essentials of Deng Tie-tao's Clinical Experience* 邓铁涛临床经验辑要. Beijing: The Medical Science and Technology Press of China, 1998. 310)

2. THE TREATMENT OF COUGH DUE TO ACCUMULATION OF COLD PHLEGM IN THE LUNG WITH *JIÉ CHUǍN TĀNG* (截喘汤) (JIANG CHUN-HUA)

【Ingredients】

佛耳草	fó ěr cǎo	1.5g	Gnaphalium Affine D.Don
碧桃干	bì táo gān	1.5g	Fructus Persicae Viride
老鹳草	lǎo guàn cǎo	1.5g	Herba Geranii
旋覆花	xuán fù huā	10g	Flos Inulae
全瓜蒌	quán guā lóu	10g	Fructus Trichosanthis
姜半夏	jiāng bàn xià	10g	Rhizoma Pinelliae Preparata
防风	fáng fēng	10g	Radix Saposhnikoviae
五味子	wǔ wèi zǐ	6g	Fructus Schisandrae Chinensis

【Indications】

Cough, copious sputum, dyspnea and panting (chronic bronchitis and emphysema).

【Formula Analysis】

Within this formula, *fó ěr cǎo* (Gnaphalium Affine D. Don), *bì táo gān* (Fructus Persicae Viride), and *lǎo guàn cǎo* (Herba Geranii) eliminate phlegm and stop cough, calm panting, and regulate the functions of the autonomic nervous system. As the assistant, *xuán fù huā* (Flos Inulae) can remove masses, transform phlegm, and downbear counterflow qi to stop cough.

(Tang Yi-xin, Wang Rui-xiang. *A Precious Manual of Secrete Prescriptions of Contemporary Famous Physicians in China* 中国当代名中医秘方临证备要. Chengdu: Sichuan Publishing House of Science & Technology, 1993. 303)

3. THE TREATMENT OF COUGH AND PANTING WITH COPIOUS SPUTUM DUE TO INVASION OF WIND-COLD WITH ZHǏ KÉ DÌNG CHUǍN TĀNG (止咳定喘汤) (YU SHEN-CHU)

【Ingredients】

炙麻黄	zhì má huáng	6g	Herba Ephedrae Praeparata
杏仁	xìng rén	5g	Armeniacae Semen Amarum
炙甘草	zhì gān cǎo	3g	Radix et Rhizoma Glycyrrhizae Praeparata
苏子	sū zǐ	10g	Fructus Perillae
白芥子	bái jiè zǐ	6g (wrapped)	Semen Sinapis Albae
葶苈子	tíng lì zǐ	6g	Semen Lepidii seu Descurainiae
炙款冬	zhì kuǎn dōng	6g	Flos Farfarae Praeparata
炙橘红	zhì jú hóng	5g	Exocarpium Citri Rubrum Praeparata
茯苓	fú líng	10g	Poria
清半夏	qīng bàn xià	6g	Rhizoma Pinelliae Praeparata

【Indications】

Acute and chronic bronchitis, bronchial asthma or mild emphysema. It is especially effective for cough and panting with copious sputum due to invasion of wind-cold.

【Formula Analysis】

In this formula, *má huáng* (Herba Ephedrae), *xìng rén* (Armeniacae Semen Amarum) and *gān cǎo* (Radix et Rhizoma Glycyrrhizae) (*Sān Niù Tāng* [三拗汤]) are acrid and warm in nature and expel the evil, diffuse the Lung and calm panting. *Tíng lì zǐ* (Semen Lepidii seu Descurainiae), *zǐ sū zǐ* (Fructus Perillae) and *bái jiè zǐ* (Semen Sinapis Albae), imitating the composing of *Sān Zǐ Yǎng Qīn Tāng* (三子养亲汤), donwbear qi and eliminate phlegm. However, Professor Yu always uses *tíng lì zǐ* (Semen Lepidii seu Descurainiae) as a substitute for *lái fú zǐ* (Semen Raphani) in the original formula. He does this in order to enhance the effects of the formula to donwbear qi, eliminate phlegm and calm panting – thus it merges with *Sān Niù Tāng* (三拗汤) to gain better results by a combination of upbearing and downbearing.

【Modifications】

➢ For cases of obvious exterior pattern manifesting with aversion to cold and fever, nasal obstruction with discharge, add *jīng jiè* (Herba Schizonepetae), *fáng fēng* (Radix Saposhnikoviae), and *zǐ sū yè* (Folium Perillae).

➢ For difficult expectation due to tenacious sputum, add *sāng bái pí* (Cortex Mori), and *zhè bèi mǔ* (Bulbus Fritillariae Thunbergii).

➢ For chest oppression, add *guā lóu* (Fructus Trichosanthis), and *yù jīn* (Radix Curcumae).

➢ For cough and panting with yellow sputum, add *huáng qín* (Radix Scutellariae), *sāng bái pí* (Cortex Mori) and *zhè bèi mǔ* (Bulbus Fritillariae Thunbergii).

(Wang Pin. *A Complete Proved Prescriptions of Famous Veteran Doctors in State Level* — Assessed by State Administration of Traditional Chinese Medicine 国家级名老中医验方大全 . Urumqi: Xingjiang People's Health Publishing House, 2003. 119)

4. The Treatment of Cough due to Yang Deficiency of the Lung and Kidney with *Fèi Qì Zhǒng Yàn Fāng* (肺气肿验方) (Li Ke-shao)

【Ingredients】

红参	hóng shēn	9g	Radix et Rhizoma Ginseng Rubra
法半夏	fǎ bàn xià	9g	Rhizoma Pinelliae Praeparatum
冬虫夏草	dōng chóng xià cǎo	9g	Cordyceps Sinensis

麦门冬	mài mén dōng	12g	Radix Ophiopogonis
核桃肉	hé táo ròu	12g	Semen Juglandis
五味子	wǔ wèi zǐ	4.5g	Fructus Schisandrae Chinensis
厚朴	hòu pò	4.5g	Cortex Magnoliae Officinalis
炙甘草	zhì gān cǎo	3g	Radix et Rhizoma Glycyrrhizae Praeparata
炒苏子	chǎo sū zǐ	3g	Fructus Perillae Tostum
桂枝	guì zhī	6g	Ramulus Cinnamomi
杏仁	xìng rén	6g	Armeniacae Semen Amarum
生姜	shēng jiāng	2 slices	Rhizoma Zingiberis Recens

【Indications】

Chronic bronchitis and emphysema during remission stage.

【Modifications】

➤ In cases with lip cyanosis and blood stasis in the Lung, remove *hòu pò* (Cortex Magnoliae Officinalis), and add *é zhú* (Rhizoma Curcumae) 9g, and *huáng jiǔ* (millet wine) 12g to invigorate blood and resolve stasis.

➤ For cases accompanied by exogenous contraction, add *sū yè* (Folium Perillae) 9g and *chén pí* (Pericarpium Citri Reticulatae) 6g to course wind and transform phlegm.

(Lu Xiang-zhi. *Famous Doctors and Their Prescriptions in China* 中国名医名方. Beijing: China Medical Scientific and Technical Publishing House, 1991. 29)

5. The Treatment of Chronic Bronchitis with *Chú Yún Zhǐ Ké Tāng* (锄云止咳汤) (Yue Mei-zhong)

【Ingredients】

荆芥	jīng jiè	6g	Herba Schizonepetae
前胡	qián hú	9g	Radix Peucedani
白前	bái qián	6g	Radix et Rhizoma Cynanchi Stauntonii
杏仁	xìng rén	9g	Armeniacae Semen Amarum
贝母	bèi mǔ	9g	Bulbus Fritillariae
化橘红	huà jú hóng	6g	Exocarpium Citri Grandis

连翘	lián qiào	9g	Fructus Forsythiae
百部	bǎi bù	9g	Radix Stemonae
紫菀	zǐ wǎn	9g	Radix et Rhizoma Asteris
桔梗	jié gěng	6g	Radix Platycodonis
甘草	gān cǎo	3g	Radix et Rhizoma Glycyrrhizae
芦根	lú gēn	24g	Rhizoma Phragmitis

【Indications】

Protracted chronic bronchitis with symptoms of cough, copious white and tenacious sputum, chest oppression, and a itching throat.

【Formula Analysis】

In the formula, *jīng jiè* (Herba Schizonepetae) courses and scatters the residual wind-cold evils, *qián hú* (Radix Peucedani) descends qi and expels phlegm, *bái qián* (Radix et Rhizoma Cynanchi Stauntonii) eliminates the deep-lying phlegm, *zhè bèi mǔ* (Bulbus Fritillariae) treats cough due to exogenously contraction — with *xìng rén* (Armeniacae Semen Amarum) they benefit the lung qi, and increase the other's actions. *Jú hóng* (Exocarpium Citri Rubrum) is surely needed for cough with a itching throat; *lián qiào* (Fructus Forsythiae) and *gān cǎo* (Radix et Rhizoma Glycyrrhizae) detoxify; *bǎi bù cǎo* (Herba Stemonae) settles cough; *jié gěng* (Radix Platycodonis) smoothes the thorax and diaphragm and eliminates phlegm; *máo gēn* (Rhizoma Imperatae Cylindricae) clears the Lung heat, and *zǐ wǎn* (Radix et Rhizoma Asteris) treats cough due to invasion by wind evil. Together, all of the medicinals function to stop cough, hence the name is "*Chú Yún Zhǐ Ké Tāng* (锄云止咳汤, Cloud-Removing and Cough-Arresting Decoction)".

(Mi Yi-e. *Essentials of Effective and Proved Secret Prescriptions of the First Group of Famous Veteran Doctors in State Level—Assessed by State Administration of Traditional Chinese Medicine · Sequel* 首批国家级名老中医效验秘方精选·续集. Beijing: China Press of Traditional Chinese Medicine, 1999. 42-44)

6. The Treatment of Cough and Panting due to Deficiency Cold of the Kidney and Du Vessel, Coagulation and Stagnation of Phlegm and Stasis with *Yáng Hé Píng Chuǎn Tāng* (阳和平喘汤) (Hu Qiao-wu)

【Ingredients】

熟地黄	shú dì huáng	30g	Radix Rehmanniae Glutinosae Praeparata
淫羊藿	yín yáng huò	20g	Herba Epimedii
当归	dāng guī	10g	Radix Angelicae Sinensis
麻黄	má huáng	6g	Herba Ephedrae
紫石英	zǐ shí yīng	30g	Fluoritum
肉桂	ròu guì	3g	Cortex Cinnamomi
白芥子	bái jiè zǐ	6g	Semen Sinapis Albae
鹿角片	lù jiǎo piàn	20g	Cornu Cervi Slice
五味子	wǔ wèi zǐ	4g	Fructus Schisandrae Chinensis
桃仁	táo rén	10g	Semen Persicae
皂角	zào jiǎo	3g	Fructus Gleditsiae Sinensis

【Indications】

Prolonged cough and panting due to deficiency cold of the Kidney and Du vessel, coagulation and stagnation of phlegm and stasis in chronic bronchitis, asthmatic bronchitis and emphysema.

【Formula Analysis】

Shú dì (Radix Rehmanniae Glutinosae Praeparata), *lù jiǎo piàn* (Cornu Cervi Slice), *yín yáng huò* (Herba Epimedii) and *ròu guì* (Cortex Cinnamomi) warm and nourish the Kidney and Du vessel to dramatically reinforce the original qi. Using *lù jiǎo piàn* (Cornu Cervi Slice) as a substitute for *lù jiǎo jiāo* (Colla Cornus Cervi) avoids stagnation of the glue in order to benefit the turbid phlegm. *Lù jiǎo* (Cornu Cervi), in addition to the actions of warming and nourishing the Kidney and Du vessel, can play a role in invigorating blood, dredging the collaterals and dispelling stagnation. It combines with *shú dì* (Radix Rehmanniae Glutinosae Praeparata) to warm and nourish essence and blood, and reduces side effect of stagnation from the combined use of *lù jiǎo jiāo* (Colla Cornus Cervi) and *shú dì* (Radix Rehmanniae Glutinosae Praeparata). *Yín yáng huò* (Herba Epimedii) supplements the Kidney and strengthens yang, *ròu guì* (Cortex Cinnamomi) warms and nourishes the fire of vital gate. *Zǐ shí yīng* (Fluoritum) is heavy in quality, red in color, and sweet and warm in nature and flavor. It has a good function to warm and nourish the original qi; it is good for treating cough and panting with copious sputum, and it comminutes with *wǔ wèi zǐ* (Fructus Schisandrae Chinensis) to more effectively stop cough. The above six medicinals function together to be warming but not dry, nourishing but not greasy, receiving the counterflow of qi and calming the hyperactive qi. This is consistent with the principle of reinforcement, essence-supplementing and original qi nourishment. *Dāng guī* (Radix Angelicae Sinensis) both nourishes and activates blood, what is more it "treats cough and dyspnea" (*Classic of Materia Medica* [本经, *Běn Jīng*]). *Táo rén* (Semen Persicae) can break blood stasis, and is a perfect medicinal for "curing cough and dyspnea" (*Miscellaneous Records of Famous Physicians* [别录, *Bié Lù*]). Thus it combines with *lù jiǎo piàn* (Cornu Cervi Slice) and *zǐ shí yīng* (Fluoritum), functioning to regulate the nutritive phase, dredge the collaterals, stop cough, calm panting. With these actions, it is an absolutely necessary agent for treating cough and panting in the condition of stagnation and blockage of the collaterals due to involvement of blood phase from qi phase. *Bái jiè zǐ* (Semen Sinapis Albae) smoothes qi and expels phlegm, and *zào jiǎo* (Fructus Gleditsiae Sinensis) removes phlegm and opens the orifices. Both are acrid and warm so as to be agents treating Lung disorders. They are the first medicinals of choice for treating blockages of the airway by accumulation of cold-phlegm in the Lung. *Má huáng* (Herba Ephedrae) can open blockages and dredge obstacles so as to stop cough and calm panting; it pairs with *wǔ wèi zǐ* (Fructus Schisandrae Chinensis), functioning to regulate Lung qi by opening and closing.

Furthermore, warming and nourishing the Lung (metal), Kidney, and Du vessel, also treats diffusing and depurating and aids recovery. This works in combination with *má huáng* (Herba Ephedrae), and *wǔ wèi zǐ* (Fructus Schisandrae Chinensis), to benefit the qi of the body to be received, and phlegm-turbidity to be transported. The whole formula is well constructed, supplementing deficiency, reducing excess, treating the Lung upward and the Kidney downward. It is a good prescription to treat cough and panting due to phlegm and stasis in the Lung (metal), and deficiency cold of the original qi.

【Modifications】

➢ For cases of yang deficiency affecting yin, subtract *ròu guì* (Cortex Cinnamomi), add *shān yào* (Rhizoma Dioscoreae) 20g and *shān zhū yú* (Fructus Corni) 10g.

➢ For cases of cold-phlegm trasforming into heat, subtract *bái jiè zǐ* (Semen Sinapis Albae), and add *tíng lì zǐ* (Semen Lepidii seu Descurainiae) 10g and *zé qī* (Herba Euphorbiae Helioscopiae) 15g.

➢ For tachypnea and severe panting, add *sū zǐ* (Fructus Perillae) 10g and *chén xiāng* (Lignum Aquilariae Resinatum) 3g (added at the end).

➢ For constipation, add *ròu cōng róng* (Herba Cistanches) 20g and *zǐ wǎn* (Radix et Rhizoma Asteris) 20g.

➢ For poor apptite with fullness of the epigatrium, add *shā rén* (Fructus Amomi) 6g and *èr yá* (Fructus Setariae Germinatus and Fructus Hordei Germinatus) 30g each.

➢ For cases with little turbid phlegm, remove *bái jiè zǐ* (Semen Sinapis Albae) and *zào jiǎo* (Fructus Gleditsiae), and add *jú hóng* (Exocarpium Citri Rubrum) 10g and *fú líng* (Poria) 20g.

(Wang Pin. *A Complete Proved Prescriptions of Famous Veteran Doctors in State Level － Assessed by State Administration of Traditional Chinese Medicine* 国家级名老中医验方大全. Urumqi: Xinjiang People's Health Publishing House, 2003. 123-124)

7. The Treatment of Cough and Panting due to Dual Deficiency of the Lung and Kidney with Jiā Wèi Mài Wèi Dì Huáng Tāng (加味麦味地黄汤) (Dong Jian-hua)

【Ingredients】

麦冬	mài dōng	10g	Radix Ophiopogonis
五味子	wǔ wèi zǐ	10g	Fructus Schisandrae Chinensis
山萸肉	shān yú ròu	10g	Fructus Corni
紫石英	zǐ shí yīng	15g (decocted first)	Fluoritum
熟地	shú dì	10g	Radix Rehmanniae Glutinosae Praeparata
山药	shān yào	10g	Rhizoma Dioscoreae
丹皮	dān pí	10g	Cortex Moutan
茯苓	fú líng	10g	Poria
泽泻	zé xiè	10g	Rhizoma Alismatis
肉桂	ròu guì	3 – 6g	Cortex Cinnamomi

【Indications】

Panting and cough in elderly patients.

【Formula Analysis】

The Lung governs depuration and downbearing, controlling respiration. The Kidney is in charge of storage and receiving qi. If the two viscera are functioning well, with normal ascent and descent of qi, then no disease will appear. A person in his old age has depleted yin and yang. If he suffers from long-standing cough and panting, he will have deficiency of both the Lung and Kidney. So in this formula, *mài dōng* (Radix Ophiopogonis) is used to nourish yin and moisten the Lung, clear heat and stop cough. *Wǔ wèi zǐ* (Fructus Schisandrae Chinensis) supplements the Kidney, secures essence, and astringes Lung qi. *Zǐ shí yīng* (Fluoritum) warms and nourishes the Kidney yang. *Ròu guì* (Cortex Cinnamomi) guides the fire back to the origin, making qi return to the Kidney. All of the medicinals join together with *Liù Wèi Dì Huáng Wán* (六

味地黄丸), functioning both to astringe Lung qi and supplement the yin and yang of the Kidney.

(Wang Pin. *A Complete Proved Prescriptions of Famous Veteran Doctors in State Level* – *Assessed by State Administration of Traditional Chinese Medicine* 国家级名老中医验方大全 . Urumqi: Xinjiang People's Health Publishing House, 2003. 125）

8. The Treatment of Cough due to Deficiency of Both Qi and Yin with *Dài Mài Yǎng Fèi Zhǐ Ké Tāng* (黛麦养肺止咳汤) (Li Bing-nan)

【Ingredients】

青黛	qīng dài	5g	Indigo Naturalis
海蛤粉	hǎi gé fěn	30g	Pulvis Concha Meretricis seu Cyclinae
人参 (党参)	rén shēn (dǎng shēn)	10g (20g)	Radix Ginseng (or Radix Codonopsitis Pilosulae)
五味子	wǔ wèi zǐ	10g	Fructus Schisandrae Chinensis
细辛	xì xīn	3g	Radix et Rhizoma Asari
炙甘草	zhì gān cǎo	10g (reduced dose for children)	Radix et Rhizoma Glycyrrhizae Praeparata

【Indications】

Cough due to deficiency of qi and yin (cough after external contraction, chronic larygopharyngitis, and tracheitis).

【Formula Analysis】

This formula is composed of *Dài Gé Sǎn* (黛蛤散) and *Shēng Mài Sǎn* (生脉散) plus some medicinals. *Shēng Mài Sǎn* (as recorded in *On Doubt-Resolving in Differentiation of Endogenous and Exogenous Injuries* [内外伤辨惑论 , *Nèi Wài Shāng Biàn Huò Lùn*]) is effective in generating fluids, and nourishing yin. It is widely used in treatment of injuries of both qi and yin in the late stage of febrile diseases. *Dài Gé Sǎn* (as recorded in

A Precious Mirror of Hygiene [卫生宝鉴, *Wèi Shēng Bǎo Jiàn*]) has effects of clearing heat from the throat, transforming phlegm, and relieving vexation. Within the formula, *rén shēn* (Radix Ginseng) is sweet and slightly bitter in flavor, and warm in nature. It has actions to supplement the original qi, secure collapse and generate fluids. Li Gao (a famous physician in the Jin dynasty) said it can tonify Lung qi. When the Lung qi is sufficient, the qi of other four viscera will all be sufficient. This is because the Lung governs qi. *Mài dōng* (Radix Ophiopogonis) is sweet and cool in flavor and nature; it can nourish yin and moisten the Lung, clear the Heart and alleviate vexation. It is a pivotal herb to treat cough due to yin deficiency. *Wǔ wèi zǐ* (Fructus Schisandrae Chinensis) is sour in flavor and warm in nature. It can astringe the Lung and generate fluids so as to treat cough and dyspnea. *The Origin of Herbal Medicinals* (本草求原, *Běn Cǎo Qiú Yuán*) says it is a key herb in treating cough. Of the three medicinals above, one nourishes, one clears, and one astringes, thus they complement one another, with perfect actions. *Qīng dài* (Indigo Naturalis) is salty and cold in flavor and nature. It can clear heat, cool blood, and detoxify. *Hǎi gé fěn* (Pulvis Concha Meretricis seu Cyclinae) is a salty agent, with a function of lowering fire and eliminating phlegm; therefore it is good at treating heat phlegm, old phlegm, or stubborn phlegm. *Xì xīn* (Radix et Rhizoma Asari) is acrid and warm in flavor and nature, with functions to eliminate the evils in the yin collaterals, dispel wind and relieve itching of the throat, and enhance the effect of settling cough. It works quickly for prolonged cough with deep-lying or latent evils. *Zhì gān cǎo* (Radix et Rhizoma Glycyrrhizae Praeparata) replenishes qi and resolves phlegm, and harmonizes all of the medicinals. As paired with *wǔ wèi zǐ* (Fructus Schisandrae Chinensis), it also engenders yin through sourness and sweetness. All of the medicinals join together to replenish qi, nourish yin, clear the throat, remove phlegm, expel wind, and stop cough.

【Modifications】

➤ For cases of copious thin and white sputum, poor appetite, and a white tongue coating, add *bái zhú* (Rhizoma Atractylodis Macrocephalae), *chén pí* (Pericarpium Citri Reticulatae) and *fǎ xià* (Rhizoma Pinelliae Ternatae Praeparata).

➤ For pharyngeal congestion, and swelling of the tonsils, add *shè gān* (Rhizoma Belamcandae), *bǎn lán gēn* (Radix Isatidis) and *jīn yín huā* (Flos Lonicerae).

➤ If accompanied by constipation, add *pàng dà hǎi* (Semen Sterculiae Lychnophorae).

➤ For dyspnea and copious sputum in cases of protracted asthma or asthmatic bronchitis, add *má huáng* (Herba Ephedrae), *guì zhī* (Ramulus Cinnamomi), *sū zǐ* (Fructus Perillae) and *tíng lì zǐ* (Semen Lepidii seu Descurainiae).

➤ If there is paroxysmal spasmodic cough, as in pertusis, add *bǎi bù* (Radix Stemonae) and *mǎ dōu líng* (Fructus Aristolochiae).

➤ For cases with occasional low fever, add *qīng hāo* (Herba Artemisiae Annuae) and *biē jiǎ* (Carapax Trionycis).

➤ For obvious spontaneous sweating, add *huáng qí* (Radix Astragali) and *fáng fēng* (Radix Saposhnikoviae).

➤ For severe itching of the throat, add *jiāng cán* (Bombyx Batryticatus) and *dǎn nán xīng* (Arisaema cum Bile), and use *xì xīn* (Radix et Rhizoma Asari) in a higer dose according to the condition.

➤ For palpitations, a pale tongue, and a thready pulse with blood deficiency, add *dāng guī* (Radix Angelicae Sinensis), *shú dì* (Radix Rehmanniae Glutinosae Praeparata), and *dān shēn* (Radix et Rhizoma Salviae Miltiorrhizae) based upon of each case.

(Zhang Feng-qiang, Zheng Ying. *Essentials of Effective and Proved Secret Prescriptions of the First Group of Famous Veteran Doctors in State Level - Assessed by State Administration of Traditional Chinese Medicine.* 首

批国家级名老中医效验秘方精选. Guangzhou: Guangdong Scientific & Technical Publishing House, 1996. 121-123)

9. The Treatment of Cough and Panting due to Kidney Deficiency Failing to Receive Qi, with Phlegm and Fluids Lodged in the Lung with Sì Zǐ Píng Chuǎn Tāng (四子平喘汤) (Lu Zhi-qing)

【Ingredients】

葶苈子	tíng lì zǐ	12g	Semen Lepidii seu Descurainiae
炙苏子	zhì sū zǐ	9g	Fructus Perillae Praeparata
莱菔子	lái fú zǐ	9g	Semen Raphani
白芥子	bái jiè zǐ	2g	Semen Sinapis Albae
北杏	běi xìng	9g	Armeniacae Semen Amarum
浙贝母	zhè bèi mǔ	12g	Bulbus Fritillariae Thunbergii
制半夏	zhì bàn xià	9g	Rhizoma Pinelliae Preparata
陈皮	chén pí	5g	Pericarpium Citri Reticulatae
沉香	chén xiāng	5g (added later)	Lignum Aquilariae Resinatum
大生地	dà shēng dì	12g	Radix Rehmanniae Glutinosae
当归	dāng guī	5g	Radix Angelicae Sinensis
丹参	dān shēn	15g	Radix et Rhizoma Salviae Miltiorrhizae

【Indications】

Cough and panting due to Kidney deficiency failing to receive qi, with phlegm and fluids lodged in the Lung. The symptoms include chest fullness and oppression, cough and panting, shortness of breath, copious white sputum, a white and greasy tongue coating, and a deep, thready and slippery pulse.

【Formula Analysis】

This formula takes Sū Zǐ Jiàng Qì Tāng (苏子降气汤) as originally recorded in Formulary of the Bureau of Medicines of the Taiping Era (太平惠民和剂局方, Tài Píng Huì Mín Hé Jì Jú Fāng) as a base, joined with modifications of Sān Zǐ Yǎng Qīn Tāng (三子养亲汤) (from Han's Treatise on Medicine [韩氏医通, Hán Shì Yī Tōng]) and Jīn Shuǐ Liù Jūn Jiān (金水六

君煎) (from *Jing-yue's Complete Works* [景岳全书, *Jǐng Yuè Quán Shū*]). The Lung governs the qi, and the Kidney is the root of qi; the Lung governs exhaling qi, and the Kidney governs receiving qi. The causes of cough and panting, if involving the Lung, are excessive turbid phlegm blockage in the Lung, leading to counterflow of qi. If the causes involve the Kidney, they are deficiency of the essence (*jing*) and qi of the Kidney, leading to disturbances of qi in exiting and entering. Therefore, though the causes of cough and panting mainly come from the Lung, they are also associated with the Kidney. Accordingly, the treatment should focus on the Lung and the Kidney. In addition, the Spleen is the source of phlegm generation, so the Spleen should also considered in the treatment. Fluids and blood share the same source, therefore, the phlegm and stasis should be treated at the same time. Doing so can obtain a remarkable clinical effect.

In this formula, *sū zǐ* (Fructus Perillae) downbears qi, transforms phlegm, and calms panting. *Bái jiè zǐ* (Semen Sinapis Albae) warms the Lung, benefits the diaphragm, and clears away phlegm. *Lái fú zǐ* (Semen Raphani) benefits qi, moves stasis, and eliminates phlegm. *Tíng lì zǐ* (Semen Lepidii seu Descurainiae) drains the Lung, transforms phlegm, and disinhibits water. The four herbs, together as the chief medicinals, function to transform phlegm. *Chén xiāng* (Lignum Aquilariae Resinatum) and *shēng dì* (Radix Rehmanniae Glutinosae) serve as the deputy medicinals. *Chén xiāng* (Lignum Aquilariae Resinatum) warms the Kidney to receive qi and calms panting. *Shēng dì* (Radix Rehmanniae Glutinosae) nourishes the Kidney in order to consolidate the root, and also to moderate the dryness of all medicinals. As the assistants, *xìng rén* (Armeniacae Semen Amarum) and *zhè bèi* (Bulbus Fritillariae Thunbergii) transform phlegm and stop cough. *Bàn xià* (Rhizoma Pinelliae) and *chén pí* (Pericarpium Citri Reticulatae) dry dampness and fortify the Spleen. Moreover, *dāng guī* (Radix Angelicae Sinensis) can be used for the "treatment of cough and dyspnea" (*Classic of Materia Medica* [本经, *Běn*

Jīng]), as well as for increasing the blood nourishing, blood invigorating, and stasis transforming functions of *dān shēn* (Radix et Rhizoma Salviae Miltiorrhizae). These two together serve as the envoy herbs. The whole formula is an efficacious prescription to treat cough and panting due to excess in the Lung and deficiency in the Kidney. This is because there are medicinals that both move and nourish, dry and moisten, descend and receive, and treat the branch and the root.

【Modifications】

➢ For intolerance of cold with cold extremities, add *ròu guì* (Cortex Cinnamomi).

➢ For severe cough, add *bǎi bù* (Radix Stemonae) and *qián hú* (Radix Peucedani).

➢ In cases of expectoration of yellow and stubborn phlegm, remove *chén xiāng* (Lignum Aquilariae Resinatum) and *shēng dì* (Radix Rehmanniae Glutinosae), and add *huáng qín* (Radix Scutellariae) and *jiāo shān zhī* (Gardeniae Praeparatus).

➢ For difficulty in expectoration, add *zhú lì* (Succus Bambusae) and *guā lóu pí* (Pericarpium Trichosanthis).

(Zhang Feng-qiang, Zheng Ying. *Essentials of Effective and Proved Secret Prescriptions of the First Group of Famous Veteran Doctors in State Level — Assessed by State Administration of Traditional Chinese Medicine.* 首批国家级名老中医效验秘方精选. Guangzhou: Guangdong Scientific & Technical Publishing House, 1996. 128-129）

10. THE TREATMENT OF DRY COUGH DUE TO LUNG-HEAT WITH *QĪNG FÈI DÌNG CHUǍN TĀNG* (清肺定咳汤) (ZHU LIANG-CHUN)

【Ingredients】

金荞麦	jīn qiáo mài	20g	Rhizoma Fagopyri Dibotryis
鱼腥草	yú xīng cǎo	15g (added later)	Herba Houttuyniae
蛇舌草	shé shé cǎo	20g	Herba Hedyotidis

天浆壳	tiān jiāng ké	12g	Rhizoma Metaplexis
化橘红	huà jú hóng	6g	Exocarpium Citri Grandis
苍耳子	cāng ěr zǐ	12g	Fructus Xanthii
枇杷叶	pí pá yè	10g (remove the hair and wrapped)	Folium Eriobotryae
生甘草	shēng gān cǎo	5g	Radix et Rhizoma Glycyrrhizae Recens

【Indications】

A pattern of bronchitis belonging to Lung heat and dry cough, with scanty and stubborn phlegm.

【Formula Analysis】

Within the formula, *jīn qiáo mài* (Rhizoma Fagopyri Dibotryis) and *yú xīng cǎo* (Herba Houttuyniae) clear and transform phlegm-heat. *Shé shé cǎo* (Herba Hedyotidis), in addition to its function of clearing and transforming phlegm heat, can also raise the resistance of the body against illness and promote recovery. *Tiān jiāng ké* (Rhizoma Metaplexis) and *pí pá yè* (Folium Eriobotryae) act as the assistants to clear the Lung and expel heat, transform phlegm and stop cough. *Cāng ěr zǐ* (Fructus Xanthii) is conventionally used as a substance to open and disinhibit the nasal orifice, scatter wind and dispel dampness. Professor Zhu uses it to guard against colds (it has anti-allergy actions). It is very beneficial to treat long term cough that does not improve. *Jú hóng* (Exocarpium Citri Rubrum) can regulate the middle jiao and transform phlegm. *Gān cǎo* (Radix et Rhizoma Glycyrrhizae) can moisten the Lung to stop cough, and harmonizes all of the medicinals. Accordingly, the formula has a definite effect in the treatment of stagnated heat in the Lung with a protracted cough and stubborn yellow sputum.

(Mi Yi-e. *Essentials of Effective and Proved Secret Prescriptions of the First Group of Famous Veteran Doctors in State Level* — *Assessed by State Administration of Traditional Chinese Medicine · Sequel* 首批国家级名老

中医效验秘方精选·续集. Beijing: China Press of Traditional Chinese Medicine, 1999. 55-56)

11. The Treatment of Acute and Chronic Bronchitis, and Bronchiectasis, with Jiā Jiǎn Zé Qī Tāng (加减泽漆汤) (Huang Ji-geng)

【Ingredients】

泽漆	zé qī	15 – 150g	Herba Euphorbiae Helioscopiae
制半夏	zhì bàn xià	10 – 30g	Rhizoma Pinelliae Preparata
陈皮	chén pí	10g	Pericarpium Citri Reticulatae
紫菀	zǐ wǎn	15g	Radix et Rhizoma Asteris
白前	bái qián	15g	Radix et Rhizoma Cynanchi Stauntonii
桂枝	guì zhī	9g	Ramulus Cinnamomi
生姜	shēng jiāng	3 slices	Rhizoma Zingiberis Recens
黄芩	huáng qín	15g	Radix Scutellariae
桔梗	jié gěng	9g	Radix Platycodonis
枳壳	zhǐ qiào	9g	Fructus Aurantii
甘草	gān cǎo	9g	Radix et Rhizoma Glycyrrhizae

【Indications】

Acute and chronic bronchitis, bronchiectasis.

【Formula Analysis】

Zé Qī Tāng (泽漆汤) is a formula from Zhang Zhong-jing's *Synopsis of Golden Chamber* (金匮要略, *Jīn Guì Yào Lüè*). Originally it had *zǐ quán* (or *zǎo xiū* [Rhizoma Paridis], *cǎo hé chē* [Rhizoma Bistortae]) in origin. Its nature is bitter cold, then *zǐ wǎn* (Radix et Rhizoma Asteris) of acrid warm nature is used in its place. Added with medicinals that have actions of relaxing the chest and regulating qi, this formula can dredge the water passage and dispel phlegm. In the formula, *zé qī* (Herba Euphorbiae Helioscopiae) acts as the chief and can expel water and eliminate phlegm. *Bàn xià* (Rhizoma Pinelliae) can dry dampness and transform phlegm. *Zǐ wǎn* (Radix et Rhizoma Asteris) and *bái qián* (Radix et Rhizoma Cynanchi Stauntonii) downbear qi and dispel phlegm. *Chén pí* (Pericarpium Citri Reticulatae), *jié gěng* (Radix Platycodonis) and *zhǐ qiào* (Fructus Aurantii) diffuse the Lung and loosen the chest, rectify qi and abduct stagnation, so that the water passage will be smooth, and phlegm-fluid retention be eliminated. *Guì zhī* (Ramulus Cinnamomi) and *shēng jiāng* (Rhizoma Zingiberis Recens) warm the Lung and transform phlegm. *Huáng qín* (Radix Scutellariae) clears and drains phlegm-heat. *Gān cǎo* (Radix et Rhizoma Glycyrrhizae) helps all of the medicinals to transform phlegm and stop cough.

【Modifications】

➢ For cases of cold panting with copious phlegm, add modified *Shè Gān Má Huáng Tāng* (射干麻黄汤).

➢ For turbid and stubborn phlegm, add *dì lóng* (Lumbricus), and use *huáng qín* (Radix Scutellariae) at a heavier dose.

➢ For cough and panting with qi deficiency, add *Yù Píng Fēng Sǎn* (玉屏风散).

➢ For phlegm-fluid retention, add modified *Qiān Jīn Mài Mén Dōng Tāng* (千金麦门冬汤).

➢ For poor appetite and diarrhea, add modified *Xiāng Shā Liù Jūn Zǐ Tāng* (香砂六君子汤).

(Mi Yi-e. *Essentials of Effective and Proved Secret Prescriptions of the First Group of Famous Veteran Doctors in State Level — Assessed by State Administration of Traditional Chinese Medicine · Sequel* 首批国家级名老中医效验秘方精选·续集. Beijing: China Press of Traditional Chinese Medicine, 1999. 51-52)

12. The Treatment of Dual Deficiency of Lung and Kidney of Chronic Bronchitis with *Pí Gōng Fāng* (脾功方) (Huang Ji-geng)

【Ingredients】

仙灵脾	xiān líng pí	15g	Herba Epimedii
菟丝子	tù sī zǐ	15g	Semen Cuscutae
功劳叶	gōng láo yè	15g	Folium Ilex

【Indications】

Chronic bronchitis transforming from a persistant phase to a remission phase, manifested by deficiency of the Lung and Kidney.

【Formula Analysis】

In the formula, *xiān líng pí* (Herba Epimedii) and *tù sī zǐ* (Semen Cuscutae) support yang and add essence (*jing*). With the assistance of *gōng láo yè* (Folium Ilex) in nourishing yin, they supplement the Lung and Kidney. Thus "yin is within the seeking of yang, then yang is ceaselessly generated and transformed from yin." The combination of these three medicinals can assist yang, boost yin, and tonify the Kidney, thus restoring the essential (*jing*) qi of the Kidney. Then the Spleen will be fortified in transportation and transformation, the Spleen qi will exuberant, and in turn, the Lung qi will also be sufficient. This allows the functioning of the Lung, Spleen, and Kidney to be healthy and vigorous, and thus phlegm turbidity is transformed.

【Modifications】

➤ For cases of chest oppression, poor appetite, and a greasy tongue coating, add *cāng zhú* (Rhizoma Atractylodis) 9g, and *hòu pò* (Cortex Magnoliae Officinalis) 6g, or modified *Liù Jūn Zǐ Tāng* (六君子汤).

➤ For severe intolerance of cold with cold limbs add *fù zǐ piàn* (Radix Aconitii Lateralis Praeparata) 5 pieces.

➤ For cases of internal heat with yin deficiency, add *shēng dì* (Radix Rehmanniae Glutinosae) 15g, and change the quantity of *xiān líng pí* (Herba Epimedii) to 9g.

(Mi Yi-e. *Essentials of Effective and Proved Secret Prescriptions of the First Group of Famous Veteran Doctors in State Level － Assessed by State Administration of Traditional Chinese Medicine · Sequel* 首批国家级名老中医效验秘方精选·续集. Beijing: China Press of Traditional Chinese Medicine, 1999. 52-53)

13. The Treatment of Phlegm-Damp Cough with Qū Tán Zhǐ Ké Chōng Jì (祛痰止咳冲剂) (Liu Wei-sheng)

【Ingredients】

党参	dǎng shēn	12g	Radix Codonopsitis
半夏	bàn xià	24g	Rhizoma Pinelliae
醋制芫花	cù zhì yuán huā	3g	Flos Genkwa Praeparata
制甘遂	zhì gān suí	3g	Radix Kansui Praeparata
白矾	bái fán	1.5g	Alumen
紫花杜鹃	zǐ huā dù juān	75g	Rhododendron mariae Hance

【Indications】

Continuous cough with a low and deep voice, especially during the night, copious thin or frothy sputum, loose stools, a white and greasy tongue coating, and a deep and slippery pulse.

【Formula Analysis】

Within the formula, *dǎng shēn* (Radix Codonopsis) fortifies the Spleen and boosts qi. *Fǎ xià* (Rhizoma Pinelliae Ternatae Praeparata) dries dampness and transforms phlegm. *Cù zhì yuán huā* (Flos Genkwa Praeparata) expels phlegm and fluids. *Bái fán* (Alumen) dries dampness, and *zǐ huā dù juān* (Rhododendron Mariae Hance) warms the Lung and stops cough. All of the medicinals together function to fortify the Spleen and dry dampness, expel phlegm and stop cough.

【Modifications】

➢ For poor appetite, add *mài yá* (Fructus Hordei Germinatus) 10g, *shān zhā* (Fructus Crataegi) 15g, and *bái dòu kòu* (Fructus Amomi Rotundus) 6g (added at the end).

➢ For copious white sputum add *bái jiè zǐ* (Semen Sinapis Albae) 10g and *gān jiāng* (Rhizoma Zingiberis) 6g.

14. The Treatment of Cough due to Accumulation of Phlegm-Heat with *Yín Huáng Hé Jì* (银黄合剂) (Liu Wei-sheng)

【Ingredients】

麻黄	má huáng	10g	Herba Ephedrae
杏仁	xìng rén	10g	Armeniacae Semen Amarum
桃仁	táo rén	10g	Semen Persicae
金银花	jīn yín huā	25g	Flos Lonicerae
鱼腥草	yú xīng cǎo	25g	Herba Houttuyniae
石膏	shí gāo	30g	Gypsum Fibrosum

【Indications】

Panting, cough with yellow sputum, accompanied by fever, chest oppression, thirst with a desire for cold drinks, scanty urine, dry stools, a red or purplish tongue with a yellow coating, and a rapid and slippery pulse.

【Formula Analysis】

Má huáng (Herba Ephedrae) and *xìng rén* (Armeniacae Semen Amarum) diffuse the Lung and calm panting. *Táo rén* (Semen Persicae) eliminates stasis and stops cough. *Jīn yín huā* (Flos Lonicerae) and *yú xīng cǎo* (Herba Houttuyniae) clear heat, transform phlegm, and stop cough. *Shí gāo* (Gypsum Fibrosum) clears heat and purge fire.

(Traditional Chinese Medical Hospital of Guangdong Province)

Selected Case Studies

1. Professor Liu Du-zhou's Case Study: Cold Fluid Retention in the Lung

Chai, male, 53 years old. Initial visit on December 3rd, 1994.

【Initial Visit】

The patient had suffered from cough and panting for more than ten years. The disease often became more severe in the winter, and milder in the summer. The patient had been to many hospitals, and was diagnosed as having chronic bronchitis or chronic bronchitis complicated with emphysema. However, treatment with Chinese medicine and biomedicine had no effect on the disease. At the first visit, the patient presented with panting, a sensation of chest oppression, breathing with shrugged shoulders, and thin white sputum. These symptoms got worse at night, and the patient could not lie flat. In the mornings he expectorated copious amounts of sputum. He also felt chilled on the back. His face appeared dark, the tongue was moist with a glossy coating, and the pulse was wiry with slippery in the *cun* position.

【Pattern Differentiation】
Latent cold fluids upwardly invading the Lung.

【Treatment Principle】
Warm the Lung and Stomach so as to scatter the cold fluids.

【Prescription】
Modified *Xiǎo Qīng Lóng Tāng* (小青龙汤)

麻黄	má huáng	9g	Herba Ephedrae
桂枝	guì zhī	10g	Ramulus Cinnamomi
干姜	gān jiāng	9g	Rhizoma Zingiberis
五味子	wǔ wèi zǐ	9g	Fructus Schisandrae Chinensis
细辛	xì xīn	6g	Radix et Rhizoma Asari
法半夏	fǎ bàn xià	14g	Rhizoma Pinelliae Praeparatum
白芍	bái sháo	9g	Radix Paeoniae Alba
炙甘草	zhì gān cǎo	10g	Radix et Rhizoma Glycyrrhizae Praeparata

【Second Visit】
After taking 7 doses of the fomula, the cough and panting were markedly decreased, and the amount of sputum was reduced. The patient could sleep at night, and no longer felt chest oppression. In order to take into consideration the treatment of both the right qi and the evil qi. *Guì*

Líng Wǔ Wèi Gān Cǎo Tāng (桂苓五味甘草汤) [as recorded in *Synopsis of Golden Chamber* (金匮要略, *Jīn Guì Yào Lüè*) plus *xìng rén* (Armeniacae Semen Amarum), *fǎ bàn xià* (Rhizoma Pinelliae Praeparatum) and *gān jiāng* (Rhizoma Zingiberis) was then taken to affect a cure.

【Comments】

Xiǎo Qīng Lóng Tāng (小青龙汤) is a famous formula for cough and panting due to cold fluid retention. Zhang Zhong-jing applied this formula in the treatment of thoracic fluid retention. It was used for conditions in which "the exterior has not been relieved after cold attack, and there is water-qi under the Heart (伤寒表不解，心下有水气)" as well as "the symptoms of cough, dyspnea, and panting with an inability to lie flat (咳逆倚息不得卧)". The conditions of this case are cough, panting, clear thin sputum, chilled back, and a moist and glossy tongue coating which results from a failure of the Lung to ascend and descend due to internal disturbances of the Lung by cold fluid retention. In the formula, *má huáng* (Herba Ephedrae) and *guì zhī* (Ramulus Cinnamomi) scatter cold evils, while at the same time calming panting. *Gān jiāng* (Rhizoma Zingiberis) and *xì xīn* (Radix et Rhizoma Asari) warm the Lung and Stomach to transform fluids, while at the same time helping *má huáng* (Herba Ephedrae) and *guì zhī* (Ramulus Cinnamomi Cassiae) to scatter cold. *Bàn xià* (Rhizoma Pinelliae) washes turbid phlegm, fortifies the Stomach and transforms fluids. *Wǔ wèi zǐ* (Fructus Schisandrae Chinensis) enriches the Kidney-water so as to astringe Lung qi. *Sháo yào* (Radix Paeoniae) nourishes yin-blood and protects Liver-yin. It also acts as a moderator to the three medicinals of *má huáng* (Herba Ephedrae), *guì zhī* (Ramulus Cinnamomi) and *xì xīn* (Radix et Rhizoma Asari), so that the evils can be expelled with out damage to the right qi. *Zhì gān cǎo* (Radix et Rhizoma Glycyrrhizae Praeparata) boosts qi and harmonizes the middle, and regulates all of the medicinals. The use of this formula can cause the cold evils to be scattered, the fluids to be expelled, and the Lung qi to be unobstructed and smooth, thereby allowing cough and panting to disappear.

It should be pointed out that this formula strongly induces diaphoresis. An inappropriate application of the formula can injure both yin and yang, and worsen the disease. Therefore, the clinical use of this formula at times when it is particularly needed should be in compliance with the several points mentioned below:

(1) Differentiation of Complexion

Cold fluid retention is a yin evil, it usually damages the yang qi. As the yang qi in the chest fails to warm, it causes the movement of the nutritive and defensive qi to be unsmooth, and thus unable to bloom up to the face. Therefore the patient presents with a dark complexion, which is described as "water colored (水色 , shuǐ sè)"; or with a dark ring around the eye, which is called "water ring"; or with dark patches on the forehead, column of nose, cheeks, and chin, which are called "water patches (水斑 , shuǐ bān)".

(2) Differentiation of Cough

There are several conditions: severe cough with mild panting, or severe panting with mild cough, or equally severe cough and panting such that there is an inability to lie flat, which is aggravated at night.

(3) Differentiation of Phlegm

Cold in the Lung (Metal) and yang deficiency will cause fluids to condense leading to production of phlegm-fluid retetion. Then the expectorative sputum is white and thin; or frothy, becoming water when it falls to the ground. Or the sputum looks like egg whites, with a cool feeling when the tongue touches it.

(4) Differentiation of the Tongue Appearance

The Lung qi is cold, and fluids congeal and stagnate and don't transform, therefore the tongue coating is commonly moist and glossy, with no obvious change of the tongue body. But if the yang qi is impaired, there will be a pale, tender, and enlarged tongue.

(5) Differentiation of the Pulse Condition

When there are cold fluid evil, the pulse usually appears wiry. This is because wiriness is governs fluid diseases. If there is exterior cold with interior fluids, then the pulse will likely be floating and wiry or floating and tight. If the disease is long standing and getting more serious by the day, with cold fluids internally hidden, then the pulse will likely be deep.

(6) Differentiation of Secondary Symptoms

Fluids in the interior of the body often moves following the qi dynamic, thus it leads to many secondary symptoms. These include choking due to cold fluids obstructing the qi, vomiting due to cold fluids attacking the Stomach, dysuria due to cold-fluids obstructing the lower jiao, and edema due to cold fluids flowing into the four limbs. If the exogenous cold cannot to be eliminated, the qi of the greater yang (*taiyang*) will stagnate, and then fever and headache may appear.

The above six points to differentiate identifying patterns are objective standards to correctly determine the use of *Xiǎo Qīng Lóng Tāng* (小青龙汤). However, not all of these six aspects must be present, but if one or two of the main patterns exist, then *Xiǎo Qīng Lóng Tāng* (小青龙汤) will be the remedy.

Zhong-jing has already explained the rules about modifications to *Xiǎo Qīng Lóng Tāng* (小青龙汤), so none of those will be repeated here. Add *fú líng* (Poria), *xìng rén* (Armeniacae Semen Amarum) and *shè gān* (Rhizoma Belamcandae) in order to strengthen the curative effect. *Xiǎo Qīng Lóng Tāng* (小青龙汤) is an efficacious formula for cough and panting due to cold fluid retention, but its power in dispersion is so strong that it can consume Lung qi in the upper jiao, and affect Kidney qi in the lower jiao. Therefore, if a patient with deficient right qi is erroneously given the formula, he will experience many side effects, including severely cold limbs, a feeling of qi rushing from the lower abdomen up to the chest and throat, and a flushed face (like being drunken). Therefore, this formula must be discontinued as soon as it affects a cure, and it cannot be taken for a long time. Once the disease condition is alleviated, use formulas with *fú líng* (Poria) and *guì zhī* (Ramulus Cinnamomi) to warm and transform cold fluid retention. This is the saying in the *Synopsis of Golden Chamber* (金匮要略 , *Jīn Guì Yào Lüè*): "The patient that suffers from phlegm-fluid retention should be given warming medicinals for harmonization".

(Chen Ming, Liu Yan-hua, Li Fang. *Quintessence of Proved Clinical Case Records from Professor Liu Du-zhou* 刘渡舟临证验案精选 . Beijing: Learning Center Press, 1995. 40)

2. Professor Gao Hui-yuan's Case Study: Dual Deficiency of Qi and Yin, With Phlegm-Heat Obstructing the Lung

Li, male, 77 years old. The initial visit was on October 17th, 1989.

【Initial Visit】

He had a repeated cough for more than forty years; in the past four years it had gotten worse and was accompanied by panting. He had dizziness for the past five months. His illness at the first office call manifested with cough, copious white or yellow sputum, panting aggravated upon exertion, dizziness, poor appetite, and cough and panting usually induced by catching a cold. The biomedical diagnosis was chronic bronchitis, and pulmonary emphysema complicated by infection. The patient presented with a red tongue with a white coating, and a slippery pulse.

【Pattern Differentiation】

Dual deficiency of qi and yin, phlegm evil obstructing the Lung and transforming into heat.

【Treatment Principle】 Boost qi, nourish yin and clear the Lung; diffuse Lung qi, transform phlegm and calm panting.

【Prescription】

生黄芪	shēng huáng qí	15g	Radix Astragali
北沙参	běi shā shēn	10g	Radix Glehniae
茯苓	fú líng	10g	Poria
法半夏	fǎ bàn xià	10g	Rhizoma Pinelliae Praeparatum
橘红	jú hóng	8g	Exocarpium Citri Rubrum
炙甘草	zhì gān cǎo	3g	Radix et Rhizoma Glycyrrhizae Praeparata
麦门冬	mài mén dōng	10g	Radix Ophiopogonis
五味子	wǔ wèi zǐ	6g	Fructus Schisandrae Chinensis
杏仁泥	xìng rén ní	10g	Armeniacae Semen Amarum Praeparata
生苡仁	shēng yì rén	15g	Semen Coicis
荷叶	hé yè	10g	Folium Nelumbinis
竹茹	zhú rú	10g	Caulis Bambusae in Taeniis
火麻仁	huǒ má rén	15g	Fructus Cannabis

【Second Visit】

After taking six doses of the formula, the cough, panting and sputum were all obviously alleviated. His appetite became a little bit better; but occasionally there was still a little bit of yellow sputum, diarrhea, a red tongue with little coating, and a wiry and slippery pulse. *Huǒ má rén* (Fructus Cannabis) was removed, and *zhì pa yè* (Folium Eriobotryae Praeparata) 10g was added so as to clear and depurate Lung qi, transform phlegm and stop cough.

【Third Visit】

After six-doses were taken again, cough, the panting and sputum were further alleviated, but dry stools appeared. The formula with slight modifications was kept for more than thirty doses. All the symptoms were gradually relieved, the spirit and appetite were markedly improved, and the cough and sputum almost disappeared. However, there was physical weakness after exertion, panting, and shortness of breath. He was told to take the formula again to slowly gain its effect.

【Comments】

The Lung belongs to Metal, and it is a delicate organ, characterized by clearing depuration. If cough and panting occur due to external contraction, the qi and yin are susceptable to injury. Too many warm-dry, cold-cool, or moistening-greasy agents are likely to injure qi and yin or obstruct Lung qi, and are thus not suitable. Therefore the formula and medicinals chosen should be clear and efficacious, with a low dosage. In this case, cough was usually induced by catching colds because of insufficient defensive qi. In addition to cough, panting and sputum, there were also symptoms of failure of the clear yang to rise, like dizziness and poor appetite. Therefore, *Shēng Mài Sǎn* (生脉散) (*shā shēn* [Radix Glehniae seu Adenophorae] is often taken as substitute for *rén shēn* [Radix Ginseng]) is taken in order to boost qi, nourish yin, and calm panting. *Èr Chén Tāng* (二陈汤) is taken to transform phlegm and stop cough, and *huáng qí* (Radix Astragali) is added so as to boost qi, consolidate the exterior, and assist *hé yè* (Folium Nelumbinis Nuciferae) in developing the clear yang. Owing to agreement of the remedy with the pattern, the patient restored his health.

(Wang Fa-wei, Yu You-shan, Xue Chang. *Quintessence of Proved Clinical Case Records from Professor Gao Hui-yuan* 高辉远临证验案精选. Beijing: Learning Center Press, 1995. 40)

3. He Yan-shen's Case Study: Warm Evil Transforming into Heat, Contending With Cold Fluids

Zhang, male, 69 years old. The initial visit was on November 21st, 1994.

【Initial Visit】

He had been addicted to alcohol and cigarettes, and suffered from cough for many years. He had been diagnosed many times (by

X-ray examination) as having senile chronic bronchitis complicated by pulmonary emphysema. This time, he was attacked by a winter-warm evil, and he had fever, panting and cough. He had been treated for nine days in a hospital with biomedicine. The fever abated slightly, but the panting and cough became more serious. The patient's physique was still healthy, with symptoms of a low fever (37.8℃), cough and panting, stubborn yellow sputum, stridor in the throat, stuffiness of the chest and epigastrium, vexation and insomnia, a dry mouth and thirst, frequent urination and oliguria, a slight yellow tongue coating, and a superficial, slippery, and rapid pulse. The treatment was based on *Treatise on Cold Pathogenic Diseases* (伤寒论 , *Shāng Hán Lùn*): "The diseases of the *yangming* channels, with a floating pulse and fever, thirst with a desire to drink, and difficult urination, should be treated with *Zhū Líng Tāng* (猪苓汤) (阳明病，脉浮发热，渴欲饮水，小便不利者，猪苓汤主之)."

【Pattern Differentiation】

Warm evil transforming into heat, contending with cold fluids.

【Treatment Principle】

Open and disinhibit the urination.

【Prescription】

Zhū Líng Tāng (猪苓汤) with modifications

泽泻	zé xiè	20g	Rhizoma Alismatis
茯苓	fú líng	25g	Poria
滑石	huá shí	30g	Talcum
阿胶	ē jiāo	15g	Colla Corii Asini
枇杷叶	pí pá yè	15g	Folium Eriobotryae
车前子	chē qián zǐ	15g	Semen Plantaginis
杏仁	xìng rén	12g	Armeniacae Semen Amarum

【Second Visit】

After taking three doses, the fever had dropped down, the pulse slowed, panting calmed, the qi became normalized, and the volume of urine increased, but there was still a productive cough, and poor appetite. He was advised to stop drinking and smoking, and to take modified *Shēn Bèi Liù Xián Sǎn* (参贝六贤散) for a long period of time:.

西洋参	xī yáng shēn	15g	Radix Panacis Quinquefolii
川贝母	chuān bèi mǔ	15g	Bulbus Fritillariae Cirrhosae
胆南星	dǎn nán xīng	15g	Arisaema cum Bile
法半夏	fǎ bàn xià	15g	Rhizoma Pinelliae Praeparatum
车前子	chē qián zǐ	15g	Semen Plantaginis
橘红	jú hóng	5g	Exocarpium Citri Rubrum
甘草	gān cǎo	5g	Radix et Rhizoma Glycyrrhizae
玄参	xuán shēn	20g	Radix Scrophulariae
蛤壳	gé ké	20g	Concha Meretricis seu Cyclinae
薏苡仁	yì yǐ rén	30g	Semen Coicis

➢ For frequent cough, add *xìng rén* (Armeniacae Semen Amarum) and *pí pá yè* (Folium Eriobotryae).

➢ For abundant expectoration and oliguria, add *guā lóu* (Fructus Trichosanthis) and *fú líng* (Poria).

The patient had taken the formula intermittently, his long-standing illness got better gradually, and no recurrence occured during two years of follow-ups.

【Comments】

In the *Synopsis of Golden Chamber* (金匮要略 , *Jīn Guì Yào Lüè*), it is said: "For shortness of breath with little fluids, one should promote diuresis (夫短气有微饮，当从小便去之)." Physicians in later ages all thought that promoting diuresis was a fundamental law in the treatment of phlegm-fliud retention. The aim of *Líng Guì Zhū Gān Tāng* (苓桂术甘汤) and *Wǔ Líng Sǎn* (五苓散) (from *Synopsis of Golden Chamber*) is to fortify the Spleen, activate yang and promote diuresis; while the aim of *Shèn Qì Wán* (肾气丸) is to strengthen the Kidney, warm yang and promote diuresis. Here the method of nourishing yin, clearing heat and promoting diuresis is needed, so *Zhū Líng Tāng* (猪苓汤) from *Treatise on Cold Pathogenic Diseases* (伤寒论, *Shāng Hán Lùn*) is added so as to make up the deficit, thus most of the time good effects are obtained. Comparing *Wǔ Líng Sǎn* (五苓散) with *Zhū Líng Tāng* (猪苓汤), it is clear that both formulas use *zhū líng* (Polyporus), *zé xiè* (Rhizoma Alismatis) and *fú líng* (Poria) to promote diuresis; however *Wǔ Líng Sǎn* (五苓散) uses *bái zhú* (Rhizoma Atractylodis Macrocephalae) to tonify the Spleen, and *guì zhī* (Ramulus Cinnamomi) to open yang; while *Zhū Líng Tāng* (猪苓汤) uses *ē jiāo* (Colla Corii Asini) to nourish yin and *huá shí* (Talcum) to purge heat. Therefore each of the two formulas has its own indications. In addition, "a person in his forties has only half of his yin-qi (人年四十，阴气自半)", and old people rest more and exercise less. Also, smoking and drinking engender fire so that an accumulation of heat will easily develop. Once exogenous evils invade the body, they trigger the latent fluids, and transform it mostly into heat. If warm and dry natured medicinals are taken, damage to the yin and fluids can also occur.

In the *Synopsis of Golden Chamber* (金匮要略, *Jīn Guì Yào Lüè*) it is said: "The patient suffering from phlegm-fluid retention should be given warming medicinals for harmonization (病痰饮者，当以温药和之)." Here, "harmonization", as used by Zhang Zhong-jing, has profound meaning. The so-called warm medicinals are not limited only to warm-nourishing, warming yang, warm-dispelling, but should also smooth the Lung qi dynamic so that phlegm-fliud retention cannot reside anywhere in the body. For example, the composition of *xìng rén* (Armeniacae Semen Amarum), *pí pá yè* (Folium Eriobotryae), *xuán fù huā* (Flos Inulae), *fǎ bàn xià* (Rhizoma Pinelliae Praeparatum), *dǎn nán xīng* (Arisaema cum Bile), *jú hóng* (Exocarpium Citri Rubrum), *gān cǎo* (Radix et Rhizoma Glycyrrhizae), *xuán shēn* (Radix Scrophulariae) and *gé ké* (Concha Meretricis seu Cyclinae) is very effctive for cases of "long-standing cough, discomfort in the chest and diaphragm, abundant expectoration, and poor appetite". This method uses warm medicinals to smooth the qi dynamic, promote fluid distribution, and transform phlegm, with replenishing qi and clearing heat as adjunctive therapies. This method is the most suitable for prolonged phlegm-fluid retention in elderly patients, accompanied by fire due to qi deficiency. The patient in this case has since taken the remedy so as to relieve disease and prolong his life.

(Liu Shi-jian, Ma Feng-bin. *Medical Collection of Double Happy Office* 双乐室医集. Guangzhou: Guangdong Higher Education Press, 1998. 24)

4. YAN ZHENG-HUA'S CASE STUDY: PHLEGM-HEAT INTERNALLY ACCUMULATING, FAILURE OF THE LUNG TO CLEAR AND DEPURATE

Zhu, male, 65 years old. The initial visit was on April 17th, 1992.

【Initial Visit】

He had suffered from chronic bronchitis for fifty years, with panting and coughing fluctuating between mild and severe. Recently, he caught a cold, which induced the symptoms of panting and cough, copious white and viscous sputum, a burning hot and stuffy feeling of the chest, excessive sweating, yellow urine, dry stools, a red tongue with a thin and yellow coating, and a wiry and slippery pulse. His blood pressure was 20/12 kPa.

【Pattern Differentiation】

Phlegm-heat internally accumulating, failure of the Lung to clear and depurate.

【Treatment Principle】

Clear the Lung and transform phlegm; stop cough and calm panting; and assist by loosening the chest and moistening the bowels.

【Prescription】

桑叶	sāng yè	10g	Folium Mori
桑白皮	sāng bái pí	10g	Cortex Mori
黄芩	huáng qín	10g	Radix Scutellariae
瓜蒌	guā lóu	30g	Fructus Trichosanthis

浙贝母	zhè bèi mǔ	10g	Bulbus Fritillariae Thunbergii
竹茹	zhú rú	6g	Caulis Bambusae in Taeniis
杏仁	xìng rén	10g (smashed)	Armeniacae Semen Amarum
苏子	sū zǐ	6g (smashed)	Fructus Perillae
橘红	jú hóng	6g	Exocarpium Citri Rubrum
清半夏	qīng bàn xià	10g	Rhizoma Pinelliae Praeparata
紫菀	zǐ wǎn	10g	Radix et Rhizoma Asteris
茯苓	fú líng	20g	Poria

He took seven doses, decocted in water for oral administration, one dose per day. He avoided pungent and greasy food.

【Second Visit】

There was no expectoration, panting was relieved and cough reduced, but there was still chest oppression, dry stools, dizziness and headache. The blood pressure was the same as before. The pattern belonged to residual phlegm-heat with hyperactivity of Liver-yang. Treatment was to clear, transform phlegm-heat, loosen the chest, check cough, and calm the Liver. The medicinals used were:

全瓜蒌	quán guā lóu	30g	Fructus Trichosanthis
清半夏	qīng bàn xià	10g	Rhizoma Pinelliae Praeparata
黄芩	huáng qín	10g	Radix Scutellariae
浙贝母	zhè bèi mǔ	10g	Bulbus Fritillariae Thunbergii
杏仁	xìng rén	10g (smashed)	Armeniacae Semen Amarum
紫菀	zǐ wǎn	10g	Radix et Rhizoma Asteris
枇杷叶	pí pá yè	10g (remove the hairs)	Folium Eriobotryae
茯苓	fú líng	20g	Poria
刺蒺藜	cì jí lì	10g	Fructus Tribuli
菊花	jú huā	10g	Flos Chrysanthemi
生牡蛎	shēng mǔ lì	30g (smashed and decocted first)	Concha Ostreae

【Third Visit】

He visited again one year later, saying that he had already taken seven doses of the formula. All of symptoms were eliminated and did not occur for about one year. Recently, because of catching a cold, there again appeared symptoms like productive cough, a bitter taste and dry mouth, yellow urine, constipation, and hemorrhoids with swelling and pain. The pattern belonged to phlegm-heat obstructing the Lung, and heat in the Large Intestine causing fluid exhaustion. The treatment was to clear Lung-heat and transform phlegm to relieve cough, and clear fire and moisten the bowels to relieve constipation. The medicinals used were:

瓜蒌	guā lóu	30g	Fructus Trichosanthis
黄芩	huáng qín	10g	Radix Scutellariae
浙贝母	zhè bèi mǔ	10g	Bulbus Fritillariae Thunbergii
杏仁	xìng rén	10g (smashed)	Armeniacae Semen Amarum
马兜铃	mǎ dōu líng	10g	Fructus Aristolochiae
槐角	huái jiǎo	10g	Fructus Sophorae Japonicae
生地榆	shēng dì yú	10g	Radix Sanguisorbae
郁李仁	yù lǐ rén	15g (smashed)	Semen Pruni
火麻仁	huǒ má rén	15g	Fructus Cannabis
陈皮	chén pí	10g	Pericarpium Citri Reticulatae
炒枳壳	chǎo zhǐ qiào	6g	Fructus Aurantii Tostum
鲜地粟 (荸荠)	xiān dì sù (bí qí)	10 pieces	Heleocharis dulcis

After taking seven doses, the phlegm and cough were relieved; and the swelling of the hemorrhoids was reduced.

【Comments】

This patient had suffered from chronic bronchitis for 50 years, and his cough and panting had fluctuated between mild and severe. On the initial visit, the symptoms were panting and cough, copious white and sticky sputum, and chest oppression, which was diagnosed as a pattern of failure of the Lung in clearing and depurating due to an obstruction of turbid phlegm in the Lung. Chest vexation and heat, yellow urine, and dry stools were ominous signs that Lung heat had scorched the fluids. *Sāng bái pí* (Cortex Mori), *huáng qín* (Radix Scutellariae), *zhè bèi mǔ* (Bulbus Fritillariae Thunbergii), *guā lóu* (Fructus Trichosanthis), *zhú rú* (Caulis Bambusae in Taeniis), *xìng rén* (Armeniacae Semen Amarum), *sū zǐ* (Fructus Perillae) and *fǎ bàn xià* (Rhizoma Pinelliae Praeparatum) were used to clear Lung heat, transform phlegm, relieve cough and calm panting. *Guā lóu* (Fructus Trichosanthis), *xìng rén* (Armeniacae Semen Amarum) and *sū zǐ* (Fructus Perillae) were taken to loosen the chest and moisten the bowels. On the second visit, the phlegm was cleared, the panting was calmed, and the cough was reduced, but there were still oppressive feelings in the chest and dry stools. This was accompanied by dizziness and headache due to residual phlegm-heat causing the qi dynamic to be unsmooth, with additional hyperactivity of Liver-yang. Therefore, *guā lóu* (Fructus Trichosanthis), *huáng qín* (Radix Scutellariae) and *zhè bèi mǔ* (Bulbus Fritillariae Thunbergii) were added again to clearing Lung heat, transform phlegm, and relieve cough. *Cì jí lì* (Fructus Tribuli), *jú huā* (Flos Chrysanthemi) and *shēng mǔ lì* (Concha Ostreae) were added to descend Liver yang. Such a remedy treats both the main and secondary symptoms, so that after taking the herbs he recovered and the disease did not recur for one year. The cough occurred again one year later, with concomitant constipation and swelling of hemorrhoids due to phlegm-heat obstructing the Lung, and impairment of fluids by fire in the Large Intestine. *Guā lóu* (Fructus Trichosanthis), *huáng qín* (Radix Scutellariae), *zhè bèi mǔ* (Bulbus Fritillariae Thunbergii), *mǎ dōu líng* (Fructus Aristolochiae), *dì yú* (Radix Sanguisorbae) and *huái jiǎo* (Fructus Sophorae Japonicae) were added to clear phlegm-heat so as to relieve cough in the upper jiao, and purge fire in the Large Intestine so as to clear hemorrhoids in the lower jiao. Thus he was completely cured again.

(Peng Jian-zhong. *Assessment of Essential Case Records in Chinese Medicine at Both Ancient and Modern Times* 中医古今医案精华评. Beijing: Learning Center Press, 1998. 585)

5. Shi Jin-mo's Case Study: Phlegm-Damp Obstructing the Middle Jiao, with Dual Deficiency of the Lung and Spleen

Zhang, male, 45 years old.

【Initial Visit】

Over the past ten or so years, he has had a cough with abundant expectoration. It is worse in the mornings and evenings, and in the fall and winter. A recent onset of illness did not resolve on its own, and he had loose stools. Several remedies had no effect. Fluoroscopy and laboratory examinations found no tuberculosis. His diagnosis was chronic bronchitis. He came to visit on a business trip. His tongue coating was white, and his pulse was moderate and weak.

【Pattern Differentiation】

Dual deficiency of both the Lung and Spleen, phlegm-damp obstruction in the middle jiao.

【Treatment Principle】

Tonify the Lung and fortify the Spleen, dry dampness, and transform phlegm.

【Prescription】

炙百部	zhì bǎi bù	5g	Radix Stemonae Praeparata
炙紫菀	zhì zǐ wǎn	6g	Radix et Rhizoma Asteris Praeparata
茯苓	fú líng	12g	Poria
炙白前	zhì bái qián	5g	Radix et Rhizoma Cynanchi Stauntonii Praeparata
炙橘红	zhì jú hóng	8g	Exocarpium Citri Rubrum Praeparata
党参	dǎng shēn	10g	Radix Codonopsis
白术	bái zhú	10g	Rhizoma Atractylodis Macrocephalae
川贝母	chuān bèi mǔ	6g	Bulbus Fritillariae Cirrhosae
北沙参	běi shā shēn	6g	Radix Glehniae
枇杷叶	pí pá yè	6g	Folium Eriobotryae
炒杏仁	chǎo xìng rén	10g	Armeniacae Semen Amarum Tostum
炙甘草	zhì gān cǎo	8g	Radix et Rhizoma Glycyrrhizae Praeparata

半夏曲	bàn xià qū	10g	Rhizoma Pinelliae Fermentata
炒远志	chǎo yuǎn zhì	10g	Radix Polygalae Tostum
南沙参	nán shā shēn	6g	Radix Adenophorae

【Second Visit】

After taking 6 doses, the cough was greatly reduced, his eating and sleeping changed for the better, and his urination and defecation were normal. *Yù zhú* (Rhioma Polygonati) 10g and *dōng chóng xià cǎo* (Cordyceps Sinensis) 10g were added into the above formula.

【Third Visit】

After 5 doses of the medication, the cough had basically stopped. The patient was allowed to go home. He was advised to increase the dosage of the formula by five, and grind the medicinals into powder. Then the powder was mixed with honey into 10g pills, and taken orally with boiled water, one pill both in the morning and the evening. He was also advised to exercise so as to prevent catching the common cold.

【Comments】

The Lung controls respiration, it is in charge of skin and hair. It is like a canopy that covers the viscera. Exogenous evils often attack the Lung first and cause cough. Endogenous damage to the five *zang* organs and six *fu* organs can involve the Lung and also cause cough. Exogenous contractions mostly occur suddenly; while endogenous injuries mostly occur slowly. Cough from exogenous contraction is excess complicated by deficiency; while cough from endogenous damage is deficiency complicated by excess. Clinically the treatment should be based on the differentiation of the new from the old, and the deficiency from the excess. This case is one of deficiency of the Spleen and Lung. First, *Yán Nián Zǐ Wǎn Sǎn* (延年紫菀散) and a modified *Sì Jūn Zǐ Tāng* (四君子汤) were used. Then a pill preparation was taken after the initially treatment.

(Zhu Chen-yu, Zhai Ji-sheng, Shi Ru-yu, et al. *Collection of Professor Shi Jin-mo's Clinical Experience* 施今墨临床经验集. Beijing: The People's Medical Publishing House, 1982. 38)

6. Liu Wei-sheng's Case Study: Lung Deficiency and Phlegm-Damp, Compounded by a Contraction of Wind-Heat

Li, male, 62 years old. The initial visit was on May 20th, 1997.

【Initial Visit】

Chief complaint: Chronic cough and expectoration for three years, and aggravation of the disease for one week.

The patient had a 3 year medical history of repeated cough and expectoration. This was aggravated with changes of the weather or external contraction of illness. During times of severe aggravation he had shortness of breath and wheezing, which could usually be alleviated by antibiotics and antiasthmatics. About one week before the first visit, his cough and expectoration were aggravated due to catching a cold. They were accompanied by fever, aversion to wind, pharyngodynia. He saw a doctor once in the out-patient department and his fever was reduced by medication with cefradine and paracetamol, but he still had a cough and yellow sputum. Therefore he came to see me. Physical examination: Hoarse respiratory sounds, along with dry and moist rales over the two lungs, were audible. A chest film revealed increased lung markings. Chronic bronchitis was considered. His tongue was red, with a thick yellow coating, and his pulse was slippery and rapid.

【Pattern Differentiation】

Lung deficiency and phlegm-damp, compounded by a contraction of wind-heat.

【Treatment Principle】

Clear heat and diffuse the Lung; transform phlegm and stop cough.

【Prescription】

Má Xìng Shí Gān Tāng (麻杏石甘汤) with modifications.

炙麻黄	zhì má huáng	9g	Herba Ephedrae Praeparata
杏仁	xìng rén	9g	Armeniacae Semen Amarum
石膏	shí gāo	20g	Gypsum Fibrosum
甘草	gān cǎo	6g	Radix et Rhizoma Glycyrrhizae
蒲公英	pú gōng yīng	20g	Herba Taraxaci
鱼腥草	yú xīng cǎo	20g	Herba Houttuyniae
牛蒡子	niú bàng zǐ	15g	Fructus Arctii
黄芩	huáng qín	15g	Radix Scutellariae
桑白皮	sāng bái pí	15g	Cortex Mori
桔梗	jié gěng	10g	Radix Platycodonis
紫菀	zǐ wǎn	15g	Radix et Rhizoma Asteris
款冬花	kuǎn dōng huā	15g	Flos Farfarae

Seven doses were decocted with water, taken orally, one dose per day.

【Second Visit】

May 27th. The cough was reduced and the phlegm changed from yellow to white and sticky, and abundant in volume. His appetite was normal, and sleep was good. The tongue was red with a slightly yellow coating, and the pulse was rapid. The pattern differentiation was turbid phlegm smoldering in the Lung, with residual heat not being cleared. The prescription was *Xiè Bái Sǎn* (泻白散) with modifications.

桑白皮	sāng bái pí	15g	Cortex Mori
地骨皮	dì gǔ pí	15g	Cortex Lycii
浙贝母	zhè bèi mǔ	15g	Bulbus Fritillariae Thunbergii
桔梗	jié gěng	9g	Radix Platycodonis
炙麻黄	zhì má huáng	9g	Herba Ephedrae Praeparata
海蛤壳	hǎi gé ké	15g	Concha Meretricis seu Cyclinae
杏仁	xìng rén	12g	Armeniacae Semen Amarum
法半夏	fǎ bàn xià	12g	Rhizoma Pinelliae Praeparatum
厚朴	hòu pò	15g	Cortex Magnoliae Officinalis
枳壳	zhǐ qiào	15g	Fructus Aurantii

| 苇茎 | wěi jīng | 30g | Coulis Phragmitis |
| 甘草 | gān cǎo | 9g | Radix et Rhizoma Glycyrrhizae |

Seven doses were decocted with water, and taken orally, one dose per day.

【Third Visit】

June 4th. The phlegm was slight and the cough mild. It was accompanied by a dry mouth, a red tongue with a slightly yellow coating, and a thready and rapid pulse. Pattern differentiation was heat damaging the Lung yin. The prescription was *Shēng Mài Sǎn* (生脉散) with modifications.

太子参	tài zǐ shēn	15g	Radix Pseudostellariae
麦冬	mài dōng	15g	Radix Ophiopogonis
五味子	wǔ wèi zǐ	10g	Fructus Schisandrae Chinensis
天花粉	tiān huā fěn	15g	Radix Trichosanthis
苇茎	wěi jīng	20g	Coulis Phragmitis
天冬	tiān dōng	15g	Radix Asparagi
石斛	shí hú	15g	Caulis Dendrobii
山药	shān yào	15g	Rhizoma Dioscoreae
桑椹子	sāng shèn zǐ	15g	Fructus Mori

Seven doses were decocted with water, and taken orally, one dose per day.

At another visit during the ten middle days of June, he was basically entirely cured.

【Comments】

In the treatment of an acute attack of chronic bronchitis, it is necessary to first clearly differentiate deficiency from excess, and heat from cold. One should treat cold patterns with warm-natured medicinals, and heat patterns with cold or cool-natured medicinals. For cough due to phlegm-heat, Professor Liu Wei-sheng attaches importance to both transforming phlegm and regulating qi. He said, "if the qi fails to be regulated, the turbid phlegm will be difficult to remove. Moistening the Lung and astringing the qi should be conducted at the later stage." He said, "the Lung is a delicate organ, being fond of moistness and averse to dryness. Therefore Lung yin is easily damaged by heat. Accordingly, moistening and nourishing the Lung, and protecting Lung qi should be stressed."

(Liu Wei-sheng, Feng Wei-bin. *Clinical Pattern Differentiation and Treatment of Tumors and Respiratory Diseases in Chinese Medicine* 中医肿瘤、呼吸病临证证治. Guangzhou: The People's Publishing House of Guangdong, 1999. 222)

7. Yang Ji-shun's Case Study: Accumulation of Phlegm-Heat Mixed with Stasis

Wang, female, 58 years old. The initial visit was on January 17th, 1985.

【Initial Visit】

Chief complaint: Repeated cough and expectoration for more than 20 years. This time, the attack had lasted for two months.

Over the past 20 plus years, the patient often had a cough and expectoration in winter and during climatic changes. The cough had become more severe dring the past two months. She had been given *Má Xìng Shí Gān Tāng* (麻杏石甘汤), *Sū Zǐ Jiàng Qì Tāng* (苏子降气汤), etc. but no effect was achieved. Therefore she turned to Professor Yang. Examination results showed cough and dyspnea, copious white and sticky sputum, left chest pain upon severe coughing, a cold appearance of the body, spontaneous sweating, loss of appetite, a dry mouth with no desire to drink, edema of lower limbs; purplish edges of the tongue with a dry yellow coating and sublingual veins, and a thready, wiry and rapid pulse. X-rays revealed chronic bronchitis and pulmonary emphysema complicated by an infection of left lower lung. An ECG showed low voltage, right axis deviation, and a pulmonary P wave.

【Pattern Differentiation】

Accumulation of phlegm-heat mixed with stasis.

【Treatment Principle】

First, clear and diffuse, and transform phlegm, then assist to invigorate blood and remove stasis.

【Prescription】

鱼腥草	yú xīng cǎo	30g	Herba Houttuyniae
金荞麦	jīn qiáo mài	30g	Rhizoma Fagopyri Dibotryis
银花	yín huā	30g	Flos Lonicerae
丹参	dān shēn	30g	Radix et Rhizoma Salviae Miltiorrhizae
车前草	chē qián cǎo	30g	Herba Plantaginis
竹沥半夏	zhú lì bàn xià	12g	Rhizoma Pinelliae cum Succus Bambusae
炙桑白皮	zhì sāng bái pí	12g	Cortex Mori Praeparata
桔梗	jié gěng	12g	Radix Platycodonis
炒枇杷叶	chǎo pí pá yè	12g	Folium Eriobotryae Tostum
桃仁	táo rén	9g	Semen Persicae
杏仁	xìng rén	9g	Armeniacae Semen Amarum
炒陈皮	chǎo chén pí	9g	Pericarpium Citri Reticulatae Tostum
鲜芦根	xiān lú gēn	30g	Rhizoma Phragmitis Communis Recens

She took 5 doses, divided into 3 portions, for 3 days.

【Second Visit】

The cough was reduced, the dyspnea was slightly alleviated, but the sputum was still sticky. Her appetite got better and the tongue coating was yellow and greasy at the root. The other symptoms were the same as before. From the primary formula, *chén pí* (Pericarpium Citri Reticulatae) and *pí pá yè* (Folium Eriobotryae) were removed, and *fú líng* (Poria) 30g was added. After 7 doses of the medication, the cough was greatly reduced, and there was just a little sputum. The dyspnea calmed down, and the appetite was good. Her tongue was red and dry, and her pulse was thready and rapid. The new treatment principle was to replenish qi and nourish yin, and to assist with clearing and diffusing the Lung qi, and removing stasis. The next formula given was:

党参	dǎng shēn	15g	Radix Codonopsis
麦冬	mài dōng	15g	Radix Ophiopogonis
北沙参	běi shā shēn	30g	Radix Glehniae
丹参	dān shēn	30g	Radix et Rhizoma Salviae Miltiorrhizae
鱼腥草	yú xīng cǎo	30g	Herba Houttuyniae
金荞麦	jīn qiáo mài	30g	Rhizoma Fagopyri Dibotryis
炒当归	chǎo dāng guī	12g	Radix Angelicae Sinensis Tostum
炒枇杷叶	chǎo pí pá yè	12g	Folium Eriobotryae Tostum
桃仁	táo rén	9g	Semen Persicae
杏仁	xìng rén	6g	Armeniacae Semen Amarum
炙款冬花	zhì kuǎn dōng huā	9g	Flos Farfarae Praeparata

14 doses.

【Third Visit】

The expectoration had already decreased, the dyspnea had been relieved, and the edema of lower limbs had disappeared. Only the cold appearance, cold limbs, and spontaneous sweating remained. Her sublingual veins had decreased and the tongue coating was yellow. Her pulse was thready and forceless. All of these signs showed that the phlegm heat had been gradually resolved, but the defensive yang was weak due to qi deficiency. Therefore a treatment to replenish qi, consolidating the defense, invigorate blood, and diffuse and descend Lung qi was prescribed:

黄芪	huáng qí	15g	Radix Astragali
防风	fáng fēng	6g	Radix Saposhnikoviae
党参	dǎng shēn	12g	Radix Codonopsitis
制川厚朴	zhì chuān hòu pò	12g	Cortex Magnoliae Praeparata
桔梗	jié gěng	12g	Radix Platycodonis
炒白术	chǎo bái zhú	9g	Rhizoma Atractylodis Macrocephalae Tostum
当归	dāng guī	9g	Radix Angelicae Sinensis
桃仁	táo rén	9g	Semen Persicae

杏仁	xìng rén	9g	Armeniacae Semen Amarum
炙紫菀	zhì zǐ wǎn	9g	Radix et Rhizoma Asteris Praeparata
炙款冬花	zhì kuǎn dōng huā	9g	Flos Farfarae Praeparata
炒枳壳	chǎo zhǐ qiào	9g	Fructus Aurantii Tostum
丹参	dān shēn	30g	Radix et Rhizoma Salviae Miltiorrhizae

【Comments】

This is a case of chronic bronchitis, pulmonary emphysema, and pulmonary heart disease combing with an infection. It belongs to a pattern of accumulation of phlegm-heat in the Lung, with a failure of the Lung to purify and descend. It is a case primarily of deficiency, and secondarily of excess. The secondary aspect is more critical than the primary aspect. First, a high dose of heat-clearing and phlegm-transforming medicinals were taken in order to drain the Lung heat and promote smoothness of the airways. The adjuvant therapy, given according to the presenting condition, was to invigorate blood and resolving stasis in order to improve the function of the Heart and Lung. After the pathogenic heat was cleared and the turbid phlegm was transformed, treatments that replenished qi, supplemented the Kidney, invigorated blood, and diffused the Lung qi were used so as to consolidate the root in order to deal with the aftermath of the illness.

(Pan Zhi-min. *Collection of One Hundred Famous Chinese Clinicians during the Century in China－Yang Ji-sun* 中国百年百名中医临床家丛书·杨继荪. Beijing: China Press of Traditional Chines Medicine, 2003. 71-72)

8. Jiao Shu-de's Case Study: Yang Deficiency with Water Flooding, Upwardly Insulting the Heart and Lung

Xue, female, 67 years old. The initial visit was on December 12th, 1969.

【Initial Visit】

Chief complaint: For over half a month, cough and panting with an inability to lie flat. The patient had suffered from cough and panting for many years; and there was an obvious aggravation due to a cold caught recently. In a hospital, her diagnosis was chronic bronchitis, pulmonary emphysema, pulmonary heart disease, and a II ~ III degree of cardiac insufficiency. Because of her poor response to biomedical treatment, she came seeking Chinese medicine. Her present symptoms were frequent cough, obvious panting, a low and weak voice, shortness of breath, palpitations, tachypnea, an inability to lie flat, insomnia at night, copious thin and frothy white sputum which could be easily expectorated, scanty urine, a yellowish-white lusterless complexion, slight edema of the lower eyelids, pitting edema of the lower limbs, loss of appetite, no desire to drink, stuffiness of the epigastrium with slight pain that was not responsive to heavy pressure, occasional nausea and vomiting, and fairly normal stools. The tongue had a white and glossy coating. The pulse was slippery and rapid at all six positions on both wrists, thready-slippery with wiry at both *cun* positions, wiry-slippery at the left *guan* position, and deep-slippery with a bit wiriness at both *chi* positions.

【Pattern Differentiation】

Yang deficiency with water flooding, upwardly insulting the Heart and Lung.

【Treatment Principle】

Donwbear qi and dispel phlegm; assist yang to transform fluids.

【Prescription】

炒苏子	chǎo sū zǐ	10g	Fructus Perillae Tostum
炒莱菔子	chǎo lái fú zǐ	9g	Semen Raphani Tostum
法夏	fǎ xià	10g	Rhizoma Pinelliae Praeparata
化橘红	huà jú hóng	10g	Exocarpium Citri Grandis
炙甘草	zhì gān cǎo	6g	Radix et Rhizoma Glycyrrhizae Praeparata
茯苓	fú líng	15g	Poria
猪苓	zhū líng	15g	Polyporus
桂枝	guì zhī	8g	Ramulus Cinnamomi

泽泻	zé xiè	10g	Rhizoma Alismatis
珍珠母	zhēn zhū mǔ	30g (decocted first)	Concha Margaritifera
藿香	huò xiāng	10g	Herba Agastachis
元胡	yuán hú	9g	Rhizoma Corydalis

It was decocted with water, and taken warm, orally, 3 doses.

【Second Visit】

December 15th. After the above medication was taken, the cough and panting were obviously relieved, and the sputum had also clearly decreased. Her urine increased, the edema was gone, and the patient was able to lie flat, and had good sleep. The tongue coating was thin, and the pulse was a bit slippery and moderate. She was again prescribed 3 doses of the formula. Her daughter then reported that her disease was cured. Another 3 doses of the formula were given after the treatment. A follow-up assesment was conducted half month later, and no relapse of the disease had appeared.

(Jiao Shu-de. *Shu-de's Chinese Internal Medicine* 树德中医内科. Beijing: The People's Medical Publishing House, 2005. 144-145)

9. Li Kong-ding's Case Study: Dual Deficiency of the Spleen

Ren, male, 49 years old, a worker with the Five Continents Electric Source Factory.

The patient had an episodic cough for four years. The episodes often occurred in winter and spring, and lasted for two or three months, with secondary symptoms including chest oppression, dizziness, physical fatigue, shortness of breath, lumbago, tinnitus, a pink tongue with a white coating, and a moderate pulse. He was diagnosed, via chest X-rays, as having chronic bronchitis. The Chinese medical pattern was a dual deficiency of the Spleen and Kidney. He began take *Ké Chuǎn Kāng Fù Jiāo Náng* (咳喘康复胶囊) on July 18th, 1994, five capsules three times per day, for forty days. With two courses of the treatment, his cough and the other symptoms disappeared. An analysis of the treatment efficacy shows that this treatment is clinically controlled. The long term the treatment efficacy was a clinical cure.

The internal cause of chronic bronchitis is an insufficiency of the right qi, and a deficiency of the Lung, Spleen and Kidney. Its external cause is a contraction of wind, cold or heat evils leading to a failure of the Lung to diffuse and ascend. In the treatment, tonification and boosting of the Lung, Spleen and Kidney is emphasized in order to treat the primary aspect of the disease. According to the fact that *Ké Chuǎn Kāng Fù Wán* (咳喘康复丸) is a proven formula from Li Kong-ding (a famous veteran physician of Chinese medicine in the Sichuan province of China) from his many years practice, the blood-invigorating and stasis-resolving treatment was modified to supplement and boost the Lung, Spleen and Kidney. It was developed into a capsule preparation. In a comparison with *Bǔ Shèn Fáng Chuǎn Piān* (补肾防喘片), 209 cases of chronic bronchitis patients were monitored for the clinical effect of the capsule preparation. The results showed that in the trial group of 152 cases, the total effective rate was 97.36%, and the long-term clinical curative rate was 20.39%. No toxic side effects were found. In the control group of 57 cases, the total effective rate was 84.21%, and the long-term clinical curative rate was 12.28%. There was a statistical difference between the two groups (P<0.01). This result suggests that *Ké Chuǎn Kāng Fù Wán* (咳喘康复丸) is of good effect to treat chronic bronchitis, with a pattern differentiation of dual deficiency of the Spleen and Kidney.

[Sheng Qi-ling, Jing Hong-gui, Li Kong-ding. Treatment of Chronic Bronchitis with *Ké Chuǎn Kāng Fù Jiāo Náng*・A Clinical Analysis of 152 Cases. *Journal of Chengdu University of Traditional Chinese Medicine* 成都中医药大学学报. 1998, 21 (2): 22-25]

10. Wang Zhi-zhong's Song Dynasty Case Study

My younger brother was drenched with rain during his ascent of the mountain. He had chest stuffiness through the night, and was almost dying. He lost control of his feelings and began to weep when he met his brothers, as if he was about to die. I suspected that he was in a sorrowful mood, so I did acupuncture at his GV 20 (*bǎi huì*), but there was no response. As I pressed his BL 13 (*fèi shù*) and he said that he got a pricking pain, so I punctured his BL 13 (*fèi shù*) with a red-hot needle and he soon recovered. Accordingly, one can puncture only BL 13 (*fèi shù*), with a bilateral insertion, and without other points, when treating asthma patients. Ignite moxa for moxibustion on the point, for patients that feel aching pain upon pressing the BL 13 (*fèi shù*), but not at other points.

(Wei Zhi-xiu of the Qing Dynasty. *A Complete Book of Clinical Skills: Panting in Supplement to Classified Case Records of Celebrated Physicians* 清·魏之琇·临床医术大全·续名医类案·喘. 1998, 21 (2): 22-25)

Discussions

1. Professor Jiao Shu-de Believes that the Concept of Two Classes, Six Patterns and Three Principles must be Grasped in Order to Treat Panting

(1) Two Classes

Panting patterns present with different clinical manifestations because of different body constitutions, etiologic factors, ages and circumstances. Panting patterns can be divided into two main classes of deficiency and excess.

Excess panting is an "exuberance of pathogenic evils resulting in excess". It is characterized clinically by forceful breathing, chest fullness, coarse breathing, loud and turbulent breathing sounds, chest expansion as if the air was not be contained, a prolonged expiratory phase; fullness and distention of the hypochondria, open mouthed gasping with the shoulders lifting, body shakes, an inflated abdomen, a yellow or white thick and greasy tongue coating, and a rapid and powerful pulse.

Deficiency panting is a "consumption of essential qi causing deficiency". It is characterized clinically by breathlessness, accompanied by forceless breathing with a low sound, panic as if qi were about to collapse, with a prolonged inspiratory phase, mental emotional weariness, a thin and white tongue coating, and a weak or deficient and powerless pulse.

Generally speaking, the excess pattern is more common than the deficient pattern. But excess and deficiency can transform into each other or intermingle with each other. For example, if an elderly person who is physically weak catches wind-cold, the external evils restrain the Lung, and panting occurs because of excess evils in the Lung. This is a deficiency pattern complicated by excess. Just like the saying in *Inner Canon of Huangdi* (内经 , *Nèi Jīng*): "If the body is invaded by exogenous evils on the base of deficiency, the illness belongs to excess (虚而受邪 , 其病则实)." Therefore the two classes of deficiency and excess must first be distinguished from the complicated signs and symptoms, and then the remedy can be prescribed according to the pattern.

(2) Six Patterns

1) Cold-excess pattern:

It is clinically characterized by susceptibility to falling ill, or having an aggravation of illness, with each encounter of catching colds or during the winter season. There is also white and thin sputum, a preference for warmth and hot drinks, a white tongue coating, a slippery or slow moderate pulse. Treatment should be to warm, diffuse, purify and descend. The formula used is a self-composed *Má Xìng Sū Chá Tāng* (麻杏苏茶汤). The ingredients are:

麻黄	má huáng	3—9g	Herba Ephedrae
杏仁	xìng rén	10g	Armeniacae Semen Amarum
苏子	sū zǐ	10g	Fructus Perillae
桔梗	jié gěng	6g	Radix Platycodonis
茶叶	Chá yè	6—10g	Folium Camelliae Sinensis
干姜	gān jiāng	3—5g	Rhizoma Zingiberis
诃子	hē zǐ	3g	Fructus Chebulae
炙甘草	zhì gān cǎo	3g	Radix et Rhizoma Glycyrrhizae Praeparata

2) Heat-excess pattern:

It is clinically characterized by panting with coarse breathing, yellow sputum, thirst, aversion to heat and preference for cool, aggravation upon invasion by heat or in summer, a yellow tongue coating, and a rapid pulse. Treatment should be to clear and diffuse Lung heat, downbear qi and clear away phlegm. The formula used is a newly-composed *Má Xìng Lóu Shí Tāng* (新拟麻杏蒌石汤). The ingredients are:

麻黄	má huáng	2—6g	Herba Ephedrae
杏仁	xìng rén	10g	Armeniacae Semen Amarum
桑白皮	sāng bái pí	10g	Cortex Mori
槟榔	bīng láng	10g	Semen Arecae
金沸草	jīn fèi cǎo	10g	Herba Inulae
地骨皮	dì gǔ pí	10g	Cortex Lycii
瓜蒌	guā lóu	20—50g	Fructus Trichosanthis
生石膏	shēng shí gāo	20—60g	Gypsum Fibrosum
葶苈子	tíng lì zǐ	6—10g	Semen Lepidii seu Descurainiae
生甘草	shēng gān cǎo	3g	Radix et Rhizoma Glycyrrhizae Recens

➤ For cases accompanied by exterior heat, remove *jīn fèi cǎo* (Herba Inulae) and add *bò hé* (Herba Menthae), *jīn yín huā* (Flos Lonicerae), and *sāng yè* (Folium Mori).

➢ For cases of severe phlegm-heat, use a larger quantity of *guā lóu* (Fructus Trichosanthis) and add *zhú lì* (Succus Bambusae), *zhú huáng* (Shiraia Bambusicola), and *jié gěng* (Radix Platycodonis).

➢ For obvious qi counterflow, add *shēng zhě shí* (Haematitum) and *xuán fù huā* (Flos Inulae).

➢ For cases with severe internal heat, pain of the throat, red eyes, constipation, halitosis, and yellow thick sputum with hot foul smell, remove *jīn fèi cǎo* (Herba Inulae), and selectively add *zhī zǐ* (Fructus Gardeniae), *huáng qín* (Radix Scutellariae), *zhī mǔ* (Rhizoma Anemarrhenae), *xuán shēn* (Radix Scrophulariae), *dà qīng yè* (Folium Isatidis), *niú bàng zǐ* (Fructus Arctii), and/or *shēng dà huáng* (Radix et Rhizoma Rhei).

3) Phlegm-excess pattern:

It is clinically characterized by chest oppression, stubborn phlegm, and difficulty in expectoration. If it is severe then there is wheezing (sounds of phlegm). If there is a lot of phlegm, then there is blockage of the airways causing panting. There is a slippery pulse, and a greasy tongue coating. Treatment should be to diffuse and eliminate phlegm and calm panting. The formula used is self-composed *Má Xìng Èr Sān Tāng* (麻杏二三汤). The ingredients are:

麻黄	má huáng	3—6g	Herba Ephedrae
杏仁	xìng rén	10g	Armeniacae Semen Amarum
法半夏	fǎ bàn xià	10g	Rhizoma Pinelliae
莱菔子	lái fú zǐ	10g	Semen Raphani Tostum
苏子	sū zǐ	10g	Fructus Perillae
橘红	jú hóng	12g	Exocarpium Citri Rubrum
茯苓	fú líng	12g	Poria
炙甘草	zhì gān cǎo	3g	Radix et Rhizoma Glycyrrhizae Praeparata
白芥子	bái jiè zǐ	3—6g	Semen Sinapis Albae

Additionally, Doctor Yang Jun-long once treated 26 cases of

asthmatic bronchitis with this prescription. The results were that 19 cases had excellently effective results, with both the clinical symptoms and the rales and wheezing over the lungs disappearing. The disease did not relapse, even when the patient was invaded by evils. 4 cases had efficacious results, with clinical symptoms disappearing or becoming obviously relieved. The rales and wheezing over the lungs were reduced. But the disease relapsed due to invasion by evils. 3 cases are had non-effective results, with the clinical symptoms not relieved, and the positive signs over the lungs not improved. The total rate of efficacy was 88.9%.

[Yang Jun-long. Asthmatic Bronchitis Treated with *Má Xìng Èr Sān Tāng* · A Clinical Analysis of 26 Cases. *Zhejiang Journal of Traditional Chinese Medicine* 浙江中医杂志. 2002, 37(12): 532]

4) Lung deficiency pattern:

It is clinically characterized by shortness of breath with panting, forceless respiration with a low sound, susceptibility to catching colds, a whitish complexion, and a deficient or soggy pulse. The treatment should be to tonify the Lung and boost qi to calm panting. The formula used is the newly-composed *Má Xìng Bǔ Fèi Tāng* (麻杏补肺汤). The ingredients are:

麻黄	má huáng	3g	Herba Ephedrae
杏仁	xìng rén	12g	Armeniacae Semen Amarum
黄芪	huáng qí	9g	Radix Astragali
党参	dǎng shēn	6g	Radix Codonopsis
陈皮	chén pí	6g	Pericarpium Citri Reticulatae
五味子	wǔ wèi zǐ	5g	Fructus Schisandrae Chinensis
熟地	shú dì	12g	Radix Rehmanniae Praeparata
紫菀	zǐ wǎn	12g	Radix et Rhizoma Asteris
桑白皮	sāng bái pí	10g	Cortex Mori
苏子	sū zǐ	10g	Fructus Perillae

➤ For damage to both qi and yin, accompanied by a dry throat and mouth, and a red tongue with little fluids, add *shā shēn* (Glehniae), *mài mén dōng* (Radix Ophiopogonis) and *wū méi* (Fructus Mume).

5) Spleen deficiency pattern:

It is clinically characterized by a yellowish complexion, tired limbs, shortness of breath, poor appetite, a swollen tongue with a white coating, and a soggy and slippery pulse. The treatment should be to fortify the Spleen, transform phlegm, and calm panting. The formula used was the newly-composed *Má Xìng Liù Jūn Zǐ Tāng* (麻杏六君子汤). The ingredients are:

麻黄	má huáng	3—5g	Herba Ephedrae
杏仁	xìng rén	10g	Armeniacae Semen Amarum
党参	dǎng shēn	10g	Radix Codonopsis
陈皮	chén pí	10g	Pericarpium Citri Reticulatae
法半夏	fǎ bàn xià	10g	Rhizoma Pinelliae
谷芽	gǔ yá	10g	Fructus Setariae Germinatus
白术	bái zhú	6g	Rhizoma Atractylodis Macrocephalae
茯苓	fú líng	10g	Poria
炙甘草	zhì gān cǎo	5g	Radix et Rhizoma Glycyrrhizae Praeparata
焦三仙	jiāo sān xiān	9g for each	Stir-fried combination of Fructus Crataegi, Massa Fermentata and Fructus Hordei Germinatus

➤ For edema with scanty urine, add *dōng guā pí* (Epicarpium Benincasae), *zé xiè* (Rhizoma Alismatis), *guì zhī* (Ramulus Cinnamomi) and *fú líng* (Poria).

6) Kidney deficiency pattern:

It is clinically characterized by dyspnea, lumbar pain, soreness of the limbs, panting induced upon exertion, a white tongue coating, and a weak pulse at the *chi* position. The treatment should be to boost the Kidney and receive qi to calm panting. The formula used was the newly-composed *Má Xìng Dū Qì Tāng* (麻杏都气汤). The ingredients are:

麻黄	má huáng	3—5g	Herba Ephedrae
杏仁	xìng rén	10g	Armeniacae Semen Amarum
山茱萸	shān zhū yú	10g	Fructus Corni
焦神曲	jiāo shén qū	10g	Massa Fermentata Praeparatus
熟地黄	shú dì huáng	20g	Radix Rehmanniae Praeparata
磁石	cí shí	20g	Magnetitum
山药	shān yào	10—20g	Rhizoma Dioscoreae
茯苓	fú líng	9—12g	Poria
泽泻	zé xiè	6—9g	Rhizoma Alismatis
牡丹皮	mǔ dān pí	3—9g	Cortex Moutan
五味子	wǔ wèi zǐ	5—10g	Fructus Schisandrae Chinensis
蛤蚧尾粉	gé jiè wěi fěn	1g (dissolved)	Exremitas Gecko Pulveratum

This is a pattern of floating yang which is caused by the impending collapse of Kidney yang. If the patient presents with a flushed face (a dark complexion with red cheeks), cold feet, panting with cold sweating, difficulty inhalation, restlessness, a black and moist tongue coating transforming from a base of white or white greasy coating, and a deep and thready pulse or feeble and hard to feel pulse at the *chi* position, then treatment should be to urgently guide the fire to return to the root, and restore the Kidney qi. Add *ròu guì* (Cortex Cinnamomi) and pill of stannum nigrum (swallowed separately) to the formula.

The above six patterns may occur alone, or in combination with each other. The doctor must flexibly choose a proper treatment according to concrete conditions.

(3) Three Principles

1) During times of disease flare up, one should primarily dispel evils, and mainly treat the excess pattern so as to eliminate the branch.

2) When there is no flare up of panting, one should primarily support the right qi, and mainly treat the deficiency pattern so as to consolidate the root.

3) When treating panting combined with wheezing (asthma), one should pay attention to adding anti-phlegmatics such as *Lěng Xiào Wán* (冷哮丸).

The ingredients are *má huáng* (Herba Ephedrae), *chuān wū* (Radix Aconiti), *xì xīn* (Radix et Rhizoma Asari), *chuān jiāo* (Pericarpium Zanthoxyli), *shēng bái fán* (Alumen), *zào jiǎo* (Fructus Gleditsiae Sinensis), *bàn xià qū* (Rhizoma Pinelliae Fermentata), *dǎn nán xīng* (Arisaema cum Bile), *xìng rén* (Armeniacae Semen Amarum), *gān cǎo* (Radix et Rhizoma Glycyrrhizae), *zǐ wǎn* (Radix et Rhizoma Asteris), *dōng huā* (Flos Farfarae), ground into a power, and mixed with ginger juice and *shén qū mò* (Pulvis Massa Medicata Fermentata), and then made into pills. 3—6g are taken orally each time. Can also use *Zǐ Jīn Dān* (紫金丹), which is composed of *pī shí* (Arsenicum), and *dàn dòu chǐ* (Semen Sojae Praeparatum), prepared into pills the size of *má rén* (Semen Cannabis Sativae), with 10—15 pills taken orally each time. Another option is *Xiǎo Luó Zào Wán* (小萝皂丸), whose ingredients are *lái fú zǐ* (Semen Raphani Tostum), *zào jiǎo* (Fructus Gleditsiae Sinensis), *nán xīng* (Rhizoma Arisaematis), *guā lóu rén* (Semen Trichosanthis), and *hǎi gé fěn* (Pulvis Meretricis seu Cyclinae), mixed with ginger juice and combined with honey, then made into 3—5g pills, with one pill melted in the mouth each time. *Bái fán* (Alumen), and *zào jiá* (Fructus Gleditsiae Sinensis) can also be taken. The above medications can be selected according to the pattern.

(Shi Yu-Guang, Shan Shu-jian. *The Clinical Essence of Contemporary Famous Physicians · Special Monograph of Asthma* 当代名医临证精华·咳喘专辑. Beijing: China Ancient Writings Publishing House, 1988. 94)

2. Professor Shao Chang-rong Believes that in the Treatment of Chronic Bronchitis, Importance should be Attached to Cold, Heat, Phlegm, Dampness, and Deficiency

Professor Shao Chang-rong believes that patients with chronic bronchitis must be weak due to their protracted course of illness. Generally the disease presents with a deficiency of the Lung, Spleen and Kidney; at the same time it is complicated by an excess of phlegm-damp. "Mixed excess and deficiency" means that patients often have manifestations of "cold, heat, phlegm, dampness and deficiency". Treatment should be to warm the Lung and transform fluids. The clinical manifestations are a cold appearance, chest oppression, thick white phlegm, and a pale and enlarged tongue with a white and purple coating. This is similar to the pattern of "phlegm-fluid retention". For this kind of case, of the treatment should be consistent with the principle stated in *Synopsis of Golden Chamber* (金匮要略 , *Jīn Guì Yào Lüè*): "The patient suffering from phlegm-fluid retention should be given warming medicinals for harmonization (病痰饮者，当以温药和之)." The ingredients are:

附子	fù zǐ	9g	Radix Aconiti Lateralis
竹茹	zhú rú	9g	Caulis Bambusae in Taeniis
葶苈子	tíng lì zǐ	9g	Semen Lepidii seu Descurainiae
五加皮	wǔ jiā pí	9g	Cortex Acanthopanacis
白术	bái zhú	9g	Rhizoma Atractylodis Macrocephalae
细辛	xì xīn	3g	Radix et Rhizoma Asari
荆芥	jīng jiè	12g	Herba Schizonepetae

The curative effect of this formula is excellent, with an effective rate of 70—80%. This formula plays a role in regulating the phlegm and fluids.

Draining the Lung and transforming phlegm is used in cases of phlegm-heat internally flourishing. The representative formula is *Sāng Bái Pí Tāng* (桑白皮汤), with a larger quantity of *huáng qín* (Radix Scutellariae). The indication of this formula is for cases of Spleen deficiency with phlegm-damp internally flourishing, which manifests as cough and panting, chest oppression, poor appetite, thin white sputum, and a dry mouth with no desire to drink. In general, transforming phlegm to calm panting is often not an efficacious treatment method. For a better effect, add *Píng Wèi Èr Chén Tāng* (平胃二陈汤). Originally, there was worry that because the nature of *cāng zhú* (Rhizoma Atractylodis) and *hòu pò* (Cortex Magnoliae Officinalis) is drying, yin might be consumed and blood injured. But it is not the case clinically, as the two medicinals have good effect on drying dampness to transform phlegm and regulating qi, and they can help the fluids to distribute, and succeed in obtaining an unanticipated effect.

There are many formulas to tonify the Spleen and Kidney, such as *Shēn Gé Sǎn* (参蛤散), *Fù Guì Bā Wèi Wán* (附桂八味丸), and *Qī Wèi Dū Qì Wán* (七味都气丸).

(Chen Ze-lin, Song Zu-dui. *Essentials of Famous Physician Special Experiences* 名医特色经验精华. Shanghai: Publishing House of Shanghai College of Traditional Chinese Medicine, 1987. 109）

3. Professor Xie Chang-ren Believes that in the Treatment of Cough and Panting Three Stages Need to be Differentiated

Professor Xie Chang-ren believes that different treatment principles and remedies should be taken in accordance with the different stages of cough and panting. Distinguish whether it is in the Lung, Spleen, or Kidney. Differentiate clearly if it is cold, hot, deficiency or excess. These are all different and thus the treatment and formulas will also be different. Carry out care systematically and then there can be success.

(1) During the Acute Episode Period, the Stress of Treatment is on the Lung, and Cold or Heat must be Differentiated

Acute attacks of cough and panting often come together and the onset is drastic and severe. It is usually induced by an external contraction of new evils, such as invasion of wind-cold, or turbid phlegm into the Lung, resulting in a failure of Lung qi to diffuse and descend. It is important to treat the Lung at this time. The formula is *Sān Niù Tāng* (三拗汤) plus *Xìng Sū Èr Chén Tāng* (杏苏二陈汤) with modifications. The medicinals are *zhì má huáng* (Herba Ephedrae Praeparata), *xìng rén* (Armeniacae Semen Amarum), *gān cǎo* (Radix et Rhizoma Glycyrrhizae), *sū zǐ* (Fructus Perillae), *tíng lì zǐ* (Semen Lepidii seu Descurainiae), *chén pí* (Pericarpium Citri Reticulatae), *fǎ bàn xià* (Rhizoma Pinelliae), *qián hú* (Radix Peucedani), *sāng bái pí* (Cortex Mori), *kuǎn dōng huā* (Flos Farfarae). These herbs are used to diffuse and depurate. If the evil is not out-thrust externally, and the phlegm is not alleviated or transformed, then cough and panting are difficult to stop. Therefore the treatment emphasizes the two aspects of diffusing the Lung to expel evils, and transforming phlegm to disinhibit qi. For cases of severe exogenous cold, add *xì xīn* (Radix et Rhizoma Asari), and *guì zhī* (Ramulus Cinnamomi) or use *Xiǎo Qīng Lóng Tāng* (小青龙汤) with modifications to dispel wind-cold and warm the Lung in order to transform fluids. For patients in the acute flare up stage, one must still at all times pay attention to cold or heat transformation or cold and heat combining. If the quality of phlegm becomes thick and yellow, and is accompanied by fever, and a yellow tongue coating, it is usually a case of chronic bronchitis complicated by infection. In Chinese medical pattern differentiation it belongs to a case of exogenous cold and internal heat or phlegm-heat accumulating in the Lung. One can change to using formulas like *Dìng Chuǎn Tāng* (定喘汤), *Xiè Bái Sǎn* (泻白散) with modifications or *Sān Niù Tāng* (三拗汤). Also use herbs that clear the Lung and drain heat such as *jīn yín huā* (Flos

Lonicerae), *huáng qín* (Radix Scutellariae), *jīn qiáo mài* (Rhizoma Fagopyri Dibotryis), *sāng bái pí* (Cortex Mori), *dōng guā pí* (Epicarpium Benincasae), *zhè bèi mǔ* (Bulbus Fritillariae Thunbergii), and *guā lóu pí* (Pericarpium Trichosanthis). For cases with severe heat, add *shēng shí gāo* (Gypsum Fibrosum). For cases accompanied by constipation, add *shēng dà huáng* (Radix et Rhizoma Rhei) to open the bowels and drain heat, often with an excellent effect.

(2) During the Chronic Protracted Period, Weigh the Relative Importance of Treating the Branch or the Root

The cough and panting is alleviated during the chronic protracted period, but the illness has not yet been cured. There are usually symptoms of deficiency of both the Lung and Spleen, such as shortness of breath and panting, breathlessness aggravated upon exertion, listlessness and lassitude, poor appetite and loose stools, and a thready and weak pulse. There are also manifestations of phlegm-damp internally smoldering, such as cough and excessive sputum, and a greasy tongue coating. If the treatment is merely concentrated on the branch, it will be difficult to recover the deficiency of the right qi. On the other hand, if the treatment aims only at the root, it is not good for elimination of the evils. During this time, one needs to weigh the relative importance of treating the branch or the root, and treat the deficiency and excess simultaneously to get results. For cases of deficiency of both the Lung and Spleen with phlegm-damp internally smoldering, modified *Liù Jūn Zǐ Tāng* (六君子汤), *Píng Wèi Sǎn* (平胃散), or *Xìng Sū Èr Chén Tāng* (杏苏二陈汤) can be used. For cases of deficiency of both the Spleen and Stomach, accompanied by turbid phlegm, use *Mài Wèi Dì Huáng Tāng* (麦味地黄汤) plus *Xìng Sū Èr Chén Tāng* (杏苏二陈汤), with the addition of herbs to receive the Kidney qi. It always has an excellent effect.

(3) During the Symptom Remission Period, the Disease is in the Spleen and Kidney, and Supplementing and Tonifying is the Proper Treatment

Every year as the climate becomes warmer, the symptoms of most patients who have cough and panting will gradually disappear as they enter a remission period. There is a saying that "the Spleen is the source for generation of phlegm", and "the phlegm is generated as the Kidney becomes deficient and fails to control water". The root is in the Spleen and Kidney, and the pattern differentiation should begin with the deficient patterns. It is proper to use methods of supplementing and tonifying the Spleen and Kidney. Modified *Liù Jūn Zǐ* (六君子) plus *Jīn Guì Shèn Qì Wán* (金匮肾气丸) can be taken continuously for several months. Clinically, the commonly used medicinals to supplement the Kidney to receive qi include *gé jiè* (Gecko), *zǐ hé chē* (Placenta Hominis), *qiàn shí* (Semen Euryales), *hú táo ròu* (Semen Juglandis Regiae), *bǔ gǔ zhī* (Fructus Psoraleae), and *chén xiāng* (Lignum Aquilariae Resinatumare). The commonly used medicinals to fortify the Spleen and replenish qi include *rén shēn* (Radix Ginseng), *dǎng shēn* (Radix Codonopsis), *huáng qí* (Radix Astragali), *shān yào* (Rhizoma Dioscoreae), *bái zhú* (Rhizoma Atractylodis Macrocephalae), and *fú líng* (Poria). Ye Tian-shi believed that "cough and panting due to a disorder of the Lung is an excessive pattern, and when it is due to the disorder of the Kidney is a deficient pattern." Therefore invigorating the Kidney is the method to treat the root for cough and panting. According to the relationship between the Spleen and Kidney, invigorating the Kidney will simultaneously reinforce the Spleen and Stomach, which can increase the source for generating qi and blood, and eliminate the cause that engenders phlegm-damp. Therefore treating the root should tonify the Spleen and Kidney at the same time. Except above medicinal decoctions, every year the medicinal extract preparations should be worked out for the patients who are in the symptomatic relief period before winter solstice. This is made from the effective formula for supplementing and tonifying the Spleen and Kidney that the patient uses in normal times. The dosage is increased 15-20 times that of the normal, decocted and filtered, with additional candy sugar added so that it is condense like an ointment. Thus an excellent effect can be achieved. For cases of a failure of the Kidney to receive qi with a prolonged cough and panting, complicated by emphysema and breathlessness upon exertion, equal portions of *hóng shēn* (Radix et Rhizoma Ginseng Rubra) or *bái shēn* (Radix Ginseng Alba), and *gé jiè* (Gecko) are often taken. These are ground into fine a powder. 3g are taken in the morning and in the evening. The effect is satisfactory if the patient is persisting in taking the medication. For cases with additional Lung deficiency, a failure of the defensive exterior to consolidate, and general susceptibility to catching colds, add *Yù Píng Fēng Sǎn* (玉屏风散). Again, take orally in small dosages for a long period of time. This treatment can obviously strengthen the physique and reduce the attacks of the cough and panting.

(Shi Yu-guang. *Clinical Mirror of Famous Physicians at Ancient and Modern · Cough, Panting and Lung Distention · Book 1* 古今名医临证金鉴·咳喘肺胀·上. Beijing: China Ancient Writings Publishing House, 1999. 339)

4. Professor Wang Zheng-gong's Opinion on the Methods to Reverse Chronic Obstructive Pulmonary Disease

(1) Treatment of the Disease should Aim at the Root

Treating this disease by aiming at the root is a basic principle of pattern differentiation and treatment in Chinese Medicine. In the treatment of chronic bronchitis and asthma, Chinese medicine talks about stopping cough, transforming phlegm, and calming panting, but the methods that are used are not simply seeing cough then stopping cough, seeing phlegm then transforming phlegm, seeing panting then calming panting [symptomatic treatments]. Moreover, the idea is to "see the root to target the origin, examine the cause to determine treatment". Chinese medicine has had a very long history of clinical practice, with the realization that a therapeutic effect gained by inhibiting cough directly, on the contrary it will result in protraction of cough, even panting and swelling.

Regarding the issue of treating phlegm: Chinese Medicine believes that "transforming phlegm" means identifying the nature of phlegm based on the factors of phlegm generation and using methods of "acting in accordance with circumstances" and "restricting the source and smoothing the flow". "Restricting the source" means reducing the source of phlegm. For example, use a method of coursing the exterior to treat excessive phlegm caused by cold damage, or use a method of fortifying the Spleen to transform dampness to treat gathering phlegm due to abundant dampness of the Spleen and Stomach. "Smoothing the flow" means strengthening the eliminating phlegm function of tracheal mucous membrane so as to reduce the secretion of phlegm and to ease expectoration. Thus the dyspnea and chest oppression will be relieved. The occurrence of secondary infections will also be reduced.

Regarding the issue of treating panting: Panting is divided into excess and deficiency types. In cases of excessive panting, the main focus is on eliminating the evil, and the treatment should concentrate on out-thrusting evils to expel phlegm. In cases of deficient panting, the treatment should concentrate on the loss of Heart and Kidney qi and blood. In addition, there can also be a contraction of evils complicated by phlegm—then the root is deficient and the branch is excess, and one should simultaneously deal with both the branch and the root, and distinguish the first from the second. These all belong to the method of treating the root of the disease.

(2) Action should be in Accordance with Circumstances, Normalizing the Generating Mechanism of the Disease

The doctor should begin by examining the whole, simultaneously seeking an understanding of the dysfunctions and imbalances of the *zang-fu* organs (viscera), channels and collaterals, and the qi and blood. By normalizing the generating mechanism, or expelling evil qi, or supporting the right qi, then the normal condition can be restored. As far as the respiratory tract is concerned, clearing and purifying are favorable and congealing and blocking are unfavorable (The Lung governs purification and descent). Cough with phlegm obstruction, due to invasion of the Lung channel by evils, should be treated by diffusing the Lung to eliminate phlegm. This follows in line with the physiological function of the respiratory tract. All other therapies are unfavorable and cannot cure the disease. Unfortunately, most modern doctors usually inhibit cough; and although the cough is not alleviated, the doctors do not think that it is harmful. Therefore there is an increase in cases of chronic bronchitis and asthma. However, the situation is not always the same. If the cough and panting is going through an acute episode, it should be treated by inhibiting cough and calming panting, as is appropriate in an emergency. However, a long-term dependency on dilating the trachea in order to calm panting and paralyzing the nerves to stop cough will not get results as expected.

"Action should be in accordance with the circumstances" is one of the most basic therapeutic principles in Chinese Medicine. From ancient times, there have been eight therapeutic methods in Chinese Medicine. The three methods of sweating, vomiting, and draining downward directly "act in accordance with the circumstances" in order to eliminate evils, thus evils are eliminated and the right qi is stable. The methods of harmonizing, warming, clearing, resolving, and tonifying are the indirect methods of regaining the balance so as to get the effect of curing diseases and out-thrusting evils. In practice there is proof that the methods of coursing and abducting are better relative to the methods of restraining and stopping. Therefore concerning respiratory system diseases, when the evils are out-thrust the cough will stop on its own, and when the phlegm is cleared then the panting will calm naturally.

(3) The Supreme Doctor Treats Disease Preventatively

Plain Questions (素问, *Sù Wèn*) says: "The sage does not treat the disease that already occurs, but treats the condition before a disease; he does not suppress the disorder that already appears, but manages to prevent the disorder (圣人不治已病，治未病，不治已乱治未乱)." To reduce the morbidity of chronic respiratory diseases, the evils should be eliminated as soon as possible before the panting and cough or panting and swelling develop. This is especially true for the acute stage when the evil initially invades the body and the right qi is not yet injured. In this way, half the work will get double the result.

Patients with chronic respiratory diseases are predisposed to secondary infections, and attention must be paid to this fact. These symptoms include expectoration of purulent sputum accompanied by fever, tachypnea, and cough. This belongs to the category of *fēng wēn* (风温, wind-warm). Treatment should be to resolve the exterior with acridity and coldness, clear the Lung and eliminate phlegm. For mild cases, use *Yín Qiào Sǎn* (银翘散) plus *qián hú* (Radix Peucedani), *sāng yè* (Folium Mori), *sāng bái pí* (Cortex Mori), *huáng qín* (Radix Scutellariae), *pú gōng yīng* (Herba Taraxaci), *yú xīng cǎo* (Herba Houttuyniae Cordatae) and, *lái fú zǐ* (Semen Raphani). For severe cases, use *Má Xìng Shí Gān Tāng* (麻杏石甘汤) plus *niú bàng zǐ* (Fructus Arctii), *qián hú* (Radix Peucedani), *jīn yín huā* (Flos Lonicerae), *lián qiào* (Fructus Forsythiae), *lú gēn* (Rhizoma Phragmitis), and *bái jiāng cán* (Bombyx Batryticatus) to control the infection. After the symptoms are relieved, the method of clearing the Lung and eliminating phlegm is used again.

Regardless of whether is it chronic bronchitis or asthma, during the remission stage the method of strengthening the right qi and cultivating the root should be used over time to reinforce the physical strength and reduce the severity of attacks. Medicine in the form of pills should be used because the action is stable and the application of medication is convenient. Extract-based medicines should be used during the winter to consolidate the effect.

(Shi Yu-guang, Shan Shu-jian. *The Clinical Essence of Contemporary Famous Physicians · Special Monograph of Asthma* 当代名医临证精华·咳喘专辑. Beijing: China Ancient Writings Publishing House, 1988. 48)

5. Professor Wu Sheng-nong Believes that in the Treatment of Chronic Bronchitis, Diffusing Lung Qi and Transforming Turbid Phlegm should be Used during the Attack Stage, and Consolidating the Defensive (*Wei*) Qi and Warming the Original Yang in the Remission Stage

In the treatment of chronic bronchitis, the therapeutic measures are to diffuse the Lung qi and transform phlegm during the attack stage, and consolidate the exterior *wei* (defensive) and warm the original yang or nourish the Lung and Kidney yin during the remission stage. The basic formula during the attack stage is *Xiǎo Qīng Lóng Tāng* (小青龙汤) plus *Shè Gān Má Huáng Tāng* (射干麻黄汤) with modifications. Because chronic bronchitis is always induced by exogenous evils, *má huáng* (Herba Ephedrae) and *guì zhī* (Ramulus Cinnamomi) are taken to diffuse the Lung and warm yang. *Xì xīn* (Radix et Rhizoma Asari) warms the Kidney to receive qi and dispels cold. *Gān jiāng* (Rhizoma Zingiberis) warms the Spleen to transform dampness in order to eliminate the source of phlegm. However *wǔ wèi zǐ* (Fructus Schisandrae Chinensis) may be omitted, because it can astringe the Lung to stop cough, but it can also astringe evils and then result in cough. The sour astringency is compatible with the acrid scattering, their effect is both opposite and complementary to each other, and they mutually control each other. Therefore *wǔ wèi zǐ* (Fructus Schisandrae Chinensis) is often pounded together with *gān jiāng* (Rhizoma Zingiberis). Panting with fullness of the chest and wheezing is caused by obstruction of the airway by phlegm and laryngeal edema. *Shè gān* (Rhizoma Belamcandae) can clear heat to smooth the throat and reduce swelling so as to dredge the airway. The medicinals such as *jú hóng* (Exocarpium Citri Rubrum), *bèi mǔ* (Bulbus Fritillariae), *bàn xià* (Rhizoma Pinelliae), and *dǎn nán xīng* (Arisaema cum Bile) are almost non-effective in chronic bronchitis patients because these patients have excessive sputum or stubborn sputum that is like glue. The commonly used medicinal is *zào jiá zǐ* (Fructus Gleditsiae Sinensis) 9—12g (pounded). If it is combined with *huà jú hóng* (Exocarpium Citri Grandis) 9g, the result will be more effective. For cases of yellow phlegm, add *shēng shí gāo* (Gypsum Fibrosum) 60g (decocted first)—this is the intent of *Xiǎo Qīng Lóng Tāng* (小青龙汤) plus *shí gāo* (Gypsum Fibrosum). For cases of chronic bronchitis complicated by secondary infections, with manifestations like fever, severe cough, copious sputum, chest oppression, and tachypnea, use the self-composed *Qī Wèi Qīng Fèi Yǐn* (七味清肺饮):

黄连	huáng lián	3g	Rhizoma Coptidis
黄芩	huáng qín	6g	Radix Scutellariae
冬瓜子	dōng guā zǐ	15g	Semen Benincasae
黛蛤散	dài gé sǎn	30g	Daige Powder
鱼腥草	yú xīng cǎo	30g	Herba Houttuyniae
大黄	dà huáng	6g	Radix et Rhizoma Rhei

The Miscellaneous Records of Famous Physicians (别录 , *Bié Lù*) says that *dà huáng* (Radix et Rhizoma Rhei) can eliminate phlegm. Indeed it has this effect. During the remission stage, the *wei* (defensive) qi should be consolidated and the original yang warmed. This is because if the *wei* qi fails to consolidate, the exogenous evils will invade the body easily; and if the original yang is deficient, the endogenous cold will generate naturally. Thus there may be a pathogenesis of "activation of latent evils by a new contraction". Therefore consolidating the *wei* qi and warming the original yang are important preventative treatment measures. Consolidating the exterior and warming yang can promote each other. The basic formula is *Liù Jūn Zǐ Tāng* (六君子汤) plus *huáng qí* (Radix Astragali), *dāng guī* (Radix Angelicae), *hēi fù kuài* (Radix Aconiti Lateralis Praeparata), powder of *zǐ hé chē* (Placenta Hominis Pulveratum) (swallowed whole). For cases of loose stools, add *dàn gān jiāng* (Rhizoma Zingiberis), *chǎo biǎn dòu* (Semen Lablab Album Tostum) in order to warm the Spleen for normal transportation. Another therapeutic measure during the remission stage is to nourish yin of the Kidney and Lung. This is because the Lung and Kidney yin will definitely become deficient in elderly patients with a prolonged course of disease. Yin deficiency will involve yang, so the patients become predisposed to invasions of external evils, resulting in a failure of Lung qi to diffuse and purify. Furthermore, it may generate internal fire making the fluids to turn to phlegm. This is another mechanism of activation of latent evils by a new contraction. Furthermore, the Lung and the Kidney are mutually engendering *zang* organs, therefore they have a big influence on the development of this disease and its recurrence. A self-composed formula is *Zī Shèn Yǎng Fèi Yǐn* (滋肾养肺饮):

南北沙参	nán běi shā shēn	12g for each	Radix Adenophorae and Radix Glehniae Littoralis
天冬	tiān dōng	9g	Radix Asparagi
麦冬	mài dōng	9g	Radix Ophiopogonis
玄参	xuán shēn	12g	Radix Scrophulariae
熟地黄	shú dì huáng	15g	Radix Rehmanniae Praeparata

当归	dāng guī	12g	Radix Angelicae Sinensis
黛蛤散	dài gé sǎn	30g (wrapped)	Daige Powder
百合	bǎi hé	15g	Bulbus Lilii
生甘草	shēng gān cǎo	9g	Radix et Rhizoma Glycyrrhizae Recens
鲜竹沥	xiān zhú lì	60ml (taken separately)	Succus Bambusae

(Chen Ze-lin, Song Zu-dui. *Essentials of Famous Physician Special Experiences* 名医特色经验精华. Shanghai: Publishing House of Shanghai College of Traditional Chinese Medicine, 1987. 109)

6. Professor Huo Jing-tang's Discussion of His Experience in Treating Panting and Cough due to Internal Damage.

Huo Jing-tang, who is a deceased veteran doctor of Chinese Medicine in Shanxi, was an expert in treating panting and cough from internal damage. He once said: "The causes of cough are divided into internal damage and external contraction. For the cough due to external contraction, its root is in the Lung. The Lung is first invaded by the evil, then other organs become involved. For the cough due to internal damage, the evil first invades other organs, then it involves the Lung. The Lung is the branch." The *Inner Canon of Huangdi* (内经, *Nèi Jīng*) says: "Both the five *zang* organs and the six *fu* organs can be the origin of cough, not merely the Lung (五脏六腑皆令人咳，非独肺也)." The root must be explored in the treatment of disease (治病必求其本)". Professor Huo summarizes the treatment methods from his clinical practice: strengthening the Earth to generate Metal, calming the Liver and purifying the Lung, and treating both the Lung and Kidney".

(1) The Method of Strengthening Earth to generate Metal

Inner Canon of Huangdi (内经, *Nèi Jīng*) states: "When cold food and drink enter into the Stomach, they go up to the Lung along the Lung channel, leading to Lung cold. The Lung cold results in the invasion of external evils, and a combination of internal and external evils affects the Lung, hence there is Lung cough (其寒饮食入胃，从肺脉 上至于肺，则肺寒，肺寒则内外合邪，因而客之，则为肺咳)." Doctor Huo believed that Stomach cold causes a failure to receive food, and Spleen deficiency causes a failure to transport food. This may make the middle qi deficient and the Lung failing to be nourished. Therefore the major causes of cough lay in the Stomach and Lung. Panting and cough become severe in winter and relieved in spring when nature returns to yang. For the panting and cough occurring in the winter, use *Fù Zǐ Lǐ Zhōng Tāng* (附子理中汤) with additions, so as to strengthen Earth to generate Metal. Dr. Huo always admonished his students: "There are four seasons in a year. The territory is divided into the north and south. There is severe cold in the winter of north China where the food and drink are crude and coarse. Therefore most of cases in the north have damage to the Spleen and Stomach. If the Spleen and Stomach are not regulated in the treatment of the Lung, it will be not a correct treatment."

(2) The Method of Calming the Liver and purifying the Lung

The stagnation of seven emotions will make the qi of the Liver fail to flow smoothly, and in turn the stagnated qi transforms into the fire and burns the Lung yin. All of these changes may cause a phlegm-heat cough, which occurs mostly among women and young adults. For the case of cough and panting followed by hypochondriac pain, abdominal distention and belching, and a wiry and surging pulse, use *Dān Zhǐ Xiāo Yáo Sǎn* (丹栀逍遥散) with modifications. Commonly prescribe *zhī zǐ* (Fructus Gardeniae), *lóng dǎn cǎo* (Radix et Rhizoma Gentianae) and *huáng qín* (Radix Scutellariae) to clear heat and purge fire, *chái hú* (Radix Bupleuri) and *xiāng fù* (Rhizoma Cyperi) to smooth the Liver and regulate qi, *dāng guī* (Radix Angelicae Sinensis) and *háng sháo* (Radix

Paeoniae Alba) to nourish blood and emolliate the Liver, *yù jīn* (Radix Curcumae), *guā lóu* (Fructus Trichosanthis) and *táo rén* (Semen Persicae) to invigorate blood and stop pain. *Mài mén dōng* (Radix Ophiopogonis), *mǎ dōu líng* (Fructus Aristolochiae), and *qīng guǒ* (Fructus Canarii), act as the assistants to purify and moisten the Lung, stop cough and panting. Thus the Lung is purified as the Liver is drained. This drains the Liver so as to purify the Lung, thus mutually clearing the metal and restraining the wood.

(3) The Method of Treating Both the Lung and Kidney

The Lung belongs to metal and Kidney to water. In the five phases doctrine, metal and water promote each, and the Lung and the Kidney share the same origin. During prolonged panting and cough, Lung yin is damaged, the pattern transforms from excess to deficiency, and the mother (Lung) fails to nourish its child (Kidney)." As metal loses its source of generation, the water will dry up". Gradually the Lung deficiency affects the Kidney, or the deficiency in the upper jiao involves the lower jiao. Kidney yin deficiency causes the turbid yin to generate phlegm accumulating in the Lung. Its clinical manifestations are prolonged cough without end, panting on exertion that is relieved in the day and aggravated at night, steaming bones and tidal fever, expectoration of bloody phlegm, lumbar soreness, and tinnitus. The treatment should be to treat both the Lung and Kidney. The formula often used by Professor Huo was *Mài Wèi Dì Huáng Tāng* (麦味地黄汤) with modifications. For cases of Kidney yang deficiency, add *ròu guì* (Cortex Cinnamomi), *shú fù zǐ* (Radix Aconiti Lateralis Praeparata), *gān jiāng* (Rhizoma Zingiberis) and *xì xīn* (Radix et Rhizoma Asari). For cases of Kidney yin deficiency, generally add *xuán shēn* (Radix Scrophulariae), *zhī mǔ* (Rhizoma Anemarrhenae) and *dì gǔ pí* (Cortex Lycii). For cases of expectoration of bloody sputum, add *bái jí* (Rhizoma Bletillae), *ē jiāo* (Colla Corii Asini) and *ǒu jié* (Nodus Nelumbinis Rhizomatis). For cases of phlegm obstruction, add *sāng bái pí* (Cortex Mori), *zhè bèi mǔ* (Bulbus Fritillariae Thunbergii) and *fú líng* (Poria). For prolonged cough without end, add *zǐ wǎn* (Radix et Rhizoma Asteris) and *kuǎn dōng huā* (Flos Farfarae) in order to moisten the Lung and downbear qi, or add *yīng sù ké* (Pericarpium Papaveris), *wū méi* (Fructus Mume) and *wǔ wèi zǐ* (Fructus Schisandrae Chinensis) in order to astringe the Lung qi and stop panting. This is consistent with the idea the branch is in the Lung, and the root is in the Kidney.

For the person who often drinks fine wine and eats rich foods, the Spleen yang is deficient and the water cannot be normally metabolized. This will result in generation of phlegm-fluid retention. If the water evil flows upward and attacks the Heart and insults the Lung, it may cause the fluid retention in the chest and hypochondria, hence *xuán yǐn* (悬饮, fluid retention in the hypochondria) develops. This *xuán yǐn* presents with panting and inability to lie flat, distending pain of the hypochondria, and general edema. Clinically, a differentiation must be made between deficiency and excess of the disease, and soundness and weakness of the body. For cases of abundant fluid retention with no decline of the right qi, use *Shí Zǎo Tāng* (十枣汤) to drastically purge fluid retention. Within the formula, *gān suí* (Radix Kansui), *yuán huā* (Flos Genkwa), and *dà jǐ* (Euphorbiae seu Knoxiae Radix) are all drastic herbs to purge fluid retention. Thus professor Huo admonished his students to pay attention to the application of *Shí Zǎo Tāng* (十枣汤). First, it only can be given to patients with strong physiques and a slippery and excess pulse. Second, the quantity of the herbs cannot be too much, and it should be discontinued as soon as the disease is cured. Third, millet gruel should be used to regulate the Stomach qi after purging. This use of millet can make the internal grain qi sufficient, and prevent the attack of evils.

(Yang Wen-ru, Huang Jie, Hong Wen-xu. *Selection of Shanxi Famous Physicians' Experiences of Chinese Medicine* 陕西名中医经验选. Xi'an: Shanxi Publishing House of Science and Technology, 1988. 40-43)

7. Professor Pu Fu-zhou's Discussion on Panting and Cough

(1) The principle for Treating Panting

Acute and serious panting belongs to an excess pattern. It is always caused by an invasion of evil qi into the Lung, leading to a failure of qi in diffusing and descending. The key of treatment is to eliminate evils and regulate the Lung. Prolonged panting belongs to a deficiency pattern. It is caused by a failure of the Lung qi in descending, and a failure of the Kidney qi in receiving qi. Thus, the essential qi becomes internally insufficient. In treatment, cultivating and tonifying the Kidney is emphasized.

For a case of panting due to wind-cold, with a floating and tight pulse, a pale tongue with a white coating, aversion to cold, and a lack of sweating, use *Sū Chén Jiǔ Bǎo Tāng* (苏陈九宝汤). The ingredients are *sū zǐ* (Fructus Perillae), *chén pí* (Pericarpium Citri Reticulatae), *má huáng* (Herba Ephedrae), *xìng rén* (Armeniacae Semen Amarum), *guì zhī* (Ramulus Cinnamomi), *gān cǎo* (Radix et Rhizoma Glycyrrhizae), *bò hé* (Herba Menthae), *sāng bái pí* (Cortex Mori), *dà fù pí* (Pericarpium Arecae) plus *hòu pò* (Cortex Magnoliae), *qián hú* (Radix Peucedani). For cases of Lung qi blocked by cold, with coughing and panting, a floating and wiry pulse, and a white tongue coating, prescribe *Sān Niù Tāng* (三拗汤) plus *hòu pò* (Cortex Magnoliae). For cases of lack of sweat due to obstruction of the exterior by the evils, add *cōng bái* (Bulbus Allii). For cases of cough and asthma due to the exterior fettered by wind-cold, with an accumulation of phlegm-heat in the interior, give *Dìng Chuǎn Tāng* (定喘汤). For cases of taiyang wind stroke, with fullness of the chest, sweating and panting, use *Guì Zhī Jiā Hòu Pò Xìng Zǐ Tāng* (桂枝加厚朴杏子汤).

For cases of panting due to exogenous cold and internal fluid retention, with a floating wiry and slippery pulse, fullness of the chest, thin and excessive sputum, and a moist tongue with white and glossy coating, use *Xiǎo Qīng Lóng Tāng* (小青龙汤), or *Shè Gān Má Huáng Tāng* (射干麻黄汤), with modifications according to the treatment method. For cases accompanied by heat signs such as restlessness and thirst, add *shēng shí gāo* (Gypsum Fibrosum).

For cases of panting due to Lung heat depression and blockage, with a floating and surging pulse or a wiry and rapid pulse, severe panting with impending desertion, perhaps sweating or no sweating, a red tongue with a white coating, and no thirst, give *Yuè Bì Jiā Bàn Xià Tāng* (越婢加半夏汤). In addition, it is good to add *sū zǐ* (Fructus Perillae). For thirst and a red tongue, prescribe *Má Xìng Shí Gān Tāng* (麻杏石甘汤) plus *sū zǐ* (Fructus Perillae), *sāng bái pí* (Cortex Mori), *qián hú* (Radix Peucedani), *lái fú zǐ* (Semen Raphani Tostum). For cases of chest fullness with a white glossy tongue coating, add *tíng lì zǐ* (Semen Lepidii seu Descurainiae), *dà zǎo* (Fructus Jujubae), and *hòu pò* (Cortex Magnoliae).

For cases of panting with neither cold nor heat, use *Èr Chén Tāng* (二陈汤) plus *sū zǐ* (Fructus Perillae), *tíng lì zǐ* (Semen Lepidii seu Descurainiae), *chǎo bái jiè zǐ* (Semen Sinapis Albae Tostum), *chǎo lái fú zǐ* (Semen Raphani Tostum), and *dà zǎo* (Fructus Jujubae).

For cases of elderly patients with prolonged panting, abundant phlegm, a deep and wiry pulse or deep and slippery pulse, use *Sū Zǐ Jiàng Qì Tāng* (苏子降气汤). *Ròu guì* (Cortex Cinnamomi) and *chén xiāng* (Lignum Aquilariae Resinatum) may be used simultaneously to warm the Kidney so as to receive qi; *bái guǒ* (Semen Ginkgo) and *wǔ wèi zǐ* (Fructus Schisandrae Chinensis) may be added to get a better effect. For cases with little phlegm, and panting aggravated with exertion, add *Shēn Gé Sǎn* (参蛤散). In short, observe the flourishing and debilitation of the Lung and Kidney, and considering whether the phlegm is more or less, deal with both of these things [Lungs and Kidneys], laying emphasis on the branch or the root.

For cases of panting due to a deficiency of Lung qi, with shortness of breath and sweating, a deficient and powerless pulse, or large and hollow pulse, consider *Shēng Mài Sǎn* (生脉散) plus *hú táo ròu* (Semen Juglandis Regiae). For profuse sweating, *lóng gǔ* (Os Draconis) and *mǔ lì* (Concha Ostreae) may be used in order to settle and contain.

For case of panting due to Kidney qi deficiency, with soreness and weakness of the waist and knees, breathlessness with a desire to pant, a short inhalation and a prolonged exhalation, panting aggravated upon exertion, cold limbs and frequent urination, *Shèn Qì Wán* (肾气丸) plus *hú táo ròu* (Semen Juglandis Regiae) may be prescribed. For thirst, add *mài dōng* (Radix Ophiopogonis) and *wǔ wèi zǐ* (Fructus Schisandrae Chinensis). For panting with vexation due to yin deficiency, along with a dry mouth and red tongue, and a thready, rapid and weak pulse, use *Mài Wèi Dì Huáng Tāng* (麦味地黄汤).

For panting due to yang deficiency and water counterflow, with palpitations, cough and panting, difficult urination, puffy limbs, a pale and swollen tongue, and a deep, thready and weak pulse, use *Zhēn Wǔ Tāng* (真武汤) plus *guì zhī* (Ramulus Cinnamomi), *tíng lì zǐ* (Semen Lepidii seu Descurainiae), and *dà zǎo* (Fructus Jujubae).

In the remission stage of panting, the emphasis should be on the Lung and Stomach. Supplementing Earth can generate Metal. Supplementing the post-heaven can replenish the pre-heaven. This is the key point to successful recuperation. For cases of panting due to exogenous contraction, use *Hòu Pò Shēng Jiāng Bàn Xià Gān Cǎo Rén Shēn Tāng* (厚朴生姜半夏甘草人参汤) with modifications. For cases of panting due to deficiency, use *Xiāng Shā Liù Jūn Zǐ Tāng* (香砂六君子汤).

The experience of Professor Pu's many decades of treating panting shows that one should have a clear and detailed treatment and pattern differentiation, and use a true and correct formula. For cases of panting due to wind-cold, use *Sān Niù Tāng* (三拗汤) plus *hòu pò* (Cortex Magnoliae), and *cōng bái* (Bulbus Allii) which can be called a milder version of *Má*

Huáng Tāng (麻黄汤). The action of this formula is moderate but not drastic. *Yuè Bì Jiā Bàn Xià Tāng* (越婢加半夏汤) and *Má Xìng Shí Gān Tāng* (麻杏石甘汤) can both treat pneumonia that is a type of panting due to an accumulation of Lung heat. The difference between the two formulas is that *Yuè Bì Jiā Bàn Xià Tāng* (越婢加半夏汤) is indicated in cases complicated by phlegm-fluid retention, but with milder heat signs. Therefore *bàn xià* (Rhizoma Pinelliae) and *shēng jiāng* (Rhizoma Zingiberis Recens) are used. On the other hand, *Má Xìng Shí Gān Tāng* (麻杏石甘汤) is indicated in cases with signs of more intense heat.

(2) Discussion on Cough

Cough is divided into two causes — exterior and interior. The Lung is like a canopy that covers the other viscera. It is in charge of the skin and fine hair. It governs respiration and communicates with the atmosphere. Exogenous evils first assail the Lung, leading to cough. Cough mostly belongs to excess patterns. The diseased qi from damage of the five *zang* organs and the six *fu* organs can upwardly steam the Lung and cause cough. This cough is often part of a deficiency pattern.

External contraction of wind-cold is the primary cause of cough. At the same time it mingles with other evils, such as fire, phlegm, food, and qi. Cough from wind attack should be treated by the methods of coursing wind and resolving the exterior. Cough from cold attack should be treated by the methods of scattering cold and resolving the exterior. Cough complicated by internal fire should be treated by the methods of clearing fire and resolving the exterior. Cough complicated by fluid retention should be treated by the methods of warming and eliminating fluid retention and resolving the exterior. Cough complicated by food retention should be treated by the methods of promoting digestion and resolving the exterior. Cough complicated by qi stagnation should be treated by the methods of normalizing qi and resolving the exterior.

Wind-cold should be treated by warm scattering remedies. Wind-heat should be treated by acrid cool (no bitter cold) remedies. These are the important principles of treating cough. The patterns of cough or panting that are caused by exogenous evils attacking Lung cannot be treated by excessively using bitter-cold medicinals. This is because they cannot eliminate the evil qi to resolve the exterior. In the initial stage evil qi is in the exterior, and the treatment should be mainly concentrated on resolving the exterior. Overly bitter and cold medicinals should be avoided, as they to seal in the evils, causing many transformed cases.

For cough due to cold damage, usually use a modified *Sū Chén Jiǔ Bǎo Tāng* (苏陈九宝汤) or *Sān Niù Tāng* (三拗汤). For cough due to wind damage, use a modified *Zhǐ Sòu Sǎn* (止嗽散) or *Xiāng Sū Yǐn* (香苏饮). For cough combined with internal fire, add *sāng bái pí* (Cortex Mori), *huáng qín* (Radix Scutellariae) and *shēng shí gāo* (Gypsum Fibrosum). For cough combined with fluid retention, add *Xiǎo Qīng Lóng Tāng* (小青龙汤). For cough combined with food retention, add *Bǎo Hé Wán* (保和丸). For cough combined with qi stagnation, use *Xiāng Sū Yǐn* (香苏饮) plus *Sì Nì Sǎn* (四逆散).

For cough caused by wind-heat, use a modified *Sāng Jú Yǐn* (桑菊饮). For cough occurring in a hot summer climate, use *Xīn Jiā Xiāng Rú Yǐn* (新加香薷饮) plus *qián hú* (Radix Peucedani), and *xìng rén* (Armeniacae Semen Amarum). For cough due to fire or dryness, use *Xiè Bái Sǎn* (泻白散), or *Qīng Zào Jiù Fèi Tāng* (清燥救肺汤). Professor Pu said: "If externally contracted cough due to wind-cold or wind-heat are treated with formulas like *Xiè Bái Sǎn* (泻白散), *Qīng Zào Jiù Fèi Tāng* (清燥救肺汤) and the like, the evils will be retained and this will cause prolonged cough. This cannot be ignored."

(Xue Bo-shou. *Comprehension in Carrying out Pu Fu-zhou's Academic and Medical Experience* 继承心悟·蒲辅周学术医疗经验. Beijing: The People's Medical Publishing House, 2000. 218-220)

8. Professor Hong Guang-xiang Believes that the Warming Method is Indispensable for Treating the Lung.

Through his studies of chronic cough and panting, Professor Hong Guang-xiang proposes the following therapeutic principle: "a warm method is indispensable for treating the Lung." He believes that the main pathological basis of cough and panting is phlegm-fluid retention. For cases of phlegm-fluid retention or phlegm-stasis in the Lung, it is appropriate to use warm medicinals because phlegm and stasis are yin evils. The main pathological bases of chronic cough and panting are Lung yang deficiency, phlegm-fluid retention in the interior, and phlegm complicated by stasis. These generally all present with heat signs for secondary symptoms. Therefore in clinical treatment, one should eliminate the erroneous appearance of the branch by using formulas and medicinals that treat the root by warmly scattering, warmly transforming, and warmly opening. Concrete applications are as follows:

(1) For Cold Fluids Transforming to Heat, the Basis is to Warmly Transform Cold Fluids

Chronic cough and panting is often induced by contraction of cold, and its course is long. Though it may present as a pattern of stagnated cold transforming into heat, with a cough with white and yellow sputum, a dark red tongue, and a yellow greasy coating, the treatment should concentrate on warming and transforming cold fluid retention according to the principle of "a warming method is indispensable for treating the Lung". At the same time, based on the fact that phlegm-stasis stagnating in the Lung is an old root of chronic cough and panting, formulas and medicinals that clear phlegm and removing stasis, regulating qi and calming panting should be used as the adjuvant treatment. An excellent result can often occur.

(2) As for Yang Deficiency and Phlegm-Stasis Turning to Heat, Primarily Warm and Tonify the Yang Qi, Flush Phlegm, and Dispel Stasis

Yang qi deficiency and phlegm-stasis in the Lung usually occur simultaneously during the remission stage of chronic cough and panting. In terms of Chinese medicine, this belongs in the category of deficiency asthma, with deficiency complicating by excess. Therefore the treatment should first concentrate on warmly-reinforcing yang qi in order to dispel phlegm-stasis, thus treating both the deficiency and the excess. After the yang qi is gradually restored and the symptoms of phlegm-stasis have improved, the next treatment method is to warmly-invigorate the Lung and Kidney yang in order to gradually achieve an effect. The causative factors of yang deficiency, in addition to being associated with insufficient pre-heaven natural endowment, are related to damage of yang qi by phlegm-stasis stagnating in the Lung, and injury of yang qi by repeated attacks of cough and panting. The deficient yang qi cannot warm and dissipate phlegm-stasis, and residual phlegm-stasis can injure yang qi, thus becoming a vicious cycle. Clinically, when the patterns of yang deficiency and phlegm-stasis transforming into heat occur at the same time, the yang deficiency is the root. Therefore the treatment should concentrate on warmly-reinforcing yang qi so as to dispel phlegm-stasis. This will achieve excellent results.

(3) As for Excess Heat with Symptoms of Cold, a Warming Method is Indispensable

An excess heat pattern with cold symptoms refers to patients with chronic cough and panting who are attacked by cold during the summer. Professor Hong abides by the principle of pattern differentiation and treatment. For cases of cough and panting with white phlegm due to the Lung yang deficiency, although the illness occurs in summer, he insists on the therapeutic principle of "warming method is indispensable for treating the Lung" and uses warmly-scattering medicinals. Professor Hong once treated a female patient with chronic asthmatic bronchitis according to the above therapeutic principle. The patient suffered from illness in July. Her clinical manifestations included paroxysmal choking cough induced by itching of the throat, with white and stubborn sputum, along with panting especially at night, inability to lie flat, susceptibility to catching colds, dark lips, normal urine and stools, a dark red tongue with a thin yellow greasy coating, and a wiry, slippery and rapid pulse. The pattern was identified as cold fluid retention stagnating in the Lung and transforming into heat. Treatment was to warm the Lung and scatter cold. The ingredients were:

生麻黄	shēng má huáng	10g	Herba Ephedrae
干姜	gān jiāng	10g	Rhizoma Zingiberis
细辛	xì xīn	3g	Radix et Rhizoma Asari
紫菀	zǐ wǎn	10g	Radix et Rhizoma Asteris
款冬	kuǎn dōng	10g	Flos Farfarae
法半夏	fǎ bàn xià	10g	Rhizoma Pinelliae
葶苈子	tíng lì zǐ	15g	Semen Lepidii seu Descurainiae
青陈皮	qīng chén pí	10g for each	Pericarpium Citri Reticulatae Viride and Pericarpium Citri Reticulatae
牡荆子	mǔ jīng zǐ	15g	Fructus Viticis Negundo

The frequency of catching colds was markedly reduced during the period of time during which the patient took the herbs. The symptoms of cough and panting did not recur after taking 40 doses.

[Zheng Jie, Hong Guang-xiang. The Clinical Research on "Warming Method Is Indispensable for Lung Disorder" in the Acute Attack of Chronic Obstructive Pulmonary Disease. *Jiangxi Journal of Traditional Chinese Medicine* 江西中医药. 2000, 31(6): 20-22]

9. Professor Yue Mei-zhong Emphasizes that the Treatment of Cough Requires Combining General Aspects with Specific Aspects

Cough is merely one kind of symptom, not one kind of disease. *Plain Questions: On Cough* (素问·咳论, *Sù Wèn · Ké Lùn*) says: "Both the five *zang* organs and six *fu* organs can be the origin of the cough, not merely the Lung (五脏六腑皆令人咳，非独肺也)." That means once diseases of five *zang* organs and six *fu* organs affect the Lung, it will cause cough. When cough occurs, the origin of the cough should be identified through the four diagnostic methods. Then treatment should aim at its root. The doctor cannot treat cough as just cough and merely treat the Lung. Li Dong-yuan selected formulas for treatment of cough patterns as discussed in *On Cough* (咳论, *Ké Lùn*). He prescribed *Xiǎo Chái Hú Tāng* (小柴胡汤) for a Liver cough; *Huáng Qín Jiā Bàn Xià Shēng Jiāng Tāng* (黄芩加半夏生姜汤) for a Gallbladder cough; *Jié Gěng Tāng* (桔梗汤) for a Heart cough; *Sháo Yào Gān Cǎo Tāng* (芍药甘草汤) for flatulence from Small Intestine disorder; *Shēng Má Tāng* (升麻汤) for a Spleen cough; *Wū Méi Wán* (乌梅丸) for vomiting of worms from the stomach; *Má Huáng Tāng* (麻黄汤) for a Lung cough; *Chì Shí Zhī Yǔ Yú Liáng Wán* (赤石脂禹余粮丸) and *Táo Rén Tāng* (桃仁汤) for diarrhea due to Large Intestine disorder — if it did not stop then he used *Zhū Pāo Tāng* (猪脬汤) to separate water; *Má Huáng Fù Zǐ Xì Xīn Tāng* (麻黄附子细辛汤) for a Kidney cough; and *Fú Líng Gān Cǎo Tāng* (茯苓甘草汤) for enuresis. For enduring and endless cough, with damage of the *San Jiao* (Triple Burner), the cough is often accompanied by abdominal fullness and a lack of desire to eat or drink. This all occurs from the Stomach affecting the Lung, which causes people to have a lot of nasal discharge, saliva, facial edema, and counterflow qi. Then *Qián Shì Yì Gōng Sǎn* (钱氏异功散) is used. If the disorders of the injured *zang-fu* organs can be resolved, then cough will follow and recover. If the doctor cannot grasp the essence of cough, and treats only the cough, it may be slightly relieved but inevitably it will recur.

Later generations of doctors used the *Inner Canon of Huangdi* (内经, *Nèi Jīng*) as a foundation and divided cough into two types— internal damage and external contraction. Zhang Jing-yue points out: "There are two main classes of cough: one is external contraction, the other is internal damage. Cough due to external contraction is from an invasion through the skin and fine hair. Because the skin and fine hair corresponds to the Lung, the external evils must first affect the Lung. If the cough persists, it transmits from the Lung to the five *zang* organs. Cough due to internal damage originates from the yin phase. In the five phases doctrine, the Lung corresponds to metal and is the mother of water (Kidney). If yin is consumed in the lower jiao, yang will stand solitarily in the upper jiao- water is dried up before metal. The Lung is susceptible to dryness, and affection of the Lung by dryness will lead to itching, and itching causes persistent cough. Between the two, yin and yang should be distinguished, and excess and deficiency should be identified (咳嗽之要，一曰外感，一曰内伤。外感之咳，必由皮毛而入。盖皮毛为肺之合，而凡外邪袭之，则必先入于肺。久而不愈，则必自肺传至五脏也。内伤之咳，必起于阴分，盖肺属金，为水之母，阴损于下，则阳孤于上，水涸金枯，肺苦干燥，肺燥则痒，痒则咳不能已也。但二者之中，当辨阴阳，当分虚实耳)." This speech by Zhang Jing-yue reveals both the general and specific characters of cough from external contraction and internal damage. This reveals that the doctor knew that there are special characteristics within general characteristics. If a doctor can identify them clearly, the curative effect will be excellent.

Cough due to external contraction is mostly caused by cold evil, regardless of the season. The cold evil invades the Lung following the seasonal climate. Thus acrid-warm agents are always used for the treatment of cough and the evils will be dispelled. It is best to use *Liù Ān Jiān* (六安煎). The ingredients are:

法半夏	fǎ bàn xià	9g	Rhizoma Pinelliae
陈皮	chén pí	4g	Pericarpium Citri Reticulatae
茯苓	fú líng	6g	Poria
甘草	gān cǎo	3g	Radix et Rhizoma Glycyrrhizae
杏仁	xìng rén	3g	Armeniacae Semen Amarum
白芥子	bái jiè zǐ	3g (subtracted for the elderly and weak)	Semen Sinapis Albae

Perhaps add *shēng jiāng* (Rhizoma Zingiberis).

➢ For all the cases from external contraction, mostly use the above formula with modifications.

➢ For cases of dryness of the Lung and Stomach with unsmooth qi dynamic, or senility with blood debility, and difficulty in coughing, add *dāng guī* (Radix Angelicae Sinensis) 6—9g to this formula.

➢ For cases of excessive cold qi or middle-cold failing to warm Lung qi, with an inability to eliminate the evil, add *xì xīn* (Radix et Rhizoma Asari) 2g or 8g to this formula.

➢ For cases of stagnation of cold qi in winter, and difficulty in dispelling the evil, add *má huáng* (Herba Ephedrae) and *guì zhī* (Ramulus Cinnamomi) or use *Xiǎo Qīng Lóng Tāng* (小青龙汤).

➢ For cases of catching colds, with alternating attacks of chills and fever, and a persistent cough, use *Chái Chén Jiān* (柴陈煎). The ingredients are:

柴胡	chái hú	9g	Radix Bupleuri
陈皮	chén pí	4g	Pericarpium Citri Reticulatae
法半夏	fǎ bàn xià	6g	Rhizoma Pinelliae
茯苓	fú líng	6g	Poria
生姜	shēng jiāng	5-7 pieces	Rhizoma Zingiberis

➢ For cases of qi counterflow and excessive cough, add *xìng rén* (Armeniacae Semen Amarum) 3g.

➢ For cases with not too much cold evil, but with excessive sputum, use *Èr Chén Tāng* (二陈汤) with modifications. It always achieves an excellent effect.

For all cases of yin deficiency and insufficient blood, or deficiency cold of the Spleen and Stomach, the patients are apt to catch colds. The following kinds of patients can all be given *Jīn Shuǐ Liù Jūn Jiān* (金水六君煎) with modifications: patients that have a weak pulse, without stasis in the chest and diaphragm; patients with Kidney qi deficiency and water overflowing to form phlegm; those with vexation, nausea and vomiting, hunger with no desire to eat; patients more than sixty years old, with blood and qi declining, and a prolonged cough. The ingredients are:

当归	dāng guī	6g	Radix Angelicae Sinensis
法半夏	fǎ bàn xià	6g	Rhizoma Pinelliae
茯苓	fú líng	6g	Poria
熟地黄	shú dì huáng	9g	Radix Rehmanniae Praeparata
陈皮	chén pí	4g	Pericarpium Citri Reticulatae
炙甘草	zhì gān cǎo	8g	Radix et Rhizoma Glycyrrhizae Praeparata
生姜	shēng jiāng	5 pieces	Rhizoma Zingiberis

➤ For cases of yang qi deficiency with a faint pulse, drowsiness, reluctance to talk, and profuse sweating, definitely add *rén shēn* (Radix Ginseng).

➤ For cases of earth deficiency failing to generate mental, and an inability to eliminate the evil, use *Liù Jūn Zǐ Tāng* (六君子汤) to strengthen the Spleen and Lung.

➤ For cases of Spleen deficiency failing to control water, with water overflowing to form phlegm, use *Lǐ Zhōng Tāng* (理中汤), *Lǐ Yīn Jiān* (理阴煎), or *Bā Wèi Wán* (八味丸) to reinforce the earth (mother). These are all good remedies. The formula selected is *Lǐ Yīn Jiān* (理阴煎). The ingredients of *Lǐ Yīn Jiān* (理阴煎) are:

熟地	shú dì	30g	Radix Rehmanniae Praeparata
炙甘草	zhì gān cǎo	9g	Radix et Rhizoma Glycyrrhizae Praeparata
当归	dāng guī	15g	Radix Angelicae Sinensis
炒干姜	chǎo gān jiāng	8g	Rhizoma Zingiberis Tostum

It should be decocted in water and taken orally. Medicinals that can eliminate the evil should be added.

For cough due to external contraction, the exterior evil is the general characteristic. Because the individual natural endowment is different, with either yang or yin predominating, or Spleen deficiency, or Kidney deficiency, and the symptoms presented are accordingly different. Therefore in the treatment, one should be aware of the combination of the general characteristics and the special characteristics. In the clinic, bronchitis often occurs in autumn and winter. This is because the cold-cool evils in autumn and winter invade the body externally and affect the Lung, hence there is cough. Since cough is a pathologic reaction of resisting diseases, the treatment should be guided according to the circumstances and the evil should be drawn out, rather than prematurely use formulas that constrain the Lung and thus imprison the evil. For cases of chronic disease, there is stagnated heat in the Lung, leading to a condition of fire being wrapped by external cold, hence there is severe cough. Treatment should be to resolve the cold, thus the internal heat also be scattered. The formula should be *Xiǎo Qīng Lóng Jiā Shí Gāo Tāng* (小青龙加石膏汤). For case of excessive heat, add *huáng qín* (Radix Scutellariae), *zhī mǔ* (Rhizoma Anemarrhenae) and so on as adjuvant herbs.

Cough due to internal damage mostly originates from the yin phase. The yin phase is the original essential qi of the five *zang* organs. The five *zang* organs all have essential qi. The Kidney is the root of original essence, and the Lung is the governor of original essence. If the essential qi of five *zang* organs are damaged, the disease will be transmitted from the lower jiao to the upper jiao, from the Kidney to the Spleen and Lung, leading to disorders of both Lung and Kidney, and then the other *zang* organs will be involved. Therefore prolonged cough should be observed carefully to determine whether it is caused by external contraction or internal damage. Cough due to external contraction is easy to deal with.

But cough due to internal damage is difficult to treat because the illness involves the root. For treatment of cough due to internal damage, the main treatment should be to nourish yin. The formulas selected are *Yī Yīn Jiān* (一阴煎), *Zuǒ Guī Wán* (左归丸) and *Liù Wèi Dì Huáng Wán* (六味地黄丸) with modifications. If the Kidney-yang is deficient in the lower jiao, the vital qi will not spread, resulting in the confinement of the Spleen in the middle jiao and Lung in the upper jiao. There then appears panting and dyspnea, stuffiness and fullness, expectoration, nausea and vomiting, diarrhea, and intolerance of cold. For all these cases of deficiency cold that manifest with a persistent cough and a thready and weak pulse, the treatment should not be to stop cough, but to reinforce yang, thus the cough will be cured. The formulas are *Yòu Guī Yǐn* (右归饮), *Yòu Guī Wán* (右归丸), *Bá Wèi Dì Huáng Wán* (八味地黄丸), *Dà Bǔ Yuán Jiān* (大补元煎), *Liù Wèi Huí Yáng Yǐn* (六味回阳饮), *Lǐ Zhōng Tāng* (理中汤), and *Jié Láo Tāng* (劫劳汤). The ingredients to this last formula are *bái sháo* (Radix Paeoniae Alba), *rén shēn* (Radix Ginseng), *zhì gān cǎo* (Radix et Rhizoma Glycyrrhizae Praeparata), *dāng guī* (Radix Angelicae Sinensis), *shú dì Huáng* (Radix Rehmanniae Praeparata), *wǔ wèi zǐ* (Fructus Schisandrae Chinensis), *fǎ bàn xià* (Rhizoma Pinelliae) and *ē jiāo* (Colla Corii Asini). These formulas can be used according to the pattern differentiation. As for what modern medicine calls emphysema, (manifesting with symptoms of cough and profuse frothy sputum, and accompanied by panting and dyspnea, a white tongue coating and a deficient pulse, and aggravated at night and relieved in daytime), this belongs to the condition of deficiency in the root and excess in the branch. The self-composed *Bǎo Fèi Tāng* (保肺汤) can be used to strengthen the right qi so as to eliminate evils. The ingredients are:

| 党参 | dǎng shēn | 12g | Radix Codonopsis |
| 黄芪 | huáng qí | 18g | Radix Astragali |

麦冬	mài dōng	12g	Radix Ophiopogonis
五味子	wǔ wèi zǐ	6g (ground)	Fructus Schisandrae Chinensis
川贝母	chuān bèi mǔ	12g	Bulbus Fritillariae Cirrhosae
百部	bǎi bù	6g	Radix Stemonae
苏子	sū zǐ	9g	Fructus Perillae
葶苈子	tíng lì zǐ	4.5g (parched, ground)	Semen Lepidii seu Descurainiae
前胡	qián hú	9g	Radix Peucedani
桔梗	jié gěng	6g	Radix Platycodonis
法半夏	fǎ bàn xià	9g	Rhizoma Pinelliae
橘红	jú hóng	6g	Exocarpium Citri Rubrum
枳壳	zhǐ qiào	6g	Fructus Citri Tostum
杏仁	xìng rén	9g	Armeniacae Semen Amarum
山药	shān yào	18g	Rhizoma Dioscoreae
炙甘草	zhì gān cǎo	6g	Radix et Rhizoma Glycyrrhizae Praeparata
红枣 (去核)	hóng zǎo	4 pieces (pit removed)	Fructus Jujubae

Decoct in water for oral use.

➢ For Kidney deficiency cases, use *gǒu qǐ zǐ* (Fructus Lycii) 2g, *tù sī zǐ* (Semen Cuscutae) 15g, and *Qīng É Wán* (Yang Maid Pill) 10g. This is a disorder of internal damage and consumptive disease, so it can be intractable to treat. The physician should study and observe it carefully.

(Xiyuan Hospital of Chinese Medical Institute. *The Collection of Yue Meizhong's Medical Record* 岳美中医案话集. Beijing: China Ancient Writings Publishing House, 1981. 129-131)

10. Professor Jiang Chun-hua's Discussion on the Treatment of Cough

Elderly patients with chronic bronchitis ordinarily present with deficiency cold constitution type patterns. In addition, the sign of profuse and thin sputum also belongs to a pattern of deficiency cold. During the infection period it may the pattern may still be one of deficiency cold, or it can transform into a pattern of excess-heat. It can also be a wind heat pattern with a deficiency cold constitution.

The traditional methods of treating cough include scattering the Lung, purifying the Lung, draining the Lung, warming the Lung, clearing the Lung, moistening the Lung, astringing the Lung, dissipating the phlegm, descending qi, tonifying the middle jiao, boosting qi, and tonifying the Kidney. Concrete measures are determined according to the concrete conditions. Scattering methods such as clearing-scattering and warming-scattering should be used during the infection period; whereas tonifying methods such as boosting qi, fortifying the Spleen, and tonifying the Kidney, are used during ordinary times. The therapeutic methods to treat phlegm include drying for damp-phlegm, scattering for wind-phlegm, warming for cold-phlegm, moistening for dry-phlegm, and eliminating for fire-phlegm. Different formulas may be given accordingly.

(1) For Ordinary Situations with Cough and Excessive Phlegm, Treat by Using "Warm Medicinals to Harmonize"

1) *Xiǎo Qīng Lóng Tāng* (小青龙汤)

麻黄	má huáng	9g (decocted first and the froth removed)	Herba Ephedrae
桂枝	guì zhī	9g	Ramulus Cinnamomi
细辛	xì xīn	3g	Radix et Rhizoma Asari
五味子	wǔ wèi zǐ	9g	Fructus Schisandrae Chinensis
干姜	gān jiāng	6g	Rhizoma Zingiberis
白芍	bái sháo	9g	Radix Paeoniae Alba
姜半夏	jiāng bàn xià	9g	Rhizoma Pinelliae Preparata

2) *Zhǐ Sòu Sǎn* (止嗽散)

百部	bǎi bù	9g	Radix Stemonae
桔梗	jié gěng	6g	Radix Platycodonis
紫菀	zǐ wǎn	9g	Radix et Rhizoma Asteris
荆芥	jīng jiè	9g	Herba Schizonepetae

白前	bái qián	9g	Radix et Rhizoma Cynanchi Stauntonii
甘草	gān cǎo	6g	Radix et Rhizoma Glycyrrhizae
陈皮	chén pí	9g	Pericarpium Citri Reticulatae

This is a formula from *Medicine Comprehended* (医学心悟, *Yī Xué Xīn Wù*). When *New Compilation of Recipes by Ma Shi* (马莳方新编, *Mǎ Shí Fāng Xīn Biān*) reprinted it, *chén pí* (Pericarpium Citri Reticulatae) and *gān cǎo* (Radix et Rhizoma Glycyrrhizae) were left out.

For cases of acute episode, add *chán tuì* (Periostracum Cicadae), *zhè bèi mǔ* (Bulbus Fritillariae Thunbergii) and *mǎ bó* (Lasiosphaerae seu Calvatia).

During ordinary times *fǎ bàn xià* (Rhizoma Pinelliae), and *chén pí* (Pericarpium Citri Reticulatae) may be added, and prepared with water into pills. The oral dose is 9g, twice daily.

(2) The Treatment of Infection

➢ For fever with aversion to cold, a red throat with itching, and a red tongue, the ingredients of the formula are:

桂枝	guì zhī	9g	Ramulus Cinnamomi
麻黄	má huáng	9g	Herba Ephedrae
金荞麦	jīn qiáo mài	9g	Rhizoma Fagopyri Dibotryis
板蓝根	bǎn lán gēn	9g	Radix Isatidis
马勃	mǎ bó	3g	Lasiosphaerae seu Calvatia
黄芩	huáng qín	9g	Radix Scutellariae
胆南星	dǎn nán xīng	9g	Arisaema cum Bile
蒲公英	pú gōng yīng	15g	Herba Taraxaci

➢ For fever with aversion to cold, no sweating, restlessness, a dry mouth, and thick sputum, use *Dà Qīng Lóng Tāng* (大青龙汤) with modifications. The ingredients are:

麻黄	má huáng	9g	Herba Ephedrae
桂枝	guì zhī	9g	Ramulus Cinnamomi

甘草	gān cǎo	6g	Radix et Rhizoma Glycyrrhizae
杏仁	xìng rén	9g	Armeniacae Semen Amarum
生姜	shēng jiāng	6g	Rhizoma Zingiberis
大枣	dà zǎo	3 pieces	Fructus Jujubae
石膏	shí gāo	15g	Gypsum Fibrosum
知母	zhī mǔ	9g	Rhizoma Anemarrhenae

➤ For fever with aversion to cold, dyspnea, and a pale tongue with a white coating, use *Guì Zhī Jiā Hòu Pò Xìng Rén Tāng* (桂枝加厚朴杏仁汤) with modifications. The ingredients are:

桂枝	guì zhī	9g	Ramulus Cinnamomi
白芍	bái sháo	9g	Radix Paeoniae Alba
杏仁	xìng rén	9g	Armeniacae Semen Amarum
厚朴	hòu pò	9g	Cortex Magnoliae
姜半夏	jiāng bàn xià	9g	Rhizoma Pinelliae Preparata
枳实	zhǐ shí	9g	Fructus Aurantii Immaturus
陈皮	chén pí	9g	Pericarpium Citri Reticulatae
甘草	gān cǎo	6g	Radix et Rhizoma Glycyrrhizae

➤ For severe cough, selectively add *bǎi bù* (Radix Stemonae) 9g, *kuǎn dōng huā* (Flos Farfarae) 9g, *zǐ wǎn* (Radix et Rhizoma Asteris) 9g, *nán tiān zhú zǐ* (Fructus Nandinae Domesticae) 6g, *tiān jiāng ké* (Rhizoma Metaplexis Japonicae) 3 pieces, *wǔ wèi zǐ* (Fructus Schisandrae Chinensis) 9g, *wū méi* (Fructus Mume) 9g, or *hē zǐ* (Fructus Terminaliae Chebulae) 9g (mostly use *kuǎn dōng huā* (Flos Farfarae), or *zǐ wǎn* (Radix et Rhizoma Asteris) as from *the Prescription Books at the Tang Dynasty* [唐人方书].

➤ For thick and yellow sputum, selectively add *zhú lì* (Succus Bambusae) 1 vial, or *zhú huáng* (Shiraia Bambusicola) 9g, or *zhú rú* (Caulis Bambusae in Taeniis) 9g, or *lóu rén* (Semen Trichosanthis) 9g.

➤ For clear and thin sputum, selectively add *dǎn nán xīng* (Arisaema cum Bile) 9g, *fǎ bàn xià* (Rhizoma Pinelliae) 9g, or *chén pí* (Pericarpium Citri Reticulatae) 9g.

➢ For cases with difficulty in expectoration, add *jié gěng* (Radix Platycodonis) 9g, *yuǎn zhì* (Radix Polygalae) 9g, *zhè bèi mǔ* (Bulbus Fritillariae Thunbergii) 9g, or *bái jiè zǐ* (Semen Sinapis Albae) and *sū zǐ* (Fructus Perillae).

➢ For cases with profuse and thin sputum, add *duàn zhōng rú shí* (Stalactitum Calcinatun) 15g, or *Èr Chén Tāng* (二陈汤).

Generally, all of the patterns that are manifestations of disease have commonalities as well as idiosyncrasies. Cough in this illness and cough in other respiratory system illnesses have things in common. But as far as the constitution and all of symptoms are concerned, each pattern and disease has its own characteristics. The characteristics of this illness are: 1) a long course of illness; 2) illness usually lasting a long time and aggravated by cold; 3) manifestations of deficiency cold in both the constitution and symptoms. This is different from the deficiency heat of pulmonary tuberculosis (This illness may also present with deficiency-heat due to other factors, but it is proportionally less common).

Insight from experience: An important key is to regulate the constitution. This is called "constitutional therapy". If the constitution is strengthened, the episodes can be reduced or relieved, or perhaps eliminated.

➢ For cases of Spleen deficiency with weakness of qi, presenting with a pale or sallow complexion, anorexia, loose stools, and debilitation, treatment should be to fortify the Spleen and boost qi. The formula selected is *Liù Jūn Zǐ Tāng* (六君子汤) with modifications.

➢ For cases of yang deficiency and water overflowing, presenting with a puffy face and feet, intolerance of cold, cyanotic lips, and a pale and swollen tongue (pulmonary heart disease), the treatment should be to warm yang and boost qi. For severe cases, use *Shēn Fù Tāng* (参附汤) with modifications. For mild cases, prescribe the formula *Fù Guì Bā Wèi Wán* (附桂八味丸) with modifications as decoction. During infection, add *jīn qiáo mài* (Rhizoma Fagopyri Dibotryis), *mǎ bó* (Lasiosphaerae seu Calvatia), *chán tuì* (Periostracum Cicadae) and *bǎn lán gēn* (Radix Isatidis seu Baphicacanthi). For cases of excessive sputum with difficulty in expectoration, add *dǎn nán xīng* (Arisaema cum Bile), *yuǎn zhì* (Radix Polygalae), *zhè bèi mǔ* (Bulbus Fritillariae Thunbergii) and *jié gěng* (Radix Platycodonis). For cases with thick sputum, add *zhú lì* (Succus Bambusae), *huáng qín* (Radix Scutellariae) and *gé fěn* (Pulvis Concha Meretricis seu Cyclinae).

(3) For Physical Weakness, Use the Listed Medicinals Below:
hóng shēn (Radix et Rhizoma Ginseng Rubra) 3g, twice daily;
wǔ wèi zǐ (Fructus Schisandrae Chinensis) 9g, three times daily;
zǐ hé chē (Placenta Hominis) 3g, three times daily;
Bǔ Zhōng Yì Qì Wán (补中益气丸) 9g, twice daily;
Liù Jūn Zǐ Wán (六君子丸) 9g, twice daily.

The question of tonifying and scattering: In the past, there have two discussions on the treatment of cough in Chinese Medicine. One is that the treatment should concentrate on tonifying, not scattering; the other is that the treatment should concentrate on scattering, not tonifying. These two perspectives are not complete. The correct treatment is that the tonifying method should be used for deficiency, and the scattering method should be used for evils. If there is a contraction of new evils, it is proper to scatter the evils. After they are scattered, the tonifying method is used again. The tonifying method is suitable to cultivate the root in ordinary times, and the scattering method is suitable to treat the branch during times of evil excess. For cases of deficiency of right qi with mild exuberance of evil qi, it is proper to tonify combined with scattering. For cases of exuberance of evil qi with mild deficiency of right qi, scattering should be primary. The Chinese medicine forefathers distinguished strictly between cough due to external contraction and cough due to internal damage. They believed that internal damage should not be treated as external contraction, and vise versa. This avoids making mistakes that would cause the deficiency to be more deficient, or the excess to be more excessive. This principle is correct, but it does not involve diseases due to the combination of internal and external causes. When the illness is initially from an external contraction, the Lung is affected and the Spleen and Kidney are involved. After this, the visceral damage becomes primary, and is complicated by the external contraction to form cough. This kind of cough is different from the cough of sheer internal damage or external contraction. Zhang Jing-yue says: "externally contracted evils are mostly exuberant. If the excess is complicated by deficiency, it is proper to do scattering with additional tonifying. Internal damage is mostly a deficiency disorder. If the deficiency is complicated by excess, it is proper to do nourishment, with additional clearing." Although this illness does not belong to the category of internal damage, the changes of organs and constitution belong to the "deficiency". Therefore Jing-yue's theory is right and reasonable.

The question of constraining and scattering: For severe and prolonged cough, astringent medicinals may sometimes be used. These include *wǔ wèi zǐ* (Fructus Schisandrae Chinensis), *hē zǐ* (Fructus Chebulae), *yīng sù ké* (Pericarpium Papaveris) and *wū méi* (Fructus Mume). The traditional prohibition is that astringent medicinals should not be used during a sudden attack of a serious illness, or in cases of external contraction. I do not approve of it. In ancient times, *wǔ wèi zǐ* (Fructus Schisandrae Chinensis) was used to treat cough with dyspnea, and also calming panting, regardless of whether it was a new or prolonged cough (Physicians during the Qing dynasty began to use *wǔ wèi zǐ* (Fructus Schisandrae Chinensis) just to treat deficieny cough, as it can retain the evil with its sour and astringent property). *Hē zǐ* (Fructus Terminaliae) is identical to *xī qīng guǒ* (Fructus Terminaliae Immaturus), which should be distinguished from *qīng guǒ* (Fructus Canarii). *Xī qīng guǒ* (Fructus Terminaliae Immaturus) is the immature *hē zǐ* (Fructus Terminaliae), and it is used to treat pharyngolaryngitis. Pharmacological research proved that *xī qīng guǒ* (Fructus Terminaliae Immaturus) can relax the smooth muscle and prevent cough. This is similar to paraverine. Thus *xī qīng guǒ* (Fructus Terminaliae Immaturus) can be used to treat cough due to external contraction. *Wū méi* (Fructus Mume) can be used to treat acute and chronic inflammation through its antibacterial action. Narcotoline is not suitable for cases of excessive phlegm, because of its anesthetic action. However, for severe cough during the acute stage, without phlegm, it can be used. People during the Song dynasty once used it, but people in modern times seldom do. Both *hē zǐ* (Fructus Terminaliae) and *wū méi* (Fructus Mume) can have an effect on reducing secretions. Ancient people believed that the sour flavor of *wǔ wèi zǐ* (Fructus Schisandrae Chinensis) and *wū méi* (Fructus Mume) can astringe, and they deduced that the two medicinals can astringe the Lung qi. The conventional idea is that evils must be scattered, and astringing agents should not be used. For Lung deficiency, without evils, the astringing method can be used. From the viewpoint of modern pharmacology, the ban on these so-called astringent medicinals can be lifted, However, if there is an exterior evil, scattering the evil is still better. For severe cough, I always simultaneously use both scattering and astringing methods.

The question of affecting a radical cure: Ancient people believe that this illness is difficult to treat. Zhang Zi-gang said: "The Lung is a delicate viscera; it is intolerant to cold and averse to heat. Therefore it is easily invaded by evil qi and is difficult to be treated." Wang Xing-zhi said: "The Lung is easily invaded, and medicine is difficult to get to the Lung." The difficulty in recovering from this illness is not only because of the infection based upon exudates of chronic inflammation, but also because of hypo-immunity due to a constitution problem. This problem especially relates to the influence of the work environment. For instance, in the countryside people walk against the wind in cold winter, or take off their clothes to air out, or catch wind-cold when they do farm work while sweating heavily, or smoke low priced cigarettes causing a choking cough. If the above factors affect the patient repeatedly, then the illness will be difficult cured. If these factors can be changed, there is hope for a radical cure.

(Jiang Chun-hua. *Collection of Medical Papers by Jiang Chun-hua* 姜春华论医集. Fuzhou: Fujian Publishing House of Science and Technology, 1985. 535-539)

11. Professor Li Ji-ren's Discussion of Clearing Phlegm and Disinhibiting Qi as the Primary Method to Treat Cough

The obstruction of the airway by phlegm is the major pathomechanism of chronic bronchitis. Thus professor Li believes that clearing the phlegm and disinhibiting qi is the primary method of treatment. He always determines the treatment according to the condition of the phlegm.

➢ For cases of scanty white and thin sputum, use *Shè Gān Má Huáng Tāng* (射干麻黄汤) with modifications. The ingredients are *shè gān* (Rhizoma Belamcandae), *má huáng* (Herba Ephedrae), *xì xīn* (Radix et Rhizoma Asari), *zǐ wǎn* (Radix et Rhizoma Asteris), *kuǎn dōng huā* (Flos Farfarae), *fǎ bàn xià* (Rhizoma Pinelliae), *jīn fèi cǎo* (Herba Inulae), *Jiāng* (Rhizoma Zingiberis Recens) and *Zǎo* (Fructus Jujubae).

➢ For cases of profuse yellow and thick sputum, use *mǎ dōu líng* (Fructus Aristolochiae), *hǎi fú shí* (Os Costaziae), *kuǎn dōng huā* (Flos Farfarae), *sāng bái pí* (Cortex Mori), *xìng rén* (Armeniacae Semen Amarum), *sū zǐ* (Fructus Perillae), *huáng qín* (Radix Scutellariae), *chǎo tíng lì zǐ* (Semen Lepidii seu Descurainiae Tostum), *qīng bàn xià* (Rhizoma Pinelliae Praeparata) and *gān dì lóng* (Lumbricus), with some modifications according to pattern differentiation.

➢ For cases of moderate or more gray and thick sputum, use *chǎo sū zǐ* (Fructus Perillae Tostum), *xuán fù huā* (Flos Inulae), *zǐ wǎn* (Radix et Rhizoma Asteris), *jú hóng* (Exocarpium Citri Rubrum), *xìng rén* (Armeniacae Semen Amarum), *fǎ bàn xià* (Rhizoma Pinelliae), *yín xìng* (Semen Ginkgo), *yuǎn zhì* (Radix Polygalae), *zhì nán xīng* (Rhizoma Arisaematis Praeparata) and *gān cǎo* (Radix et Rhizoma Glycyrrhizae) with modifications.

This illness always occurs among the elderly whose constitutions are often weak. Thus, except for cases of severe internal heat with yellow sputum, I often add *Guì Fù Bā Wèi Wán* (桂附八味丸) or *Tāi Pán Wán* (胎盘丸) to evenly invigorate Kidney yin and yang at the same time that I treat phlegm. This method of administering both a decoction and a pill for reduction and tonification will affect an excellent cure. In addition, when both a decoction and a pill are given, I carefully choose the time when the medicines are taken. *Guì Fù Bā Wèi Wán* (桂附八味丸) is taken at daybreak to promote Kidney qi to develop by making use of the ascending power of yang qi of both nature and body at dawn. The decoction is taken to clear the phlegm and disinhibit qi so as to get rid of the accumulation of last night. The decoction, when taken one hour before bedtime, can bring the medicinal actions into full play just at the point of panting and coughing attack. The pill, taken at bedtime, can invigorate the declining yang qi at night so as to relieve the panting and cough at night. I believe that if the curative effect is not clinically obvious, the formula should not to be entirely blame. It may be caused by either the mistaken method of administration or the unsuitable time of taking medicine. Good doctors should change the medicinals according to the changed disease, and it will affect a cure.

(Chen Ze-lin, Song Zu-dui. *Essentials of Famous Physician Special Experiences* 名医特色经验精华 . Shanghai: Publishing House of Shanghai College of Traditional Chinese Medicine, 1987. 108)

12. Professor Chao En-xiang's Discussion on the Failure of the Kidney to Receive Qi, and the Internal Obstruction of Turbid Phlegm

Chao En-xiang believes that this illness often occurs among the elderly whose Kidney qi declining, or in those who have a prolonged disease that involves the Kidney. Therefore there must be Kidney deficiency. First the focus of this illness is in the Lung, and then in turn the Lung deficiency causes a transformation in the pathomechanism. The deficiency of both the Lung and Kidney is the foundation at the onset. Although clinically, the disease is induced by external evils invading the Lung, this is a very transient period. The patterns of qi deficiency of both the Lung and Kidney and internal obstruction of turbid phlegm may appear very quickly. At this time the right qi deficiency and the evil qi excess are marked. The harm of anoxia is more serious than that of carbon dioxide retention for this illness, therefore it is extremely important to receive qi and drain the Lung.

(Wang Yong-yan, Chao En-xiang. *Today's Chinese Internal Medicine* 今日中医内科. Beijing: The People's Medical Publishing House, 2000. 231)

13. Professor Zhang Zhen-ru: Determine the Treatment of Lung Distention (Emphysema) According to the Deficiency and Damage of the Five *Zang* Organs from Phlegm Turbidity, Water Fluids, and Blood Stasis

(1) Lung Qi Deficiency and Weakness, Sneak Attack by External Evils

Lung distention (emphysema) often occurs in the cold season, or it is induced by an indulgence in eating and drinking cool food and cold drinks, with an invasion by wind-cold which trigger the interior phlegm-fluid retention. It can also be from an invasion of a dampness transforming into heat, with the heat burning the fluids into phlegm. In turn the phlegm blocks the Lung qi, resulting in the Lung distention. Its symptoms are panting and cough, aversion to cold, profuse sticky white and frothy sputum, general pain, fullness of the chest, vomiting and hiccup, stridor in the throat, a floating and tight pulse, or a floating and moderate pulse, and a pale dark tongue with a thin and white coating, or a glossy and moist coating. Treatment should be to resolve the exterior, scatter cold, warm the Lung, and transform fluids. The formula selected is *Xiǎo Qīng Lóng Tāng* (小青龙汤) plus *Shè Gān Má Huáng Tāng* (射干麻黄汤) with modifications. Professor Zhang believes that the Lung distention has right qi deficiency as its root. However, do not hesitate to dispel the evil as soon as possible when the evil invades the body. Only when the evil is removed, can the disease be cured. Then the right qi is reinforced again. If the Lung qi is ordinarily deficient, and the defensive qi not consolidated, there is susceptibility to catch external evils. Professor Zhang often uses *Bǔ Fèi Tāng* (补肺汤) plus *Yù Píng Fēng Sǎn* (玉屏风散) with modifications to replenish qi and consolidate the exterior, thus preventing invasions of evils when the right qi is deficient.

(2) Dual Deficiency of the Lung and Kidney, Abnormal Exhaling and Receiving qi

The Lung is the governor of qi and the Kidney is the root of qi. In prolonged diseases involving the Kidney, the Kidney deficiency fails to aid the Lung to receive qi, in turn the clear qi is difficult to inhale and the turbid qi is difficult to exhale. The Lung qi fails to descend, resulting in the Lung distention. Its symptoms are fullness of the chest, shortness of breath, a low voice, panting aggravated upon exertion, paroxysmal cough and panting at night, salty and thin sputum, inability to lie flat, sweating, frequent urination, a deep and thready pulse, and a pale and dark tongue with a thin white coating. Treatment should be to tonify the Kidney to receive qi, and astringe the Lung to transform phlegm. The formula selected is *Mài Wèi Dì Huáng Tāng* (麦味地黄汤) with modifications. If the Lung deficiency fails to spread the fluids, it will gather to generate phlegm, resulting in a blockage of the airway by phlegm. In addition, if the deficient Kidney fails to receive qi, Lung distention will occur. Its symptoms are cough and panting, excessive and thick sputum, difficulty in expectoration, a dry mouth with no desire to drink, a deep and thready pulse, and a red and dark tongue with a thin white coating or a greasy coating. Treatment should be to tonify the Lung and Kidney, dispel dampness and transform phlegm. The formula selected is *Jīn Shuǐ Liù Jūn Jiān* (金水六君煎) with additions.

(3) Dual Deficiency of the Lung and Spleen, Phlegm-Damp Internally Obstructed

The Spleen is the source for the generation of phlegm and the Lung is the container for storage of the phlegm. The Spleen in deficiency fails to transport, leading to the stagnation of water-damp in the middle jiao and forming phlegm. The phlegm goes up to the Lung and blocks the airway. Its symptoms are panting, inability to lie flat, general lassitude, stuffiness and fullness of the chest and abdomen, excessive sputum difficult in expectoration, poor appetite, a deep thready and powerless pulse, and a pink tongue with a white or greasy coating. Treatment should be to fortify the Spleen to transform dampness. The formula selected is *Liù Jūn Zǐ Tāng* (六君子汤) with modifications. If there is also a puffy complexion, distention and fullness of the chest and hypochondria, vertigo and palpitations, or oppression and fullness, loose stools, shortness of breath, and debilitation, prescribe *Líng Guì Zhú Gān Tāng* (苓桂术甘汤) plus *Zhēn Wǔ Tāng* (真武汤) with modifications.

(4) Involvement of the Heart by Lung illness with a Combination of Phlegm and Stasis

The prolonged disease causes turbid phlegm retention. This may make the Lung fail in its regulatory function and cause the Heart-blood to be stagnated. Thus there appears a case of the disease of the Lung involving the Heart, with phlegm complicated by stasis obstructing the airway and the blood vessels. Its symptoms are cough with shortness of breath, profuse white and thick sputum, palpitations and vexation, chest oppression, a puffy complexion, cyanosis of the lips and tongue, and a deep and thready or knotted and intermittent pulse. Treatment should be to transform phlegm and remove stasis, descend qi and calm panting. The formula should be *Xuè Fǔ Zhú Yū Tāng* (血府逐瘀汤) with modifications. If the phlegm combines with stasis and the Heart *ying* is unsmooth, this leads to obstruction of the orifice, and confusion of Heart-spirit. Its symptoms are mental wandering, vexation and agitation, insomnia, perhaps indifferent expression (apathy), gradually becoming sleepy, unconscious murmuring and delirious speech, even coma. Treatment should be to resolve the blood stasis and open the orifice. The formula selected is *Wēn Dǎn Tāng* (温胆汤) with modifications.

(5) Lung Yin Insufficiency with Wood and Fire Torturing Metal

Lung distention with a prolonged cough may damage yin and consume qi, leading to a failure of the Lung to be moistened and nourished. This may cause deficient fire to internally burn the yang collaterals. Its symptoms are cough with panting, sputum with blood, a dry mouth with a desire to drink, emaciation, an itching throat and a hoarse voice, and a feverish feeling in the palms and soles. Treatment should be to nourish the Lung and moisten the collaterals. The formula selected is *Bǎi Hé Gù Jīn Tāng* (百合固金汤) with modifications.

(6) Three-Yin Combination Disease, Water Flooding into the Flesh and Skin

Because of panting and cough in prolonged diseases, the Lung becomes deficient and cannot regulate the waterways, the Spleen becomes deficient and cannot transport and transform the *jing* (essence), and the Kidney becomes deficient and fails to steam and transform the water fluids. All of these deficiencies — of the Lung, Spleen and Kidney — will lead to internal generation of water fluids, and water will flood to the flesh and skin. The symptoms include a puffy complexion and swollen limbs, palpitations and shortness of breath, frequent cough and panting, distention and fullness of the chest and abdomen, soreness and weakness of the waist and knees, scanty urine and difficult urination, and even panting and tachypnea because of the fluid retention in the hypochondria upwardly affecting the Lung. Treatment should be to fortify the Spleen and warm the Kidney, diffuse the Lung and transform fluids. The formula selected is *Jīn Guì Shèn Qì Tāng* (金匮肾气汤) plus *Sān Zǐ Yǎng Qīn Tāng* (三子养亲汤) with modifications.

In summary of the above, professor Zhang determines the treatment of Lung distention based on the deficiency of five *zang* organs. He advocates that "the branch should be treated during the attack stage, and the root should be treated during the remission stage." The treatment should concentrate on regulating and tonifying the five *zang* organs for their deficiency, accompanying by eliminating phlegm, dissolving fluid retention, and expelling stasis so as to treat the branch.

(Zhang Zhen-ru. *Clinical Experience Collection of the Famous Veteran Physicians in Chinese Medicine · Essential Compilation of Zhang Zhen-ru's Clinical Experience* 章真如临床经验辑要 . Beijing: China Press of Medical Science and Technology, 2000. 163-166)

14. Professor Yu Shen-chu's Discussion of His Experience Treating Cough and Panting

Clinically, for the treatment of cough and panting, external contraction or internal damage should first be distinguished, then the conditions of *zang-fu* organs should be observed clearly and the pathomechanism should be judged carefully. The treatment should be determined flexibly according to whether it is a condition of cold or heat, deficiency or excess, branch or root, and slow or urgent.

(1) First Diffuse the Lung and Eliminate Phlegm in the Treatment of Cough due to Wind-Cold

Cough and panting is usually caused by catching external evils. The Lung governs qi and belongs to the defensive (*wei*) phase, controlling respiration and functioning to diffuse the defensive (*wei*) qi. Because the Lung corresponds to the skin and fine hair, when the external evils invade the skin and fine hair, they often affect the Lung, leading to its failure to purify. If the external evils trigger the internal turbid phlegm, this can result in phlegm obstruction, qi counterflow, and a failure of the Lung to diffuse and descend. Thus there appears both cough and panting because the cough is induced by phlegm, and the panting is induced by cough. Clinically, besides the repeated cough, there are often symptoms of tachypnea, panting, and wheezing. Doctor Yu begins treatment by diffusing the Lung and eliminating the phlegm. The formula selected is a self-composed *Zhǐ Ké Dìng Chuǎn Tāng* (止咳定喘汤). The ingredients are *zhì má huáng* (Herba Ephedrae Praeparata), *xìng rén* (Armeniacae Semen Amarum), *sū zǐ* (Fructus Perillae), *bái jiè zǐ* (Semen Sinapis Albae), *tíng lì zǐ* (Semen Lepidii seu Descurainiae), *zhì kuǎn dōng* (Flos Farfarae Praeparata), *zhì jú hóng* (Exocarpium Citri Rubrum Praeparata), *fú líng* (Poria), *bàn xià* (Rhizoma Pinelliae) and *zhì gān cǎo* (Radix et Rhizoma Glycyrrhizae Praeparata). This formula has the function of diffusing the Lung, calming panting, eliminating phlegm, and stopping cough, with a good effect for the treatment of cough and panting due to wind-cold. This formula is often used clinically to treat acute and chronic bronchitis, bronchial asthma or mild emphysema. In terms of the clinical application of *Zhǐ Ké Dìng Chuǎn Tāng* (止咳定喘汤): for an obvious exterior pattern, with aversion to cold and fever, nasal obstruction with nasal discharge, add *jīng jiè* (Herba Schizonepetae), *fáng fēng* (Radix Saposhnikoviae) and *zǐ sū yè* (Folium Perillae); for thick phlegm, and difficulty in expectoration, add *sāng bái pí* (Cortex Mori) and *zhè bèi mǔ* (Bulbus Fritillariae Thunbergii); for chest oppression, add *guā lóu* (Fructus Trichosanthis) and *yù jīn* (Radix Curcumae); for cases of wind-cold fettering the exterior, and phlegm-heat blocking the Lung, with cough, yellow sputum, panting, vexing heat, and a dry mouth, use *Dìng Chuǎn Tāng* (定喘汤) plus *tíng lì zǐ* (Semen Lepidii seu Descurainiae) and *bái jiè zǐ* (Semen Sinapis Albae).

(2) Treatment of Many Kinds of Cough with Modified *Zhǐ Sòu Sǎn* (止嗽散)

Based on the principle of composing *Zhǐ Sòu Sǎn* (止嗽散), as found in the *Medicine Comprehended* (医学心悟, *Yī Xué Xīn Wù*), Doctor Yu modified this original formula and made *Jiā Jiǎn Zhǐ Sòu Sǎn* (加减止嗽散). Modified *Zhǐ Sòu Sǎn* (加减止嗽散) consists of seven medicinals: *jīng jiè* (Herba Schizonepetae), *bǎi bù* (Radix Stemonae), *xìng rén* (Armeniacae Semen Amarum), *zhè bèi mǔ* (Bulbus Fritillariae Thunbergii), *kuǎn dōng huā* (Flos Farfarae), *chén pí* (Pericarpium Citri Reticulatae) and *gān cǎo* (Radix et Rhizoma Glycyrrhizae). It has a good effect to expel wind, stop cough, regulate qi and transform phlegm. Clinically, Doctor Yu often takes this formula as the basic formula and modifies it according to the pattern. It is extensively applied to treat many kinds of cough. For example, for cases of cough due to wind-heat, prescribe this formula plus *Sāng Jú Yǐn* (桑菊饮) or *Yín Qiào Sǎn* (银翘散). For cases of cough due to wind-cold, prescribe this formula plus *fáng fēng* (Radix Saposhnikoviae) and *zǐ sū yè* (Folium Perillae). For cases of cough due to turbid phlegm, prescribe this formula plus *Èr Chén Tāng* (二陈汤). For cases of cough due to adverse rising of qi, prescribe this formula plus *Sān Zǐ Yǎng Qīn Tāng* (三子养亲汤); For cases of cough due to Lung-heat, add *sāng bái pí* (Cortex Mori), *huáng qín* (Radix Scutellariae) and *pí pá yè* (Folium Eriobotryae). For cases of impairment of the Lung and consumption of body fluids by dry evil, manifesting as cough with scanty sputum, add *shā shēn* (Glehniae), *mài dōng* (Radix Ophiopogonis), *zhī mǔ* (Rhizoma Anemarrhenae) and *xuán shēn* (Radix Scrophulariae).

(3) Pay Attention to Drying Dampness and Transforming Phlegm for Phlegm Turbidity Assailing the Lung

The Spleen functions to transport and transform the *gǔ jīng* (谷精, essence of food) and water-damp. Overstrain or improper diet can injure the Spleen and Stomach, leading to the failure of the Spleen to transform and transport. Then the *gǔ jīng* and water-damp cannot be distributed normally, hence phlegm will form through gathering of dampness. If the turbid phlegm goes up and affects the Lung, this can lead to a failure of the Lung to diffuse and descend, hence cough and panting will appear. This is what is meant when the ancestors said "the Spleen is the source for generation of phlegm, and the Lung is the container for storage of the phlegm." This disease is of both the Lung and Spleen, presenting with repetitive episodes of cough, or persistent panting, stridor in the throat, lassitude and poor appetite, a white and greasy coating, and a slippery pulse. Treatment should be to fortify the Spleen to dry dampness, and transform phlegm to stop cough. For cough with excessive and white phlegm, professor Yu usually uses *Qián Xìng Èr Chén Tāng* (前杏二陈汤). This is *Èr Chén Tāng* (二陈汤) plus *qián hú* (Radix Peucedani) and *xìng rén* (Armeniacae Seme Amarum). For cough with fullness and oppression of the chest and epigastrium, use *Pò Xìng Èr Chén Tāng* (朴杏二陈汤). This is *Èr Chén Tāng* (二陈汤) plus *hòu pò* (Cortex Magnoliae) and *xìng rén* (Armeniacae Semen Amarum). For severe cough with excessive and white phlegm, use *Kuǎn Xìng Èr Chén Tāng* (款杏二陈汤). This is *Èr Chén Tāng* (二陈汤) plus *kuǎn dōng huā* (Flos Farfarae) and *xìng rén* (Armeniacae Semen Amarum). For panting due to qi counterflow, add *tíng lì zǐ* (Semen Lepidii seu Descurainiae), *bái jiè zǐ* (Semen Sinapis Albae) and *zǐ sū zǐ*

(Fructus Perillae). For lassitude, debility, and poor appetite, add *Liù Jūn Zǐ Tāng* (六君子汤). For yellow and thick sputum, breathlessness and a dry mouth, add *sāng bái pí* (Cortex Mori), *guā lóu* (Fructus Trichosanthis) and *zhè bèi mǔ* (Bulbus Fritillariae Thunbergii).

(4) Lay Emphasis on Coursing the Liver and Diffusing the Lung for Cough and Panting due to Qi Depression

There is a very close relationship between the Liver and Lung. Their channels are related and their functions can influence each other. The Liver qi governs ascent and dispersion and the Lung qi governs purification and descent. If the Liver qi and the Lung qi can coordinate with each other and restrict each other, the qi dynamic of body will ascend and descend as normal. If a person becomes distressed, worried or angry, the Liver qi will be bound and constrained, failing in ascent and dispersion and free coursing. This may affect the purification and descent of Lung qi, resulting in cough and panting. To treat this kind of coughing, Professor Yu often treats the Liver and Lung simultaneously by using the methods of coursing the Liver and diffusing the Lung, relieving cough and panting. The formula selected is *Sì Nì Sǎn* (四逆散) plus *Sān Niù Tāng* (三拗汤), with additions of *zhì kuǎn dōng* (Flos Farfarae) and *xiāng fù* (Rhizoma Cyperi). If Liver qi depression transforms into fire which then adversely affects the Lung, it will cause failure of the Lung to purify. Its symptoms are dyspnea, persistent cough and panting. For this case, use *Sì Nì Sǎn* (四逆散) plus *Xiè Bái Sǎn* (泻白散), with additional *xìng rén* (Armeniacae Semen Amarum), *pí pá yè* (Folium Eriobotryae), *zhè bèi mǔ* (Bulbus Fritillariae Thunbergii) and *huáng qín* (Radix Scutellariae).

(5) For Prolonged Cough, Treatment should be Aimed mostly at the Lung and Kidney

Prolonged cough and panting may affect the Lung and Kidney, and there will appear symptoms of Lung and Kidney deficiency, especially

Kidney deficiency. Cough and panting due to Lung deficiency always presents with panting and shortness of breath, sweating and intolerance of wind, and a deficient and powerless or hollow pulse. Professor Yu treats it clinically with methods of boosting qi and stopping panting, often using *Shēng Mài Sǎn* (生脉散) plus *huáng qí* (Radix Astragali) and *hú táo ròu* (Semen Juglandis Regiae). There is a saying from ancient times that says that the Lung governs exhalation and Kidney governs reception of qi. If the deficient Kidney fails to consolidate in the lower jiao, it will lead to a failure of the Kidney in receiving qi, then qi adversely ascends, hence cough and panting appear. The symptoms are panting, prolonged exhalation and short inspiration, panting aggravated upon exertion, accompanied by soreness and weakness of the waist and knees, lassitude and debility, a deep and thready pulse, and a pale tongue with a white coating. Professor Yu treats this by the methods of descending qi and calming panting, combined with boosting the Kidney and astringing qi. He uses *Sū Zǐ Jiàng Qì Tāng* (苏子降气汤) from the *Collected Exegesis of Recipes* (医方集解 , *Yī Fāng Jí Jiě*), plus *shān yú ròu* (Fructus Corni), *xuán fù huā* (Flos Inulae) and *dài zhě shí* (Haematitum). For cases of panting due to deficiency of both qi and yin, use *Shēng Mài Sǎn* (生脉散) plus *Shēn Zhě Zhèn Qì Tāng* (参赭镇气汤). Professor Yu likes to use *shān yú ròu* (Fructus Corni) to treat panting due to the Kidney deficiency. He always use *shān yú ròu* (Fructus Corni) 60g, simmered singly and taken orally, to get a good affect. He holds that *shān zhū yú* (Fructus Corni) can not only boost the Kidney and replenish the essence but also astringe qi. The effect is excellent for treating panting due to Kidney deficiency. For cases of Kidney yang deficiency, use *Sū Zǐ Jiàng Qì Tāng* (苏子降气汤) plus medicinals to help receive qi, such as *hú táo ròu* (Semen Juglandis Regiae), *bǔ gǔ zhī* (Fructus Psoraleae) and *ròu guì* (Cortex Cinnamomi), or add *Rén Shēn Gé Jiè Sǎn* (人参蛤蚧散) to assist. For cases of Kidney yin deficiency, use *Mài Wèi Dì Huáng Wán* (麦味地黄丸) for nourishing the Kidney to receive qi.

(Liu De-rong, Yu Ding-fang. *Collection of One Hundred Famous Chinese Clinicians during the Century in China · Yu Shen-chu* 中国百年百名中医临床家丛书·俞慎初. Beijing: China Press of Traditional Chinese Medicine, 2001. 7-15)

15. Professor Li Shi-qing: Treatment of Cough in Bronchitis

Cough in bronchitis mostly belongs to the Chinese medical category of cough due to external contraction. "Wind is the chief evil of all diseases". Of the six evils that externally contract, wind evil is often the first. The wind often comes carrying cold, and moreover can transform into dryness or heat. If the wind evil invades and binds the exterior of the body, it will usually affect the diffusion of Lung qi, with a resultant obstruction of the qi dynamic, and a failure of fluids to spread. In turn, the fluids can gather to form phlegm and block the qi dynamic. When wind-phlegm stagnates in the Lung, it will lead to Lung qi counterflow, hence there is cough. The beginning of bronchitis always presents with cough, itching of the throat, a choking feeling in the throat and chest, or a frequent dry cough, and difficulty in coughing. At this time, cold and heat are not obvious, and the pattern mostly belongs to obstruction by wind evil in the Lung, mixed with phlegm and stasis. If a person with a predominantly yang constitution ordinarily catches wind-cold, and the wind-cold cannot be dispelled in time, it can transform into heat. If a doctor does not identify whether there is an evil, and only treats cough, or clears the Lung with bitter-cold medicinals for inflammation, this will lead to stagnation of wind-phlegm, and the cough will not disappear. Clinically, I find that the initial cough is not severe among most patients, but due to either delayed or mistaken treatment, it will result in a failure of dissipation of the stagnating wind and phlegm. The evils stagnate and obstruct the Lung collaterals, thus various kinds of deteriorating cases will occur. Therefore the nature of cough should be clearly distinguished, and characteristics of stagnating wind, phlegm, and the transformation of wind-cold into depressed heat should all be recognized. The chief therapeutic principle is to expel the wind evil from the exterior by using medicinals that are light and have actions of clearing, diffusing and transforming. Thus the progression of the illness can be checked quickly, and the evil qi cannot spread from the exterior to the interior, or lead to stubborn complications. Just as Chen Shi-duo, of the Qing dynasty, said: "At the beginning of cough, must first scatter wind-cold, and slightly assist with fire scattering medicinals. One cannot excessively use cold and cool medicinals to restrain the fire, and also cannot excessively use dry and hot medicinals, lest they aid the evil."

Based on the above information, Professor Li Shi-qing created *Fèi Níng Hé Jì* (肺宁合剂). Within this formula, *má huáng* (Herba Ephedrae) diffuses the Lung qi to scatter wind-cold, and *kǔ xìng rén* (Armeniacae Semen Amarum) courses and downbears the Lung qi to downbear the phlegm counterflow. In combination with *shēng gān cǎo* (Radix et Rhizoma Glycyrrhizae Recens), these to function to open the exterior and expel evils, diffuse the Lung and downbear counterflow. Together, the above three medicinals are called *Sān Niù Tāng* (三拗汤), and they act to reinforce within the diffusion. As the deputy medicinals, *qián hú* (Radix Peucedani) and *jié gěng* (Radix Platycodonis) strengthen the effect of diffusing the Lung to resolve phlegm and remove stagnation. *Jié gěng* (Radix Platycodonis) plus *gān cǎo* (Radix et Rhizoma Glycyrrhizae) can diffuse the Lung to disinhibit the throat. They are the necessary medicinals for an initial cough with throat itching and soreness. *Guā lóu pí* (Pericarpium Trichosanthis) is light and can clear and transform phlegm, disinhibit the qi dynamic to relax the chest, as well as moisten the Lung, generate fluids, course the Liver, and harmonize the collaterals. Furthermore it can prevent the side effect of diffusion damaging the fluids. Clinically *guā lóu pí* (Pericarpium Trichosanthis) is especially suitable for cough due to wind-cold binding the exterior, heat stagnating in the channels, stasis of the Lung collaterals, cough with difficulty in expectoration, and chest oppression. The Lung governs diffusion, and it is a fragile organ of clearing and purifying, thus *pí pá yè* (Folium Eriobotryae), which is slightly bitter in nature, is used as an assistant to purify the Lung and transform phlegm. With its clearing nature, it also can have the effect of normalizing the Stomach. This is consistent with the principle written in *Inner Canon of Huangdi* (内经 , *Nèi Jīng*) "The Lung is apt to suffer from adverse rising of qi, and bitter medicinals should be used immediately to drain the counterflow of qi (肺苦气上逆，急食苦以泄之)." Together, all of the medicinals have the actions of coursing wind and outthrusting evil, diffusing the Lung, and transforming phlegm, downbearing counterflow and stopping cough."

In order to systematically observe the clinical effect of *Fèi Níng Hé Jì* (肺宁合剂), the Chinese Medical Hospital of Jiangshu Province carried out the initial clinical observation of treatment of 1200 cases of bronchitis type cough with this remedy. The research was done in the clinical from 1989 to 1996. Its total effective rate was 97.1％. It was especially good for cough in acute bronchitis and upper respiratory infection. Clinically it has been proved that *Fèi Níng Hé Jì* (肺宁合剂) is better to treat cases of wind evils invading the Lung, with a tendency of wind-cold to transform into heat. Clinically the curative rates were 95.7% and 91.6% respectively.

[Shi Suo-fang, Li Nai-yu, Zhu Jia. Bronchitis Treated with *Fèi Níng Hé Jì* · A Clinical Observation of 1200 Cases. *Jiangshu Journal of Traditional Chinese Medicine* 江苏中医药 . 1997, 18(1): 9-10]

PERSPECTIVES OF INTEGRATIVE MEDICINE

Around the world, COPD is the main chronic disease that leads to death. COPD is characterized by partially reversible airflow limitation, which is usually gradually progressive. In the advanced stage, the obstruction of peripheral airways, destruction of lung parenchyma, and abnormality of pulmonary blood vessels can all reduce the lung's gas exchange capacity. This leads to hypoxemia and hypercapnia (respiratory failure). COPD in the advanced stage is often complicated by pulmonary artery hypertension and pulmonary heart disease. The prognosis is mostly unfavorable. Lung damage in COPD is slowly progressive, and the patient's quality of life is obviously affected even in the middle-to-advanced stages. At present, the management of COPD includes four parts: 1) the evaluation and monitoring of disease; 2) reducing risk factors; 3) rehabilitative treatment with integrative medicine during the stable stage; 4) treatment of COPD in the acute exacerbation stage. Even with the thorough continuous knowledge of COPD, there are still many challenging aspects of COPD treatment. These issues include: the treatment of respiratory failure; how to efficiently treat the acute exacerbation; how to prevent relapse, preventing the progression of disease; how to change the tendency of the lung function to decrease over time; how to prevent and treat complications. All of these problems need urgently to be researched and resolved.

Challenges and Solutions

CHALLENGE #1: TREATMENT OF RESPIRATORY FAILURE

Airway obstruction is main cause of respiratory failure. Airway obstruction can cause aggravation of pulmonary artery hypertension, an increase on the load of the heart, and a reduction of the oxygen supply to the tissues and organs of the whole body, thereby inducing heart failure and multiple organ failure, which are of serious injuries that should be actively treated. Treatment principles: In the acute aggravation stage, the treatment should use integrative medicine to concentrate on actively controlling the infection of the respiratory tract and lungs, using antispasmodics and anti-asthmatics, and clearing the respiratory tract excretions to keep it smooth. If necessary, respiratory stimulants or artificial mechanical ventilation should also be considered. In this stage the Chinese medical patterns belong mainly to the conditions of phlegm, heat and stasis accumulating in the Lung. The treatment should begin with purging Lung excess and eliminating stagnation. The concrete measures have been dealt with in the treatment section, and it is unnecessary to go into detail here. Clinically, some COPD patients during the protracted and remission stages mainly present with chronic respiratory failure. This pattern belongs to one of panting, with symptoms including chronic cough, expectoration, and dyspnea, which seriously affects daily life and work. This type of chronic respiratory failure is every difficult to treat, and the chief strategies have two aspects: eliminating evils, and strengthening the right qi to stop panting.

(1) Correctly Using Evil-Eliminating Medicinals to Stop Panting

1) Medicinals that eliminate wind to stop panting include: *má huáng* (Herba Ephedrae), *zǐ sū* (Folium Perillae), *chán tuì* (Periostracum Cicadae), *jīng jiè* (Herba Schizonepetae), *fáng fēng* (Radix Saposhnikoviae), *sāng yè* (Folium Mori), *jú huā* (Flos Chrysanthemi), *xì xīn* (Radix et Rhizoma Asari), etc.. Among these medicinals, *má huáng* (Herba Ephedrae), is the principal herb, with its acrid warm flavor, to expel wind and dispel cold, diffuse the Lung to calm panting, and affect both diffusing and descending actions. Modern pharmacologic research shows that ephedrine has a marked and lasting effect on the relaxation of tracheal smooth muscle. The volatile oil of *má huáng* (Herba Ephedrae) has a remarkable in vitro effect of inhibiting the influenza virus, and it has an effect of killing staphylococcus aureus.

2) Medicinals that downbear qi to stop panting include: *sū zǐ*

(Fructus Perillae), *lái fú zǐ* (Semen Raphani Tostum), *bái jiè zǐ* (Semen Sinapis Albae), *tíng lì zǐ* (Semen Lepidii seu Descurainiae), *sāng bái pí* (Cortex Mori), *kuǎn dōng huā* (Flos Farfarae), *xìng rén* (Armeniacae Semen Amarum), *bǎi bù* (Radix Stemonae), etc.. Modern researches reveal that amygdalin from *xìng rén* (Armeniacae Semen Amarum) can inhibit the respiratory center to prevent the cough and calm panting. *Tíng lì zǐ* (Semen Lepidii seu Descurainiae), with a bitter flavor and very cold nature, has a cardio-tonic function. *Zǐ wǎn* (Radix et Rhizoma Asteris) is often used in combination with *kuǎn dōng huā* (Flos Farfarae). Experiments have proved that the ether extract of *kuǎn dōng huā* (Flos Farfarae) can relieve bronchial spasms caused by histamine, but the effect is certainly not the same as that of aminophylline. In addition, it can stimulate respiration, just like coramine. *Bǎi bù* (Radix Stemonae), with a bitter flavor and slightly warm nature, can moisten the Lung to stop cough, and transform phlegm to calm panting. It is effective for both the new and prolonged cough. Experiments prove that the alkaloid of *bǎi bù* (Radix Stemonae) has the effect of relaxing bronchial spasms caused by histamine, and its effect is similar to that of aminophylline, but it is slower and more lasting.

3) Medicinals that remove stasis to stop panting include: *dān shēn* (Radix et Rhizoma Salviae Miltiorrhizae), *táo rén* (Semen Persicae), *mǔ dān pí* (Cortex Moutan), *chì sháo* (Radix Paeoniae Rubra), *dāng guī* (Radix Angelicae Sinensis), etc.. Modern pharmacologic researches prove that these medicinals can resist viruses and bacteria, remove oxygen free radicals, improve microcirculation, and block calcium channels, so as to get the effect of removing stasis to stop panting. If the above medicinals are selectively used based on pattern differentiation and treatment, a better curative affect will be achieved.

(2) Attach Importance to Supporting the Right Qi to Stop Panting
1) Medicinals that boost qi and fortify the Spleen include: *rén*

shēn (Radix Ginseng), bái zhú (Rhizoma Atractylodis Macrocephalae), fú líng (Poria), gān cǎo (Radix et Rhizoma Glycyrrhizae), shān yào (Rhizoma Dioscoreae), etc.. Research over many years reveals that both single medicinals and compound preparations, such as Bǔ Zhōng Yì Qì Tāng (补中益气汤) and Sì Jūn Zǐ Tāng (四君子汤), can raise immunity of the body. The mechanisms of these medicinals include fortifying the Spleen to improve the nutritional status of the body so as to raise immunity of the body, increasing the contractibility of respiratory muscle, and improving the fatigue of respiratory muscle. They have a better therapeutic effect on respiratory failure caused by respiratory muscle fatigue. Their applications open a new route for the treatment of COPD.

2) Medicinals that boost the Kidney and consolidating the root include: shēng dì huáng (Radix Rehmanniae Recens), shān zhū yú (Fructus Corni), shān yào (Rhizoma Dioscoreae), shú fù zǐ (Radix Aconiti Lateralis Praeparata), bǔ gǔ zhī (Fructus Psoraleae), dōng chóng xià cǎo (Cordyceps Sinensis), gé jiè (Gecko), etc.. Research has found that formulas that support the right qi and consolidating the root have some antispasmodic and anti-asthmatic effects, and they can regulate the immune and adrenal cortex functions. These formulas can be used for a long time without obvious toxic and side effects. Uses of these formulas over a long time are effective in calming panting during the remission stage. Emphasizing the treatment during the remission stage can prevent repetitive attacks of COPD, being helpful delaying the progression of disease and pulmonary function damage.

Challenge #2: Treatment of Respiratory Tract Infection is the Key Point to Relieving Acute Exacerbation

The treatment of acute and chronic respiratory tract infection is a difficult issue in the treatment of an acute exacerbation of COPD. The main reason that this is a challenge is that it is difficult to control, and there are multiple drug resistances. At this time, Chinese medicine should be brought into full play because of its superiority to reduce inflammation. Respiratory tract infection is the chief inducing factor of an acute exacerbation of COPD. Some respiratory infections begin with a viral infection. When a respiratory tract infection occurs, usually one of the below formulas are used to resist the virus. For cases of external contraction by wind-cold, usually use *Jīng Fáng Bài Dú Sǎn* (荆防败毒散). For cases of external contraction by wind-heat, usually use *Yín Qiào Sǎn (Tāng)* (银翘散/汤). For cases of dry-heat, usually use *Qīng Zào Jiù Fèi Tāng* (清燥救肺汤). If the medicinals are correctly selected and used the development of infection can be checked early on, and there can be a good clinical curative effect.

Viral infections are usually followed by bacterial infections. The herbal determination based on pattern identification can also be used for the treatment of bacterial infections. The beginning of infection usually presents with symptoms of blockage of the Lung by phlegm-heat. At this time it is proper to use *huáng qín* (Radix Scutellariae), *yú xīng cǎo* (Herba Houttuyniae) and *shè gān* (Rhizoma Belamcandae) to clear Lung-heat; and *guā lóu* (Fructus Trichosanthis), *zhè bèi mǔ* (Bulbus Fritillariae Thunbergii) and *zhú huáng* (Shiraia Bambusicola) to clear heat and transform sputum. The Lung and the Large Intestine have an interior exterior relationship. For cases of Lung heat blazing, use *dà huáng* (Radix et Rhizoma Rhei) and *qín pí* (Cortex Fraxini) to clear the Intestine and drain heat so as aid in removing Lung-heat. Clinically, we find that draining the *fu* organs can get rid of toxins and reduce inflammatory damage to the body, therefore they are also chief anti-inflammatory measures.

With further developments of pulmonary inflammatory infection, there may appear manifestations of stasis resulting from heat. At this moment *Xiān Fāng Huó Mìng Yǐn* (仙方活命饮) can be used. While clearing

Lung-heat, medicinals that invigorate blood, such as *táo rén* (Semen Persicae), *sháo yào* (Radix Paeoniae) and *dān shēn* (Radix et Rhizoma Salviae Miltiorrhizae) should be added to promote the absorption of inflammatory substances.

Biomedical antibiotics need to be used to treat severe infections. At this time our therapeutic strategy is to use biomedical drugs for antibacterial treatments, and to use Chinese medicinals for strengthening the right qi. Chinese medicine can regulate the patient's constitution and physical state, promote the absorption of inflammatory substances, increase the curative effect of biomedicine, and reduce the toxic side effects of biomedical antibiotics. Chinese Medicine, combined with biomedicine, can overcome the crisis of infection. For example, in the clinical treatment of some severe cases of pulmonary infection with antibiotics, there are also gastrointestinal reactions, manifesting as Spleen qi deficiency with poor appetite. For this case, use *Xiāng Shā Liù Jūn Zǐ Tāng* (香砂六君子汤) plus *lái fú zǐ* (Semen Raphani Tostum) and *mài yá* (Fructus Hordei Germinatus) to fortify the Spleen, boost qi, and promote digestion. Again, for severe cases of infection, there can be low immune function, presenting as qi deficiency or yang deficiency. At this time, the effect of biomedical antibiotics is not good, so one can also use *Sì Jūn Zǐ Tāng* (四君子汤), *Bǔ Zhōng Yì Qì Tāng* (补中益气汤), *Dú Shēn Tāng* (独参汤) and *Shēn Fù Tāng* (参附汤) in order to strengthen the right qi, and elevate the curative effect of biomedical drugs.

For infections with multiple drug resistances, our strategy is to use integrative medicine. Based on conventional biomedical anti-inflammatory medicine, on can use Chinese antibiotic medicinals, For example, using *Yú Xīng Cǎo Zhù Shè Yè* (鱼腥草注射液) or *Shuāng Huáng Lián Zhēn Fěn Jì* (双黄连针粉剂), in combination with Chinese medicinals that can be tonifying and anti-inflammatory, such as *Běi Qí Zhù Shè Yè* (北芪注射液), *Shēn Mài Zhù Shè Yè* (参麦注射液) or single medicinal like *dāng guī* (Radix Angelicae Sinensis), *huáng jīng* (Rhizoma Polygonati), *qín pí* (Cortex Fraxini), *bái tóu wēng* (Radix Pulsatillae) and *dān shēn* (Radix et Rhizoma Salviae Miltiorrhizae), can have anti-inflammatory effects and synergetic results when used with integrative medicine.

For cases of protracted pulmonary infection, our strategy is to strengthen the right qi and eliminate evils, selectively using the antibiotic medicinals with tonifying actions. Modern researches indicate that some Chinese medicinals, such as *huáng qí* (Radix Astragali), *dāng guī* (Radix Angelicae Sinensis), *bái sháo* (Radix Paeoniae Alba) and *huáng jīng* (Rhizoma Polygonati), not only have tonifying actions to elevate the immune function of the body, but also have direct antibiotic actions. Thus it will get the effect of killing two birds with one stone.

CHALLENGE #3: PREVENTING THE ACUTE EXACERBATION OF COPD AS AN IMPORTANT KEY IN DELAYING THE PROGRESSION OF COPD

COPD patients are susceptible to developing respiratory tract infections because they often have lowered immune function. Respiratory tract infections can induce acute exacerbation and further damage to lung function, leading to the respiratory failure. Therefore preventing relapse is one of the most important keys to delaying the progression of COPD. To prevent relapse, the measure taken is to elevate the immunity of the body and thus reduce the chance of respiratory tract infection. Clinically we adopt the below methods:

(1) Treatment with Chinese Medicinals Based on Pattern Differentiation

Many Chinese medicinals that tonify the Lung, fortify the Spleen and consolidate the Kidney have a good effect to elevate the immunity of the body. These medicinals can be used based on pattern differentiation, such as *huáng qí* (Radix Astragali), *dǎng shēn* (Radix Codonopsis), *bái zhú*

(Rhizoma Atractylodis Macrocephalae), *bǔ gǔ zhī* (Fructus Psoraleae), *líng zhī* (Gamoderma Lucidim), *huáng jīng* (Rhizoma Polygonati) and *gǒu qǐ zǐ* (Fructus Lycii). For the pattern of dual deficiency of the Lung and Spleen, usually use *Yù Píng Fēng Sǎn* (玉屏风散), or *Bǔ Zhōng Yì Qì Tāng* (补中益气汤) to tonify the Lung and fortify the Spleen. For cases of dual deficiency of the Spleen and Kidney, use *Liù Wèi Dì Huáng Wán* (六味地黄丸) or *Shèn Qì Wán* (肾气丸) to fortify the Spleen and consolidate the Kidney.

(2) Acupuncture Therapy

Acupuncture, moxibustion or pustulating moxibustion at ST 36 (*zú sān lǐ*) have good effects of elevating immunity, so they deserve merit and popularization.

(3) External Application

Illnesses of the winter may be treated in the summer. At the greatest heat days in summer, use external application with *bái jiè zǐ* (Semen Sinapis Albae) as recorded in *Zhang's Treatise on Medicine* (张氏医通 , *Zhāng Shì Yī Tōng*). Grind *bái jiè zǐ* (Semen Sinapis Albae), *gān suí* (Radix Kansui), *xì xīn* (Radix et Rhizoma Asari) and *yán hú suǒ* (Rhizoma Corydalis) into a fine powder. The sieved powder is then mixed with ginger juice into a paste. This paste is put on BL 13 (*fèi shù*), BL 15 (*xīn shù*) and BL 23 (*shèn shù*) etc. On the first day of the first days, do the application once, then do it once again during the first day of the second and third period of the greatest heat days respectively, for 4—6 hours each time. It can not only elevate the immunity of the body but also effectively prevent and reduce respiratory tract infection.

(4) Nutritional Supportive Therapy

Because low immune function is closely related to malnutrition in patients with pulmonary heart disease, nutrients such as proteins and fats should be given to elevate the immunity of the body. However, it should be noted that COPD patients are predisposed to suffer from gastrointestinal dysfunction and hypofunction in terms of digestion and absorption. This is because of long-term hypoxia and carbon dioxide retention. At this time, Chinese medicinals that tonify the Spleen and Stomach and promote digestion should be used based on pattern differentiation. In combination with nutritional therapy, these medicinals can boost the effect of nutritional support. In addition, carbohydrate metabolism will generate a large amount of carbon dioxide, which can increase respiratory load and induce the respiratory failure. Thus nutritional support should depend mainly on fats to supply energy to respiratory failure patients, and should avoid using carbohydrates to supply energy.

CHALLENGE #4: TREATMENT OF PULMONARY ARTERY HYPERTENSION

Pulmonary artery hypertension is a main cause of pulmonary heart disease. Pulmonary artery hypertension accompanied by pulmonary heart disease belongs to pre-capillary pulmonary artery hypertension. The key link of the pathogenesis is pulmonary blood vessel spasms and contractions due to hypoxia. The pathogenesis also relates to the extensive affection of lung parenchyma which reduces the pulmonary vascular bed areas. Clinical researches prove that the severity of pulmonary microcirculation obstruction correlates with the severity of blood stasis. This means that if the pulmonary microcirculation is severely blocked, the pulmonary arterial pressure is higher, and there are more serious the clinical symptoms of blood stasis. These include a dark grey complexion, cyanosis of lips and nails, and a dark or dark purple tongue. Clinically, this is very difficult to treat. Our strategies include the following:

(1) Continuous Oxygen Therapy

Oxygen therapy is an important measure to reduce pulmonary blood vessel spasms and contractions due to hypoxia. Continuous oxygen therapy in the hospital or at home may result in continuous and beneficial changes of pulmonary hemodynamics, and improve the condition of pulmonary microcirculation obstruction. Generally we advocate the time of oxygen therapy to be no less than 15 hours every day.

(2) The Selection of Biomedical Vasodilators

Vasodilator agents have certain therapeutic effects on primary pulmonary hypertension and postcapillary pulmonary hypertension in a few cases, especially by improving the left heart function. However, because pulmonary hypertension caused by COPD has pathological physiological changes from diminished oxygen supply, the clinical effects of vasodilator agents to treat pulmonary hypertension needs to be further researched. We often use the following drugs: those that directly expand the blood vessels, such as phentolamine, glycerol trinitrate, dinitrosorbide; Ca^{2+} channel inhibitors such as adalat; and angiotensin converting enzyme inhibitors, such as captopril. Clinically, these drugs have some effect in improving right-sided heart failure and reducing pulmonary arterial pressure. Generally, we use only one drug, at most we use only two in as a therapeutic alliance.

(3) Reducing Pulmonary Artery Hypertension with Chinese Remedies

As there has been advances in the research of invigorating blood and transforming stasis, in recent years it has been gradually found that blood stasis is an important link of pulmonary artery hypertension and runs through the whole course of disease. Thus, invigorating blood and resolving stasis will be regarded as the main method to treat pulmonary artery hypertension. More and more attention has been paid to the studies on using Chinese medicinals to reduce COPD pulmonary artery hypertension. It has now been proved that all of the following drugs have a certain effect to reduce pulmonary artery hypertension. They are: medicinals that invigorate blood and resolve stasis, like *Chuān Xiōng Qín Zhù Shè Yè* (川芎嗪注射液), *Dān Shēn Zhù Shè Yè* (丹参注射液), *Chì Sháo Zhù Shè Yè* (赤芍注射液), *Sān Qī Zhù Shè Yè* (三七注射液); medicinals that nourish blood, like extract of *dāng guī* (Radix Angelicae Sinensis); medicinals that transform phlegm, like *qián hú* (Radix Peucedani); medicinals that dissipate dampness, like *hàn fáng jǐ* (Radix Stephaniae Tetrandrae); and medicinals that promote digestion, like *lái fú zǐ* (Semen Raphani Tostum). Their effective mechanism is that they can directly expand pulmonary blood vessels and improve blood viscosity. Some of the medicinals also affect calcium antagonistic actions, such as *hàn fáng jǐ* (Radix Stephaniae Tetrandrae), *chuān xiōng* (Rhizoma Chuanxiong), *dāng guī* (Radix Angelicae Sinensis), *chì sháo* (Radix Paeoniae Rubra), *dān shēn* (Radix et Rhizoma Salviae Miltiorrhizae) and *qián hú* (Radix Peucedani). In addition, *lái fú zǐ* (Semen Raphani Tostum) has an additional action to inhibit the angiotensin converting enzyme, and can be used according to the pattern differentiation. Clinically, we often use methods of boosting qi and invigorating blood to treat pulmonary artery hypertension. We use *Shēn Mài Zhù Shè Yè* (参麦注射液) combined with *Dān Shēn Zhù Shè Yè* (丹参注射液) or *Chuān Xiōng Qín Zhù Shè Yè* (川芎嗪注射液), in an intravenous drip, with a good effect on reducing pulmonary artery hypertension and improving right-sided heart function.

To sum up, for COPD complicated by pulmonary artery hypertension, treatment based on the primary flare-up and oxygen therapy using the above mentioned Chinese and western integrative medicine methods of applying medicinals and can obtain very good curative effects. Modern researches indicate that COPD complicated by pulmonary artery hypertension is not irreversible, and active treatment is the key point to stop further aggravation of pulmonary heart disease.

Insight from Empirical Wisdom

1. When Encountering Any of the Below, Quickly Treat with Combined Western and Chinese Medicine

(1) Acute respiratory failure

(2) Pneumoniae gravis

(3) Pulmonary encephalopathy

(4) Cor pulmonale

(5) Alimentary tract hemorrhage

The most severe COPD patients in community clinics should be transferred to a better hospital as soon as possible.

2. Treatment of Respiratory Muscle Fatigue

In COPD patients, the increase of airway resistance also increases the load of respiratory muscles. Also, the energy supply is lessened, thus resulting in respiratory muscle fatigue. This fatigue belongs to *xū chuǎn* (虚喘 , deficiency panting) or *chuǎn tuō* (喘脱 , panting collapse). The clinical manifestations are breathlessness with an elongated expiratory phase, panting induced by physical exertion, gasping with the shoulders raised, a bluish complexion, cyanosis of the face and lips, sweating, and lassitude. This is often accompanied by poor appetite, emaciation, frequent urination and nocturia, lumbar soreness and intolerance of cold, cold limbs, susceptibility to catch colds, a pale and dusky tongue with a thick and greasy coating or a yellow or scanty coating, and a slippery, thready, rapid, or knotted and intermittent pulse, which is forceless when pressed heavily.

The pathomechanism of COPD respiratory muscle fatigue is associated with qi deficiency of the Lung, Spleen and Kidney, especially depletion and sinking of gathering qi in the thorax. Gathering qi, also named great qi in the thorax, is a combination of the clear qi inhaled by the Lung and the essential qi of water and grain transported and transformed by the Spleen and Stomach. *Inner Canon of Huangdi* (内经 , *Nèi Jīng*) says "it cumulates in the thorax, permeates into the Heart and vessels, and promotes respiration." The Kidney is the root of congenital constitution and the source of all qi. The Kidney grows first to generate the original qi, or the minor fire generates the right qi. So the gathering qi originates from the Kidney. Therefore the gathering qi takes the original qi of the Kidney as its basis, the essential qi of water and grain its nourishment, and the thorax as its residence, and combines with the clear qi. Thus the strength of the Lung, Spleen and Kidney qi directly influence the ascending and descending of the gathering qi. Because of the prolonged course of the illness, the Lung, Spleen and Kidney in COPD patients are functioning below normal levels, which leads to insufficiency of the gathering qi. The recurrent flare ups consume the gathering qi, and result in the decline and sinking of qi in severe cases, hence there is respiratory muscle fatigue. Therefore patients with respiratory muscle fatigue present with qi deficiency of both the Lung and Spleen. This manifests as short and forceless breathing, panting accompanied by poor appetite, emaciation, even all the skin and bones, and repetitively external contractions; and an insufficiency of the original qi, such as intolerance of cold, lumbar soreness and knee weakness, poor appetite, sloppy or hard stools, abdominal distention, poor digestion, and acral coldness.

    We observed the maximal inspiratory pressure (MIP) and the maximal expiratory pressure (MEP) in three groups of COPD patients. The results were as followed. In the patients with Lung qi deficiency, MIP is lower and MEP is normal; while in the patients with Spleen qi deficiency and Kidney qi deficiency, both MIP and MEP were lower, especially in the patients with Kidney qi deficiency. This suggests that, viewed from the angle of respiratory muscle function, the changes from Lung qi deficiency to Kidney qi deficiency is a process of gradual aggravation of the condition. Therefore qi deficiency of the Lung, Spleen and Kidney is closely associated with the degree of respiratory muscle fatigue.

To treat respiratory muscle fatigue with Chinese Medicine, we emphasize the reinforcement of the gathering qi, putting focus on tonifying the qi of the Lung and Spleen, and assisting by warming the Kidney. The common types of patterns seen in clinic are as follows:

(1) Lung, Spleen, and Kidney Deficiency, Phlegm-Stasis Obstruction in the Lung

This type usually appears in the acute exacerbation and persistent phases.

Manifestations: cough, panting, dyspnea, gasping with the shoulders raised, aggravation upon exertion, excessive sticky sputum, chest oppression, a dry mouth, cyanosis of the lips and nails, normal appetite, a dark red or slightly dark tongue with a yellowish, white, thick and greasy coating, and a deficient slippery rapid pulse that is forceless when pressed heavily.

Treatment: Simultaneously tonify deficiency and eliminate obstruction.

Prescriptions: *Bǔ Zhōng Yì Qì Tāng* (补中益气汤), *Shēng Mài Sǎn* (生脉散), *Dìng Chuǎn Tāng* (定喘汤), *Wǔ Zǐ Píng Chuǎn Tāng* (五子平喘汤), *Wěi Jīng Tāng* (苇茎汤), or *Guì Zhī Fú Líng Wán* (桂枝茯苓丸). Select the prescriptions according to the severity of the condition.

(2) Sinking of the Gathering Qi

Manifestation: forceless cough, panting, sinking of qi, breathlessness, panting induced by physical exertion, a faded and weak voice, palpitations or fearful palpitations, spontaneous sweating, fatigue and weakness, emaciation, poor appetite, abdominal distention, bowel movements and urination without strength, a pale tongue with a white coating, and a deep and weak pulse that is forceless when pressed heavily.

Treatment: Tonify qi and lift sinking.

Prescriptions: *Bǔ Zhōng Yì Qì Tāng* (补中益气汤) with modifications.

(3) Deficiency of Both Yin and Yang

This type usually appears in *chuǎn tuō* (喘脱 , panting collapse) and cases of severe respiratory muscle fatigue.

Manifestations: breathlessness, panting induced by physical exertion, cough and expectoration, chest oppression, a pale complexion, a dry mouth with no desire to drink, poor appetite and digestion, tidal fever, palpitations or fearful palpitations, insomnia and dream-disturbing sleep, vexation and agitation, tremor of the limbs, profuse sweating, weak and cold limbs, especially the lower limbs, frequent urination, a dark, pale and tender tongue, and a wiry, slippery, weak and rapid pulse that fades when pressed heavily.

Treatment: Tonify qi and astringe yin, settle counterflow and stop panting.

Prescriptions: *Shēn Zhě Zhèn Qì Tāng* (参赭镇气汤) and *Sì Nì Tāng* (四逆汤). The ingredients are *shú fù zǐ* (Radix Aconiti Lateralis Praeparata), *gān cǎo* (Radix et Rhizoma Glycyrrhizae), *gān jiāng* (Rhizoma Zingiberis), *zhě shí* (Haematitum), *huái shān* (Rhizoma Dioscoreae), *shān yú ròu* (Fructus Corni), *qiàn shí* (Semen Euryales), *lóng gǔ* (Os Draconis), *mǔ lì* (Concha Ostreae), *sū zǐ* (Fructus Perillae), plus *gāo lì shēn* (Radix Ginseng) 10g (simmered separately and mixed into decoction). *Bǔ Zhōng Yì Qì Tāng* (补中益气汤) can also be used.

Regimen: Take *Shēn Zhě Zhèn Qì Tāng* (参赭镇气汤) plus *Sì Nì Tāng* (四逆汤) first to warm the lower jiao and lift the gathering qi. After two hours, continue to take *Bǔ Zhōng Yì Qì Tāng* (补中益气汤) to nourish and lift the gathering qi.

In short, the pathomechanism of COPD respiratory muscle fatigue has a connection with qi deficiency of the Lung, Spleen and Kidney, and especially depletion and sinking of gathering qi in the thorax. In treatment, the focus should be on tonifying deficiency, especially fortifying the Spleen. *Secret Records of Stone Chamber* (石室秘录 , *Shí Shì Mì Lù*) says: "For the method of treating the Lung, routine treatment is very difficult. One should in turn treat the Spleen, for if the Spleen qi has nourishment, then Earth will generate Metal."

We have made it a principle to "build up earth to generate metal", and have used the self-composed *Jiàn Pí Bú Fèi Chōng Jì* (健脾补肺冲剂), (*dǎng shēn* [Radix Codonopsis], *bái zhú* [Rhizoma Atractylodis Macrocephalae], *fú líng* [Poria], *sāng bái pí* [Cortex Mori], *mài dōng* [Radix Ophiopogonis], and *shān yào* [Rhizoma Dioscoreae]), with *Shēn Mài Zhù Shè Yè* (参麦注射液) 4ml into ST 36 (*zú sān lǐ*). This was done once a day. The result demonstrated that MIP, MEP and FEV_1 improved after treatment, and the clinical effect was satisfactory, with a total effective rate of 81.6%.

3. The Pathogenesis and Treatment of Blood Stasis in COPD

In the development of researches on COPD and the invigoration of blood and transformation of stasis, it has been gradually uncovered that blood stasis is a fundamental link of the pathomechanism of COPD, and it runs through the entire process. Consequently, treatments that invigorate blood and transform stasis are the methods to treat COPD and its complication of pulmonary artery hypertension.

The causes of blood stasis include: 1) Stasis due to phlegm obstruction: The Lung is the container to store phlegm. The phlegm turbidity collects and obstructs the ascending, descending, exiting, and entering movement of qi, so that the Lung qi is depressed and stagnated, and the Heart vessels are not open, thus leading to stasis.

Modern studies have shown that blood stasis patterns in Lung disease are characterized by a decrease of hemorrheologic indexes, an increase of blood coagulability, a disturbance of microcirculation, pulmonary hypertension, etc.. 2) Stasis due to qi deficiency: In a prolonged disease of cough and panting, the Lung qi is deficient and damaged, and it fails to permeate into the Heart and converge all the vessels so as to assist the Heart in propelling blood flow. The gathering qi is a combination of the clear qi inhaled by the Lung and the essential qi of water and grain transported up to the Lung by the Spleen. Therefore Lung qi deficiency will lead to gathering qi deficiency, and further affects normal blood flow in the vessels. 3) Stasis due to yang deficiency: The Lung qi deficiency leads to yang qi deficiency in the thorax, which over time may involve the Spleen and Kidney. Yang deficiency of the Spleen and Kidney gives rise to a decline of yang qi, and then the Heart loses its warmth. Thus the Heart fails to propel blood flow in the vessels, and as a result stasis forms. Chinese medicinals that invigorate blood and transform stasis can expand blood vessels, dredge stagnation to improve microcirculation, increase hemoperfusion volume of the lung tissues, and thus relieve pathological changes. Adding Chinese medicinals that invigorate blood and transform stasis in various prescriptions can increase the curative effect in treating COPD. These medicinals include *táo rén* (Semen Persicae), *dān shēn* (Radix et Rhizoma Salviae Miltiorrhizae), *dāng guī* (Radix Angelicae Sinensis), *guì zhī* (Ramulus Cinnamomi Cassiae), *dà huáng* (Radix et Rhizoma Rhei), *chì sháo* (Radix Paeoniae Rubra), *chuān xiōng* (Rhizoma Chuanxiong), *fáng jǐ* (Radix Stephaniae Tetrandrae), *máo dōng qīng* (Radix Ilicis Pubescentis). In addition, ligustrazine (the extract of *chuān xiōng* [Rhizoma Chuanxiong]), *Dān Shēn Zhù Shè Yè* (丹参注射液) and Ilexonin A (the extract of *máo dōng qīng* [Radix Ilicis Pubescentis]) have been extensively used to lower the pulmonary hypertension of COPD, with a notable effect.

4. Pay attention to opening the *Fu* Organs, Draining Heat, and Downbearing the Lung to Calm Panting

According to the *zang-fu* theory of Chinese medicine, the Lung is internally-externally correlated with the Large Intestine. These two organs have a close physiological and pathological relationship and interact with each other. In the acute stage of COPD, especially for the types of phlegm-heat and phlegm clouding the mental orifices, Lung heat is transmitted to the Large Intestine, and the heat generates dryness. Thus there are often blockages of *fu* qi and stagnation of Lung qi. This is characterized by chest oppression, abdominal distention, and constipation. In this case, the illness of the Lung affects the Large Intestine, resulting in diseases of both of the correlated *zang-fu* organs. Because the dry-heat in the Large Intestine cannot be purged downward, the Lung qi will fail in its diffusion and descent. These two aspects influence each other to form a vicious cycle. Modern medicine has proved that hypoxia, carbon dioxide retention, and heart failure can cause gastrointestinal congestion, dysfunction of the digestive tract, decreased enterokinesic function, and destruction of intestinal mucosa, and even ulcers of alimentary canal. This creates fermentation and putrefaction in the intestines, abdominal distention and constipation, etc.. Abdominal distention can influence the upward and downward movement of the diaphragmatic muscles, thus leading to limitation of respiratory movement, dyspnea, and aggravation of pulmonary infections. The obstructed drainage of toxins in the intestinal tract will cause deterioration and general toxic symptoms, as well as pulmonary encephalopathy and DIC. Therefore clearance of the intestinal tract achieves the purpose of diffusing the upper jiao through purging the lower jiao, and is an important link in the treatment of COPD. Nevertheless, the application of purgation must be based on pattern differentiation, or if there is an indication to purge while treating

COPD, otherwise a mistaken treatment can easily occur. For phlegm-heat obstructing the Lung, with dry and hard stools, add *dà huáng* (Radix et Rhizoma Rhei), and *máng xiāo* (Natrii Sulfas). For loose stools with unsmooth defecation or abdominal distention, add *dà huáng* (Radix et Rhizoma Rhei), *máng xiāo* (Natrii Sulfas), and *zhǐ shí* (Fructus Aurantii Immaturus). For constipation accompanied by sticky sputum, add *Měng Shí Gǔn Tán Wán* (礞石滚痰丸). For constipation due to yin deficiency, caused by a failure of the Lung to diffuse and descend, leading to a disorder of body fluid distribution so that the Large Intestine cannot be moistened, add *shēng dì huáng* (Radix Rehmanniae Glutinosae), *mài mén dōng* (Radix Ophiopogonis), *xuán shēn* (Radix Scrophulariae), *huǒ má rén* (Fructus Cannabis), *yù lǐ rén* (Semen Pruni), *bǎi zǐ rén* (Semen Platycladi), and *táo rén* (Semen Persicae). Bitter and cold natured medicinals with purging actions and side effects that damage the yin should be avoided.

Summary

In recent years, there have been considerable researches within Chinese medicine on the clinical practice and mechanism of treating COPD. Certain clinical affects have been achieved. However, there are a few reports on treating COPD during the acute attack stage with single Chinese medicinals. Most Chinese medicinals are used along side comprehensive biomedical therapy, and the effect is better than that of routine treatment with only biomedicine. For COPD during the remission stage, Chinese medicinals have good results in stopping its progression and aggravation, and improving and increasing patient's quality of life. The advantages of Chinese medicinals in treating COPD include regulating the functions of immune and endocrine systems, improving microcirculation, affecting anti-inflammation and spasmolysis, exerting antitussive and expectorant actions, and improving nutritional status. It has been reported that the effective mechanism of Chinese medicinals in treating COPD consists of inhibiting inflammatory cells and mediators, decreasing airway hyper-reactivity and pulmonary hypertension, improving pulmonary ventilation functions and blood circulation, and adjusting organic immunity. The unique superiority of Chinese medicine has been shown for the treatment of COPD. However at the present time, researches into new substances of Chinese medicine and their ability to treat the respiratory system shows that the absolute majority can be used to treat diseases like upper respiratory infections, bronchitis, and bronchial asthma. Yet researches on COPD are still in the beginning stages. The key points of studying new species of Chinese medicinals are to establish COPD models that feature Chinese medicine, select appropriate aspects of clinical treatment, formulate standards to assess the patterns, and evaluate the Chinese medicinals. COPD is a gradually progressive disease, so an early prevention is important in the treatment of COPD. With Chinese medicine, the principle of "prevention before a disease arises and treatment before a disease develops" should be fully emphasized. The effects and mechanisms of Chinese medicinals at every stage of COPD should be the focus of researches. The substantial basis of their actions and functions should be thoroughly researched, and Chinese patent medicines should be developed for precise treatment efficacy and convenience in clinical treatment. Chinese medicine can play an active role in the prevention and treatment of COPD.

SELECTED QUOTES FROM CLASSICAL TEXTS

Plain Questions - On the Most Important and Abstruse Issues (素问·至真要大论篇, *Sù Wèn · Zhì Zhēn Yào Dà Lùn Piān*):

"诸气愤郁，皆属于肺。"

"All qi rushing and depression belongs to the Lung."

Plain Questions - On the Most Singularity (素问·大奇论篇, *Sù Wèn ·*

Dà Qì Lùn Piān):

"肺之雍，喘而两胠满。"

"If the Lung channel is stagnated, there will be panting and fullness of both flanks".

Plain Questions - On Genuine - Zang (素问·玉机真脏论篇 , *Sù Wèn · Yù Jī Zhēn Zàng Lùn Piān*):

"秋脉……不及则令人喘，呼吸少气而咳。"

"If the floating pulse ... is weak, there will be panting, shortness of breath and cough."

Miraculous Pivot - On Distention (灵枢·胀论 , *Líng Shū · Zhàng Lùn*):

"肺胀者，虚满而喘咳。"

"As for Lung distention, there is deficiency fullness and panting and cough."

Jing-yue's Complete Works - On Panting and Dyspnea (景岳全书·喘促 , *Jǐng Yuè Quán Shū · Chuǎn Cù*):

"实喘者，气长而有余；虚喘者，气短而不续。实喘者胸胀气粗，声高息涌，膨膨然若不能容，惟呼出为快也。虚喘者，慌张气怯，声低息短，惶惶然若气欲断，提之若不能升，吞之若不相及，劳动则甚，而惟急促似喘，但得引长一息为快也。"

"As for excess panting, the breath is long and in surplus; as for deficiency panting, the breath is short and not continuous. As for excess panting, the chest is distended and the breathing is rough, the sounds are high and the breath is turbulent, it expands as if it cannot be contained, only the exhalation is fast. As for deficiency panting, it is hurried and the breath is timid, the sounds are low and short, there is panic as if the breath is about to cease. Breathing is difficult both in and out which is aggravated upon exertion. Only the shortness of breath apparently indicates panting. It appears that the patient will feel better when there is a drawn out and long breath."

Synopsis of Golden Chamber - Patterns and Treatment on Consumptive Disease of the Lung, Lung Carbuncle, Cough and Dyspnea (金匮要略·肺痿肺痈咳嗽上气病脉证治, *Jīn Guì Yào Lüè · Fèi Wěi Fèi Yōng Ké Sòu Shàng Qì Bìng Mài Zhèng Zhì*):

"上气喘而躁者，属肺胀，欲作风水，发汗则愈。"

"As for shortness of breath and agitation, these belong to Lung distention, which can lead to wind water. Inducing sweating will bring a cure."

Supplement Recipes to Effective Recipes from Renzhai House - Pantig and Cough (仁斋直指附遗方论·喘嗽, *Rén Zhāi Zhí Zhǐ Fù Yí Fāng Lùn · Chuǎn Sòu*):

" 有肺虚寒而喘者；有肺实夹热而喘者；有水气乘肺而喘者……如是等类，皆当审证而主治之。"

"As for Lung deficiency cold and panting; as for Lung excess with heat and panting; as for water qi overwhelming the Lung with panting... and so forth, all should have the pattern identified and treated accordingly."

General Treatise on Causes and Manifestations of All Diseases - Symptoms of Cough, Dyspnea and Shortness of Breath (诸病源候论·咳逆短气候, *Zhū Bìng Yuán Hòu Lùn · Ké Nì Duǎn Qì Hòu*):

"肺虚为微寒所伤则咳嗽，嗽则气还于肺间则肺胀，肺胀则气逆，而肺本虚，气为不足，复为邪所乘，壅否不能宣畅，故逆短乏气也。"

"If there is Lung deficiency and slight cold then the damage will cause cough; cough then the qi in the Lungs is trapped and causes distention. Lung distention leads to qi counterflow. The Lung is original deficiency and qi is not sufficient, again evils assail, then causing obstruction and no diffusing and opening, therefore there is counterflow and short breathing."

General Treatise on Causes and Manifestations of All Diseases - Symptoms of Dyspnea and Wheezing (诸病源候论·上气鸣息候, *Zhū Bìng Yuán Hòu Lùn · Shàng Qì Míng Xī Hòu*):

"肺主于气，邪乘于肺则肺胀，胀则肺管不利，不利则气道涩，故上气喘逆，鸣息不通。"

"The Lung governs qi. Evils assail the Lung, then there is Lung distention presenting with unsmooth Lung airway. Therefore there is shortness of breath and counterflow, and the breath sounds obstructed."

Necessary Readings of Medicine - Panting (医宗必读·喘, *Yī Zōng Bì Dú · Chuǎn*):

"治实者攻之即效，无所难也。治虚者补之未必即效，须悠久成功，其间转折进退，良非易也。故辨证不可不急，而辨喘为尤急也。"

"As for treating excess, attacking immediately brings results, without difficulty. As for treating deficiency, tonfication does not necessarily bring results, and it should take a long time to have effects, for during that time there are changes and advances and retreats as the disease changes. Therefore, excess-deficiency dierentiatetion is much more urgent than pattern differentiation."

Necessary Readings of Medicine - Cough (医宗必读·咳嗽, *Yī Zōng Bì Dú · Ké Sòu*):

"肺胀嗽而上气，鼻扇抬肩，脉浮大者，越婢加半夏汤主之，无外邪而内虚之肺胀，宜诃子、海藻、香附、瓜蒌仁、青黛、半夏、杏仁、姜汁为末，蜜调噙之。"

"For Lung distention with cough and dyspnea, flaring nose with the shoulders rising up, and a floating and large pulse, *Yuè Bì Jiā Bàn Xià*

Tāng (越婢加半夏汤) is effective. For Lung distention due to internal deficiency with no external evil, the remedy should be *hē zǐ* (Fructus Terminaliae), *hǎi zǎo* (Herba Sargassi), *xiāng fù* (Rhizoma Cyperi), *guā lóu rén* (Semen Trichosanthis), *qīng dài* (Indigo Naturalis), *bàn xià* (Rhizoma Pinelliae), *xìng rén* (Armeniacae Semen Amarum), and *jiāng zhī* (juice of Rhizoma Zingiberis Recens). The medicinals are ground into a powder, and then mixed with honey. It is taken by melting one in the mouth."

Compendium of Patterns: Panting (诸证提纲·喘证, *Zhū Zhèng Tí Gāng · Chuǎn Zhèng*):

"凡喘至于汗出如油，则为肺喘，而汗出发润，则为肺绝……气雍上逆而喘，兼之直视谵语，脉促或伏，手足厥逆乃阴阳相背，为死证。"

"In general, if panting is with sweating like oil, then this is Lung panting, and if excessive sweats comes out dripping wet, then this is Lung exhaustion... if the panting is from qi counterflow, with staring eyes and delirious speech, an urgent or hidden pulse, and severe coldness of hands and feet, then yin and yang are separating, and there will be death."

Luo's Convention and Mirror of Medicine: On Panting, Dyspnea and Wheezing (罗氏会约医镜·论喘、促、哮三证, *Luó Shì Huì Yuē Yī Jìng · Lùn Chuǎn, Cù, Xiào Sān Zhèng*):

"三证相似，而实不同。须清析方可调治。喘者，气急声高，张口抬肩，摇身撷肚，惟呼出一息为快。……促者，即经之所谓短气者也，呼吸虽急，而不能接续，似喘而无声，亦不抬肩，劳动则甚，此肾经元气虚也……。哮者，其病似喘，但不如喘出气之多，而有呀呷之音。"

"The three patterns appear similar, but actually they are different. Therefore one must clearly analyze them and then administer the treatment. As for panting, with short breathing that is anxious and with a high sound, an open mouth and lifting shoulders, body shakes and abdominal inflation. It appears that only there is a drawn out and long breath can the patient will feel better... As for urgency, as called in the classics is shortness of breath, although the breathing is urgent, it is not continuous, and it is similar to panting but without sound, and without shoulders lifting. It is aggravated upon exertion, and this is deficiency of the Kidney channel's original qi... As for wheezing, this disease is similar to panting, but with less exhalations, and the sounds of inhalation and exhalation".

Recipes Worth a Thousand Gold - Deficiency and Excess in Lung Distention (千金要方·肺胀·肺虚实 , *Qiān Jīn Yào Fāng · Fèi Zàng · Fèi Xū Shí*):
"右手寸口气口以前脉阴实者,手太阴经也,病苦肺胀汗出,若露上气喘,咽中塞,如欲呕状,名曰肺实热也。"
"As for yin-excess pulse before the *cun* position of the right wrist, its pattern belongs to hand Taiyin channel, and the patient has Lung distention and sweating, and if there is dyspnea, panting, obstructed swallowing and seemingly have a desire to vomit, this is called Lung excess heat."

Dan-xi's Mastery of Medicine - Cough (丹溪心法·咳嗽 , *Dān Xī Xīn Fǎ · Ké Sòu*):
"肺胀而嗽,或左或右,不得眠,此痰夹瘀血碍气而病。"
"Lung distention with cough, and an inability to lie down on either the left or right side, this is a disease of phlegm with static blood obstructing the qi."

Treatment Based on Symptoms, Etiology and Pulse - On Panting (症因脉治·喘证论 , *Zhèng Yīn Mài Zhì · Chuǎn Zhèng Lùn*):
"肺胀之因,内有郁结,先伤肺气,外复感邪,肺气不得发泄,则肺胀作矣。"

"The cause of Lung distention is internal depression and binding that first damages the Lung qi, and there are external repeated contractions of evils, so that the Lung qi cannot be vented, and then there is Lung distention."

Records of Traditional Chinese Medicine and Biomedicine in Combination-Formulas for Treating Panting (医学衷中参西录·治喘息方·咳嗽, *Yī Xué Zhōng Zhōng Cān Xī Lù · Zhì Chuǎn Xī Fāng · Ké Sòu*):

"心有病可以累肺作喘，此说诚信而有证……由是言之，心累肺作喘之证，亦即肾虚不纳气之证也。"

"If the Heart has disease it can wear out the Lung and cause panting, this is actually and reliably... from this, is a pattern of the Heart wearing out the Lung and causing panting, namely it is a pattern of Kidney deficiency not receiving the qi."

Compilation and Supplement to Diagnosis and Treatment - On Cough (证治汇补·咳嗽, *Zhèng Zhì Huì Bǔ · Ké Sòu*):

"如痰夹瘀血，宜养血以流动乎气，降火以利其痰，用四物汤加桃仁、枳壳、陈皮、瓜蒌、竹沥。又风寒郁于肺中，不得发越，喘嗽胀闷者，宜发汗以祛邪，利肺以顺气，用麻黄越婢加半夏汤。有停水不化，肺气不得下降者，其症水入即吐，宜四苓散加葶苈、桔梗、桑皮、石膏。有肾虚水枯，肺金不敢下降而胀者，其症干咳、烦冤，宜六味丸加麦冬、五味。又有气散而胀者，宜补肺，气逆而胀者，宜降气，当参虚实而施治。"

"For cough due to phlegm mixed with blood stasis, use the methods of nourishing blood to promote qi flow, and descending fire to disinhibit phlegm. Select *Sì Wù Tāng* (四物汤) plus *táo rén* (Semen Persicae), *zhǐ qiào* (Fructus Aurantii), *chén pí* (Pericarpium Citri Reticulatae), *guā lóu* (Fructus Trichosanthis), and *zhú lì* (Succus Bambusae). For panting, cough, oppression and fullness of the chest due to accumulation of wind-cold in the Lung, use the methods of promoting sweating to expel evils, and disinhibit the Lung to downbear qi. Use *Má Huáng Yuè Bì Jiā Bàn Xià Tāng* (麻黄越婢加半夏汤). For a failure of the Lung qi to descend due to water amassing and not transforming, which is characterized by vomiting upon drinking, prescribe *Sì Líng Sǎn* (四苓散) plus *tíng lì* (Semen Lepidii seu Descurainiae), *jié gěng* (Radix Platycodonis), *sāng pí* (Cortex Mori), and *shí gāo* (Gypsum Fibrosum). For Lung distention due to a failure of the Lung qi to descend with Kidney deficiency and fluid exhaustion, characterized by dry cough and restlessness, use *Liù Wèi Wán* (六味丸) plus *mài dōng* (Radix Ophiopogonis), and *wǔ wèi* (Fructus Schisandrae Chinensis). One should identify excess or deficiency to determine treatment. For Lung distention due to qi scattering, one should tonify the Lung. For Lung distention due to qi counterflow, one should downbear qi. Thus all the treatments should be based upon the differentiation of excess from deficiency."

Zhang's Treatise on General Medicine - Lung Wilting (张氏医通 · 肺痿, *Zhāng Shì Yī Tōng · Fèi Wěi*):

"肺胀而发其汗，即《内经》开鬼门之法，一汗而令风邪外泄于肌表。水无风战，自顺趋而从下出也。咳而上气，此为肺胀，其人喘，目如脱状，脉浮大者，越婢加半夏汤主之。肺胀，咳而上气，烦躁而咳，脉浮者，心下有水气，小青龙加石膏汤主之。……上气面浮动肩，其脉浮大，不治。又加利，尤甚。……肺胀而咳，左右不得卧，此夹瘀血碍气而胀，当归、丹皮、赤芍、桃仁、枳壳、桔梗、半夏、甘草、竹沥、姜汁。如外邪去后，宜半夏、海石、香附、瓜蒌、甘草为末，姜汁蜜调噙之。"

"For Lung distention with sweating, the *Inner Canon* (内经, *Nèi Jīng*) says to open the ghost gates (pores) to induce sweating. Sweating can cause the wind evil to drain to the exterior flesh. Water is nothing without wind to battle; on its own it will quickly drain from the lower jiao. As for cough with dyspnea, this is Lung distention. The patient has cough, and the eyes stare as if about to leave the sockets, and the pulse is floating and large, then *Yuè Bì Jiā Bàn Xià Tāng* (越婢加半夏汤) governs. As for cough with vexation and agitation, and a floating pulse, under the Heart there is water qi, then *Xiǎo Qīng Lóng Jiā Shí Gāo Tāng* (小青龙加石膏汤) governs. … If there is dyspnea accompanied by shrugging of the shoulders, and a floating and large pulse, it is difficult to treat; if there occurs diarrhea, the condition would be more serious. …For Lung distention with cough, and inability to lie down on either the left or right side, that is caused by obstruction of qi by phlegm and stagnant blood, use *dāng guī* (Radix Angelicae Sinensis), *dān pí* (Cortex Moutan), *chì sháo* (Radix Paeoniae Rubra), *táo rén* (Semen Persicae), *zhǐ qiào* (Fructus Aurantii), *jié gěng* (Radix Platycodonis), *bàn xià* (Rhizoma Pinelliae), *gān cǎo* (Radix et Rhizoma Glycyrrhizae), *zhú lì* (Succus Bambusae), and *jiāng zhī* (juice of Rhizoma Zingiberis Recens). If the external evils have been eliminated, prescribe *bàn xià* (Rhizoma Pinelliae), *hǎi shí* (Os Costaziae), *xiāng fù* (Rhizoma Cyperi), *guā lóu* (Fructus Trichosanthis), and *gān cǎo* (Radix et Rhizoma Glycyrrhizae). Grind the medicinals into a powder, then mix them with honey, and take by melting one in the mouth."

Exposition on Source and Course of Miscellaneous Diseases - Origin and Development on Lung Diseases (杂病源流犀烛·肺病源流, *Zá Bìng Yuán Líu Xī Zhú · Fèi Bìng Yuán Liú*):

"肺胀本为肺经气分之病，故宜以收敛为主，宜诃子青黛丸、清化丸；即夹痰夹血者，亦不离乎气，不得专议血专议痰也。"

"The root of Lung distention is a Lung channel qi phase disease. Therefore should primarily astringe and contain. Use *Hē Zǐ Qīng Dài Wán* (诃子青黛丸) and *Qīng Huà Wán* (清化丸). Even if the illness is mixed with phlegm and stagnant blood, it is still a disorder associated with qi. It cannot be treated only from the aspect of phlegm and stagnant blood."

MODERN RESEARCH

Clinical Research

Within the field of Chinese medicine, it is so far generally believed that the pathogenesis of COPD is deficiency of the root and excess of the branch. The deficiency of the root is due to deficiency of the Lung, Spleen and Kidney. The excess in the branch is due to wind (cold), heat, and phlegm mixed with blood stasis. In any of the pathological stages of COPD, the deficiency of the Lung, Spleen and Kidney is the most essential, and the turbid phlegm and static blood is significant. Chinese medicinal remedies are all based on the recognition of deficiency of the root and excess of the branch, and they focus on both supporting the right qi and eliminating evils. Eliminating evils is often focused on during the acute stage, and supporting the right qi often focused on during the stable stage.

1. Pattern Differentiation and Corresponding Treatment

(1) Treatment during the Acute Aggravation Stage

1) Phlegm-stasis obstructing the Lung type or Phlegm-heat depressed in the Lung type

In the acute aggravation stage of COPD, the pathomechanism is phlegm and qi mutually bound with obstruction of phlegm, and heat and blood stasis in the Lung. Therefore the treatment should be to invigorate blood, transform stasis, clear the Lung, and transform phlegm. Cui Yan et al.[1] treated COPD during the acute aggravation stage with *Huó Xuè Huà Yū Fāng* (活血化瘀方). The ingredients were *dān shēn* (Radix et Rhizoma Salviae Miltiorrhizae) 30g, *táo rén* (Semen Persicae) 15g, *chì sháo* (Radix Paeoniae Rubra) 20g, *chuān xiōng* (Rhizoma Chuanxiong) 20g, *hóng huā*

(Flos Carthami) 10g, *tíng lì zǐ* (Semen Lepidii seu Descurainiae) 20g, *dāng guī* (Radix Angelicae Sinensis) 15g, and *yì mǔ cǎo* (Herba leonuri) 30g, with modifications according to pattern differentiation. In comparison with the control group, the results were all very satisfactory in terms of the improvement of symptoms, clinical effects, and the improvement of pulmonary function. The formula also reduced blood viscosity. Shi Ke-hua et al.[2] used the treatment methods of clearing the Lung, transforming phlegm, invigorating blood, fortifying the Spleen, and eliminating dampness to treat COPD belonging to the pattern phlegm and stasis mutually bound in the Lung or phlegm-heat depressed in the Lung. The treatment had actions of clearing the Lung, transforming phlegm, and invigorating blood. It was composed of *sāng bái pí* (Cortex Mori) 15g, *bèi mǔ* (Bulbus Fritillariae) 15g, *fú líng* (Poria) 15g, *zǐ sū zǐ* (Fructus Perillae) 15g, *nán shā shēn* (Radix Adenophorae) 15g, *táo rén* (Semen Persicae) 15g, *dān shēn* (Radix et Rhizoma Salviae Miltiorrhizae) 15g, *huáng qín* (Radix Scutellariae) 9g, *gān cǎo* (Radix et Rhizoma Glycyrrhizae) 9g, *jīn qiáo mài gēn* (Rhizoma Fagopyri Dibotryis) 30g, *yú xīng cǎo* (Herba Houttuyniae) 30g, *yì yǐ rén* (Semen Coicis) 30g, *chén pí* (Pericarpium Citri Reticulatae) 12g, and *hòu pò* (Cortex Magnoliae) 12g. He combined this formula with biomedical anti-infection medication. In comparison with the group treated only with biomedicine, the symptoms of cough, expectoration and panting were markedly relieved, the PaO_2 and $PaCO_2$ in the arterial blood were noticeably improved, and the hematocrit was clearly decreased. Li Su-yun et al.[3] used *Tōng Sè Kē Lì* (通塞颗粒) to treat elderly patients with a phlegm heat depressed in the Lung type of COPD. It was composed of *tíng lì zǐ* (Semen Lepidii seu Descurainiae), *dì lóng* (Lumbricus), *chì sháo* (Radix Paeoniae Rubra), *chuān bèi mǔ* (Bulbus Fritillariae Cirrhosae), *shēng shài shēn* (Radix Ginseng), *mài dōng* (Radix Ophiopogonis), *zhì má huáng* (Herba Ephedrae Praeparata), *zhì dà huáng* (Radix et Rhizoma Rhei Praeparata), and *shí chāng pú* (Rhizoma Acori Tatarinowii), in 1g (1 granule = 5.78g of crude medicinals). After treatment, the levels of serum collagen Ⅰ, Ⅲ and Ⅳ, soluble intercellular adhesion molecule-1, and selectin-E decreased markedly. These results suggested that reducing the levels of extracellular matrix and adhesion molecules may be one of the main mechanisms for *Tōng Sè Kē Lì* (通塞颗粒) to treat elderly patients with COPD.

2) Qi deficiency, blood stasis and phlegm obstruction type

According to the pathomechanisms of qi deficiency, blood stasis and phlegm obstruction that cause COPD pulmonary hypertension, Zhang Li-shan et al.[4] used *Fèi Kāng Fāng* (肺康方) decoction to treat 30 patients with COPD pulmonary hypertension during the acute aggravation stage. The ingredients were *shēng huáng qí* (Radix Astragali) 30g, *shān zhū yú* (Fructus Corni) 15g, *dān shēn* (Radix et Rhizoma Salviae Miltiorrhizae) 12g, *tíng lì zǐ* (Semen Lepidii seu Descurainiae) 15g, *Dài Gé Sǎn* (黛蛤散) 12g (wrapped), *shuǐ zhì* (Hirudo) 3g, and *bái qián* (Radix et Rhizoma Cynanchi Stauntonii) 10g. The total effective rate was 83.33%, and clinical symptoms were markedly improved. In addition, the formula was also able to adjust the balance between blood vessel endothelin and calcitonin gene-related peptide, decrease pulmonary hypertension, improve pulmonary ventilation function, correct anoxia, and decrease blood viscosity.

3) The type of yin cold internally blocking

Lin Jian[5] used *Yáng Hé Tāng* (阳和汤) with modifications to treat COPD belonging to the type of yin cold internally blocking, with a failure of the Lung to diffuse. Its ingredients are *shú dì* (Radix Rehmanniae Glutinosae Praeparata) 15g, *lù jiǎo jiāo/ shuāng* (Colla Cornus Cervi or Cornu Cervi Degelatinatum) 10g, *bái jiè zǐ* (Semen Sinapis Albae) 10g, *ròu guì* (Cortex Cinnamomi) (ground into powder and swallowed) 3g, *pào jiāng* (Rhizoma Zingiberis Praeparatum) 3g, *gān cǎo* (Radix et Rhizoma Glycyrrhizae) 6g, and *má huáng* (Herba Ephedrae) 6g. For cases of excessive sputum and serious dyspnea, he added *sū zǐ* (Fructus Perillae) 10g and *lái fú zǐ* (Semen Raphani) 10g. For cases of qi deficiency of the Lung and Spleen, he added *dǎng shēn* (Radix Codonopsis) 20g and *huáng qí* (Radix Astragali) 30g. For cases with a dark purple tongue, he added *táo rén* (Semen Persicae) 12g and *dān shēn* (Radix et Rhizoma Salviae Miltiorrhizae) 20g. The remedy was given for 2 courses of treatment, 15 days per course. Compared with the group treated only with biomedicine, it was able to increase the total effective rate.

(2) Treatment during the Stable Stage

Common patterns during the stable stage of COPD include deficiency of the Lung, Spleen and Kidney, and deficiency of both qi and yin. The treatments are to tonify the Lung, fortify the Spleen and boost the Kidney, or boost qi and nourish yin.

1) Tonify the Lung, fortify the Spleen, and boost the Kidney

Li Su-yun et al.[6] used *Bǔ Fèi Yì Shèn Kē Lì* (补肺益肾颗粒) to treat COPD of Lung and Kidney qi deficiency type. It was composed of *rén shēn* (Radix Ginseng), *huáng qí* (Radix Astragali), *bái zhú* (Rhizoma Atractylodis Macrocephalae), *fáng fēng* (Radix Saposhnikoviae), *mài mén dōng* (Radix Ophiopogonis), *wǔ wèi zǐ* (Fructus Schisandrae Chinensis), *bǔ gǔ zhī* (Fructus Psoraleae), *gé jiè* (Gecko), *shān zhū yú* (Fructus Corni), *dōng chóng xià cǎo* (Cordyceps Sinensis), *chén xiāng* (Lignum Aquilariae Resinatum), *lú jīng* (Coulis Phragmitis), *quán xiē* (Scorpio), *xìng rén* (Armeniacae Semen Amarum), *zhè bèi mǔ* (Bulbus Fritillariae Thunbergii), and *chuān xiōng* (Rhizoma Chuanxiong). The formula was able to decrease the serum level of collagen Ⅰ, Ⅲ, and Ⅳ of the patients, suggesting that the medicinals could tonify the Lung, boost the Kidney, invigorate blood, and transform stasis so as to relieve chronic inflammation of the airway during the remission stage of COPD. It was also able to adjust metabolism of collagen. Zheng Hong et al.[7] treated

COPD during the stable stage according to the pattern differentiation. For Lung qi deficiency, he used *tài zǐ shēn* (Radix Pseudostellariae) 30g, *huáng qí* (Radix Astragali) 30g, *bǎi hé* (Bulbus Lilii) 30g, *wǔ wèi zǐ* (Fructus Schisandrae Chinensis) 20g, and a pair of *gé jiè* (Gecko) (about 10g). For type of Spleen yang deficiency, he used *huáng qí* (Radix Astragali) 30g, *dǎng shēn* (Radix Codonopsis) 30g, *yún líng* (Poria) 30g, *bái zhú* (Rhizoma Atractylodis Macrocephalae) 20g, *gān jiāng* (Rhizoma Zingiberis) 15g, and *dà zǎo* (Fructus Ziziphi Jujubae) 10 pieces (about 20g). For type of Kidney yang deficiency, he used *shān yú ròu* (Fructus Corni) 30g, *yún líng* (Poria) 30g, *zé xiè* (Rhizoma Alismatis) 15g, *shú dì* (Radix Rehmanniae Glutinosae Praeparata) 30g, *ròu guì* (Cortex Cinnamomi) 10g, *fù zǐ* (Radix Aconiti Lateralis Praeparata) 10g, *xiān líng pí* (Herba Epimedii) 15g, *máo gēn* (Rhizoma Imperatae Cylindricae) 30g, and *yuǎn zhì* (Radix Polygalae) 15g. After treatment, the scores of St. George's respiratory questionaire (SGRQ) were all improved, and the improved levels were obviously higher than those of the control group. The level of sputum IL-8 was lower than before treatment ($P<0.05$); while the ratio of FEV_1/FVC was higher than before treatment and higher than the control group's ($P<0.05$). Through the treatment of a whole winter, there were obvious improvements in both of the groups, in both the degree and frequency of attacks, the frequency of catching colds, and the average time of interval and persistence of attack ($P<0.01$). The results of the treatment group were better than that of the control group ($P<0.05$).

2) Boost qi and nourish yin

Ji Hong-yan et al.[8] used a method of boosting qi and nourishing yin to treat COPD with malnutrition during the remission stage. This type of COPD belongs to a Chinese medicine pattern of deficiency of both qi and yin, with turbid phlegm and stasis. The ingredients of formula were *fǎ bàn xià* (Rhizoma Pinelliae Praeparatum) 10g, *yún líng* (Poria) 10g, *chuān xiōng* (Rhizoma Chuanxiong) 6g, *chǎo èr yá* (Fructus Setariae Germinatus Tostum and Fructus Hordei Germinatus Tostum) 10g, *bǎi hé* (Bulbus Lilii) 20g, *shān yào* (Rhizoma Dioscoreae) 30g, *nán shā shēn* (Radix Adenophorae) 30g, *fó shǒu* (Fructus Citri Sarcodactylis) 10g, *shān zhā* (Fructus Crataegi) 15g, *jīn fèi cǎo* (Herba Inulae) 10g, and *dà bèi* (Bulbus Fritillariae Thunbergii) 10g. It was taken orally five days per week, for three months. Compared with the control group, the body weight and quality of life of the patients in the Chinese medicinal group had increased; while the chance of respiratory infection had decreased. For six months, Wu Qi-biao et al.[9] used methods of boosting qi, nourishing yin, invigorating blood, and transforming phlegm to treat COPD patients during the stable stage. The formula was composed of *rén shēn* (Radix Ginseng), *huáng qí* (Radix Astragali), *shān yào* (Rhizoma Dioscoreae), *fáng fēng* (Radix Saposhnikoviae), *mài dōng* (Radix Ophiopogonis), *wěi jīng* (Phragmites), *dān shēn* (Radix et Rhizoma Salviae Miltiorrhizae), *táo rén* (Semen Persicae), *quán guā lóu* (Fructus Trichosanthis), and *zhè bèi mǔ* (Bulbus Fritillariae Thunbergii). Both the cellular and humoral immune functions of the patients were enhanced and regulated.

3) Boost qi, invigorate blood and transform phlegm

Feng Cui-ling[10] used methods of boosting qi, invigorating blood, and transforming phlegm to treat COPD with qi deficiency, blood stasis, and phlegm obstruction. Based on biomedical treatment methods, she prescribed a formula to boost qi, invigorate blood, and transform phlegm. The ingredients were *huáng qí* (Radix Astragali) 10g, *shuǐ zhì* (Hirudo) 6g, *bèi mǔ* (Bulbus Fritillariae) 10g, *guǎng dì lóng* (Lumbricus) 6g plus *Bǎi Lìng Jiāo Náng* (百令胶囊) (the essential component is the fermented Cordyceps bacterial filament), or *Fèi Kāng Chōng Jì* (肺康冲剂), which is composed of *huáng qí* (Radix Astragali), *shuǐ zhì* (Hirudo), *huáng jīng* (Rhizoma

Polygonati), *dāng guī* (Radix Angelicae Sinensis), *chén pí* (Pericarpium Citri Reticulatae) plus *Bǎi Lìng Jiāo Náng* (百令胶囊). The course of treatment was three months. Compared with the biomedical control group, the symptoms of patients with COPD during the stable stage were improved and the quality of life was elevated.

2. Specific Formulas

(1) *Yǎng Yīn Qīng Fèi Zhú Yū Táng Jiāng* (养阴清肺逐瘀糖浆)

Wang Zhi-gang, et al.[11] treated patients with COPD complicated by pulmonary heart disease with *Yǎng Yīn Qīng Fèi Zhú Yū Táng Jiāng* (养阴清肺逐瘀糖浆). This formula is founded upon medicinals that clear the Lung, and also uses medicinals that invigorate blood and transform stasis. This treatment was carried out along with biomedical treatment. After treatment, patients had obvious improvement in clinical symptoms and platelet activation.

(2) *Zhǐ Ké Qīng Fèi Kǒu Fú Yè* (止咳清肺口服液)

Che Hong-zhu, et al.[12] treated COPD patients during the stable stage with *Zhǐ Ké Qīng Fèi Kǒu Fú Yè* (止咳清肺口服液) for six weeks. This formula was composed of *jīn yín huā* (Flos Lonicerae), *huáng qín* (Radix Scutellariae), *lián qiào* (Fructus Forsythiae), *bǎn lán gēn* (Radix Isatidis), *kuǎn dōng huā* (Flos Farfarae), *zǐ wǎn* (Radix et Rhizoma Asteris), *yú xīng cǎo* (Herba Houttuyniae), *jié gěng* (Radix Platycodonis), *má huáng* (Herba Ephedrae), *pí pa yè* (Folium Eriobotryae), *huáng qí* (Radix Astragali), and *gān cǎo* (Radix et Rhizoma Glycyrrhizae). The results were better than those of conventional therapy in improving clinical symptoms and lung function, and inhibiting chronic airway inflammation.

(3) *Shān Ěr Hé Jì* (山耳合剂)

He Xin, et al.[13] treated COPD with *Shān Ěr Hé Jì* (山耳合剂). The formula was *shān hǎi luó* (Radix Codonopsis Lanceolatae) 15g, *fó ěr cǎo* (Gnaphalium Affine D.Don) 12g, *chē qián cǎo* (Herba Plantaginis) 15g, *yú xīng cǎo* (Herba Houttuyniae) 30g, *yín xìng yè* (Folium Ginkgo) 12g, *shān dòu gēn* (Radix et Rhizoma Sophorae Tonkinensis) 15g, and *gān cǎo* (Radix et Rhizoma Glycyrrhizae) 6g. The above dosage was for one day. The medicinals were decocted with water to 150ml, and divided into three portions, with 50ml taken orally, three times a day. The effect of transforming phlegm and stopping cough was better than that of the brown mixture (compound glycyrrhiza mixture).

(4) *Jǐ Jiāo Lì Huáng Tāng* (己椒苈黄汤) with Additions

Lin Lin, et al.[14] treated patients with COPD pulmonary artery hypertension with *Jǐ Jiāo Lì Huáng Tāng* (己椒苈黄汤) with additions. It was composed of *hàn fáng jǐ* (Radix Stephaniae Tetrandrae), *chuān jiāo mù* (Semen Zanthoxyli Bungeani), *tíng lì zǐ* (Semen Lepidii seu Descurainiae) (decocted first), *zhì dà huáng* (Radix et Rhizoma Rhei Praeparata), *shú fù piàn* (Radix Aconiti Lateralis Praeparata), and *chuān xiōng* (Rhizoma Chuanxiong). The results showed that the total effective rate, decrease in pulmonary pressure, and improvement of clinical symptoms were all better than those of the group that was treated with nifedipine.

(5) *Bǎo Fèi Dìng Chuǎn Chōng Jì* (保肺定喘冲剂)

Based on biomedical treatments, Luo Xian-fang, et al.[15] used *Bǎo Fèi Dìng Chuǎn Chōng Jì* (保肺定喘冲剂) to treat patients with COPD in the chronic persistent stage. This formula has actions to boost qi, invigorate blood, nourish yin, clear the Lung, transform phlegm ,and stop cough, Compared with biomedicinal therapy, these granules can effectually increase arterial partial pressure of oxygen, decrease pulmonary alveolararterial difference of oxygen pressure, and decrease the concentration of plasma endothelin-1.

(6) Qīng Yuán Huà Tán Kē Lì (清源化痰颗粒剂)

Shi Suo-fang, et al.[16] used single-blind, random and matched-pair principles to conduct a clinical research on treatment of acute attack stage of COPD (pattern of a phlegm-heat accumulated in the Lung, with Lung and Spleen qi deficiency) with *Qīng Yuán Huà Tán Kē Lì Jì* (清源化痰颗粒剂). The effects of these granules in improving symptoms, signs, lung function, and pulmonary arterial pressure were better than those of the control group. In addition, it was also able to elevate the level of serum nitric oxide, and decrease the levels of plasma ET-1, serum IL-8 and IL-2R.

(7) Yì Fèi Jiàn Pí Fāng (益肺健脾方)

In addition to conventional treatment methods, Wang Sheng, et al.[17] used *Yì Fèi Jiàn Pí Fāng* (益肺健脾方). This formula was composed of *huáng qí* (Radix Astragali) 30g, *dǎng shēn* (Radix Codonopsis) 15g, *bái zhú* (Rhizoma Atractylodis Macrocephalae) 15g, *fú líng* (Poria) 15g, *fáng fēng* (Radix Saposhnikoviae) 10g, *bàn xià* (Rhizoma Pinelliae) 15g, *chén pí* (Pericarpium Citri Reticulatae) 10g, *dì lóng* (Lumbricus) 8g, *kuǎn dōng huā* (Flos Farfarae) 10g, and *gān cǎo* (Radix et Rhizoma Glycyrrhizae) 10g. Eight weeks was a course of treatment Compared with the group treated only with biomedicine, the effects of the group treated with *Yì Fèi Jiàn Pí Fāng* (益肺健脾方) were better in decreasing the numbers of polymorphonuclear neutrophils (PMN), and the levels of IL-8 and TNF-α in the sputum, and in improving lung function.

(8) Jiàn Pí Yì Fèi Chōng Jì (健脾益肺冲剂)

Lin Lin, et al.[18] treated patients who had respiratory muscle fatigue during the stable stage of COPD with *Jiàn Pǐ Yì Fèi Chōng Jì* (健脾益肺冲剂). The ingredients were *rén shēn* (Radix Ginseng) 20g, *bái zhú* (Rhizoma Atractylodis Macrocephalae) 15g, *fú líng* (Poria) 15g, *mài dōng* (Radix Ophiopogonis) 15g, *sāng bái pí* (Cortex Mori) 15g, and *huáng qí* (Radix Astragali) 10g. The effects were better than those of the control group in terms of symptoms, comprehensive therapeutic effects, lung function, and blood gas analysis.

(9) *Tiáo Bǔ Fèi Shèn Jiāo Náng* (调补肺肾胶囊)

Based on the recognition that dual deficiency of Lung and Kidney is the chief pathomechanism of COPD during the stable stage, Zhang Hong-chun, et al.[19] treated thirty patients with *Tiáo Bǔ Fèi Shèn Jiāo Náng* (调补肺肾胶囊). The effective rate for the therapeutic effects of combined treatment and those of treatment based on Chinese medical patterns are 93.33% and 96.67% respectively. In addition, it also improved shortness of breath and pulmonary ventilation function, increased PaO_2, and decreased $PaCO_2$.

(10) *Jiā Wèi Yòu Guī Wán* (加味右归丸)

Yu Xia, et al.[20] used *Jiā Wèi Yòu Guī Wán* (加味右归丸) to treat the patients with COPD during the stable stage. It was composed of *shú dì* (Radix Rehmanniae Glutinosae Praeparata) 240g, *zhì fù zǐ* (Radix Aconiti Lateralis Praeparata) 60g (decocted first) 120g, *lù jiǎo jiāo* (Colla Cornus Cervi) 120g (melted by heat), *tù sī zǐ* (Semen Cuscutae) 120g, *shān yào* (Rhizoma Dioscoreae) 120g, *shān zhū yú* (Fructus Corni) 90g, *dāng guī* (Radix Angelicae Sinensis) 90g, *ròu guì* (Cortex Cinnamomi) 60g, *gǒu qǐ* (Fructus Lycii) 90g, *dù zhòng* (Cortex Eucommiae) 120g, *huáng qí* (Radix Astragali) 60g, *sān qī* (Radix et Rhizoma Notoginseng) 30g, *zhì má huáng* (Herba Ephedrae Praeparata) 20g, *lì zǐ* (Semen Lepidii seu Descurainiae) 20g, *lái fú zǐ* (Semen Raphani) 20g, *yú xīng cǎo* (Herba Houttuyniae) 20g, *huáng qín* (Radix Scutellariae) 20g, and *zhì gān cǎo* (Radix et Rhizoma Glycyrrhizae Praeparata) 20g. All of the medicinals were crushed and ground into a fine powder, then prepared with honey into 9g pills. One pill was taken three times daily. A course of treatment was one month, and the medication was taken for a total of six courses. If there was an acute episode or complication by other disease during the treatment, symptomatic treatment was given. Compared with the group treated only with biomedicine, this formula elevated the effective rate, and delayed the speed at which the lung function decreased.

3. ACUPUNCTURE AND MOXIBUSTION

(1) Scalp Acupuncture

Ni Wei-min, et al.[21] observed the extent to which scalp acupuncture can improve anoxia in patients of chronic bronchitis during acute stage. According to the *International Standard Scheme for Scalp Acupuncture Acupoints,* they needled the lateral line 1 of forehead (located at the site lateral to the median line of forehead, directly opposite to the medial canthus, 0.5 *cun* above and below the hair line, totally 1 *cun*) bilaterally. They selected four stainless steel needles, 0.30mm in diameter and 25mm in length, and inserted the needles oppositely at the two sides of hair line to form an angle of 15 to 30 degrees with the scalp. The depth of insertion was 1 *cun*. A rotating method was used. After the arrival of qi, they used electroacupuncture apparatus G6805 to carry out electric stimulation (with sparse-dense waves, and a current intensity according to patient tolerance). The needles were retained for thirty minutes. After treatment, compared with the control group, the indexes of heart rate, respiratory frequency, PaO_2, $PaCO_2$, and pH, in the scalp acupuncture group are obviously improved ($P<0.001$); while the indexes of heart rate, PH, $PaCO_2$, and respiratory frequency and PaO_2, in the scalp acupuncture group and medicinal groups are notably improved ($P>0.05$).

(2) Acupuncture plus Chinese Medicinals

Doctor Zhang[22] used *Yì Qì Fú Zhèng Tāng* (益气服正汤), with functions to boost qi, clear heat, transform phlegm, and invigorate blood, plus needling at *dǐng chuǎn*, BL 15 (*xīn shù*), BL 17 (*gé shù*), BL 23 (*shèn shù*), LU 1 (*zhōng fǔ*), LU 5 (*chǐ zé*), LU 6 (*kǒng zuì*), RN 17 (*dàn zhōng*), and RN 4 (*guān yuán*) to treat 288 COPD patients with Spleen and Lung qi deficiency, and phlegm obstruction. The total effective rate was 93.1%. The symptoms of qi deficiency and phlegm obstruction were obviously relieved or completely disappeared, the levels of serum CD_3, CD_4, and CD_8 were markedly increased, and the ratio of CD_4/CD_8 was corrected.

(3) Point Injection

Shi Hong[23] conducted the following study: In the acute attack stage of COPD draw 2ml of *Yú Xīng Cǎo Zhù Shè Yè* (鱼腥草注射液), 2ml of *Chuān Hǔ Níng Zhù Shè Yè* (穿琥宁注射液) and 2ml of vitamin-B_1 injection into a syringe. Choose DU 14 (*dà zhuī*), BL12 (*fēng mén*) (bilaterally), and BL 13 (*fèi shù*) (bilaterally) and, for cases of excessive phlegm, add ST 40 (*fēng lóng*) (bilaterally), and then use the injection needle for acupuncture. After arrival of qi, inject 0.5 – 1ml of the above medicine into every acupoint. In the chronic persistent stage: draw 2ml of *Huáng Qí Zhù Shè Yè* (黄芪注射液), 2ml of *Sī Qí Kāng Zhù Shè Yè* (斯奇康注射液 , Polysaccharide Nucleic Acid Fraction of Bacillus Calmette Guerin for Injection) and 2ml of vitamin-B_1 injection into a syringe. Choose BL 13 (*fèi shù*) (bilaterally), BL 20 (*pí shù*) (bilaterally), BL 23 (*shèn shù*) (bilaterally) and then use the injection needle for acupuncture. After the arrival of qi, every point is injected with 1ml of the medicinals. For the acupuncture group: During the acute attack stage: the points selected were the same as those in the point injection group. After the arrival of qi, drainage method was used, and then the needles were retained for twenty minutes. During the needle-retaining period, the manipulation was performed once every five minutes. During the chronic persistent stage the points selected were the same as those in the point injection group. After the arrival of qi, even supplementation and drainage method was used, and then the needles were retained for twenty minutes. During the needle-retaining period, the manipulation was performed once every five minutes. The clinical therapeutic effect of the point injection group was better than that of the acupuncture group.

(4) Point Application

According to the Chinese medical theory of "treating interior disease with external treatment", Xu Xin-yi, et al.[24] treated 36 COPD patients with their self-composed Chinese medicinal extract *Zhĭ Ké Píng Chuăn Gāo* (止咳平喘膏). They based this treatment on the routine treatment according to the pattern differentiation. *Zhĭ Ké Píng Chuăn Gāo* (止咳平喘膏) is made from *huáng qí* (Radix Astragali) 150g, *ròu guì* (Cortex Cinnamomi) 100g, *dāng guī* (Radix Angelicae Sinensis) 120g, *zé lán* (Herba Lycopi)120g, *shēng dì* (Radix Rehmanniae Glutinosae) 80g, *shā shēn* (Radix Glehniae seu Adenophorae) 100g, *wŭ wèi zĭ* (Fructus Schisandrae Chinensis) 100g, *zhì fù zĭ* (Radix Aconiti Lateralis Praeparata) 50g, *zhì nán xīng* (Rhizoma Arisaematis Praeparata) 50g, *sū zĭ* (Fructus Perillae) 100g, *tíng lì zĭ* (Semen Lepidii seu Descurainiae) 100g, and *dì lóng* (Lumbricus) 100g. The medicinals were ground into a powder, mixed with vaseline into a paste, and then placed onto a 2.5cm×2.5cm aseptic dressing which was covered with a plaster. A plaster was put on every point and fixed with adhesive tape. The basic points were BL 13 (*fèi shù*), BL 20 (*pí shù*), BL 23 (*shèn shù*), BL 17 (*gé shù*), BL 43 (*gāo huāng*), ST 40 (*fēng lóng*), LU 6 (*kŏng zuì*), and *dìng chuăn*. For cases complicated by Spleen yang deficiency, they added RN 6 (*qì hăi*), KI 3 (*tài xī*). For cases complicated by Lung qi deficiency, they added ST 36 (*zú sān lĭ*). For cases complicated by phlegm-heat, they added LU5 (*chĭ zé*), For cases complicated by spontaneous sweating, they added HT 6 (*yīn xì*). For cases complicated by panting, they added *băi láo*. For cases complicated by difficulty in expectoration, a dry throat, dizziness and tinnitus, they added SP 6 (*sān yīn jiāo*). They replaced the plasters once every two days. Compared with only biomedical treatment, this therapy was superior in raising the total effective rate, and improving blood gas levels and lung function.

(5) Needle Embedding in Ear Points

Sun Shu-qi, et al.[25] used the method of acupuncture needle embedding in ear points to treat thirty COPD patients with mild hemoptysis. The following points were used with press-tact plasters: Lung (CO14), *Shenmen* (TF4), Adrenal gland (TG2p), Spleen (CO13), Liver (CO12), and Large intestine (CO7). Before embedding the needle they, kneaded and pinched the points for 1−2 minutes first in order to make them congested, tender and easy to find. They then sterilized the tender points and embedded the needles, and fixed them with adhesive plasters. A course of treatment was 3−7 days and the next course was conducted at intervals of five days. The points of the Lung, Trachea (CO16), Shenmen, and Adrenal gland have effects of purifying Lung fire, tranquilizing and quieting the collaterals, harmonizing qi and blood, fortifying the Spleen, and tonifying the Kidney. For cases of constipation with difficult defecation, poor appetite and abdominal distention, Spleen and Large intestine points were added so as to purge *fu* organs and eliminate heat. For cases of the Lung affected by Liver fire, the Liver point was added so as to calm the Liver and downbear fire. The total effective rate was 73.3%.

(6) Combined Therapy

During the hottest days of summer, Chu Wen-hao, et al.[26] conduct prophylactic treatment and follow-up for 125 patients. They used medical point applications, point injections, and medicinal cupping. For the medical point application: the used DU 14 (*dà zhuī*), BL 13 (*fèi shù*), or BL 43 (*gāo huāng*) BL 17 (*gé shù*), and BL 18 (*dăn shù*). The two sets of points were used alternately. The herbs selected were *má huáng* (Herba Ephedrae), *bái jiè zǐ* (Semen Sinapis Albae), *xì xīn* (Radix et Rhizoma Asari), *xìng rén* (Armeniacae Semen Amarum), *bàn xià* (Rhizoma Pinelliae), *gān suí* (Radix Kansui), *gān jiāng* (Rhizoma

Zingiberis), and *dì lóng* (Lumbricus). After grinding the medicinals into a fine powder, they were mixed with enough honey so as to prepare into pills. The pill was used as a moxa paste fixed on the point. The time of application was 6-8 hours. For the point injection they used ST 36 and LU 5, alternately. The medicine was nucleic acid and casein hydrolysate composite injection 2ml per point, totally 4ml. As for medicinal cupping, they used DU 14, BL 13, and BL 43; or BL 20 and BL 23. The two sets of points were used in alternation. The medicals used were *qiāng huó* (Rhizoma et Radix Notopterygii), *dú huó* (Radix Angelicae Pubescentis), *fáng fēng* (Radix Saposhnikoviae), *ài yè* (Folium Artemisiae), *sū yè* (Folium Perillae), *dāng guī* (Radix Angelicae Sinensis), and *cōng* (Bulbus Allii). These were decocted and then a bamboo cup was soaked into the decoction. The decoction temperature was kept at 60℃. Each cup was retained for five minutes. The therapy began for the trial group on the first period of the greatest heat days each summer, twice per week, for a total of ten times. The symptoms of cough and expectoration were markedly improved, and the frequency of catching colds had obviously decreased. He Yingchun, et al[27] added acupuncture and cupping therapy to a base of conventional therapy. The main points for acupuncture were BL 23, BL 26 (*guān yuán shù*), BL 27 (*mìng mén shù*), DU 3 (*yāo yáng guān*), *bǎi láo*, RN 17 (*dàn zhōng*), and SP 6. The following were additional points: for cases of obvious Kidney deficiency, KI 3 was added. For cases of deficiency of both the Lung and Kidney, BL 13 was added. For cases of deficiency cold, ST 36, and DU 12 (*shēn zhù*) were added. For cases of profuse turbid phlegm, ST 40 was added. For cases of phlegm-fire, DU 14 was added. The manipulation was as follows: after routine sterilization, 1.5 *cun* needles were used, with a even supplementation and drainage method. After the arrival of qi, the needles were connected to electroacupuncture apparatus (G6805-2A), and stimulated with a continuous wave for 30min. This was done once per day, and 10 times made up a course of treatment. As for the cupping therapy, after acupuncture was finished, vaseline was put on the mouth of the cup, and the cup was placed on on *bǎi láo*. Then the cup was moved along the first lateral line of the foot *Tai*yang (Bladder) channel to BL 26. This was done on both sides back and forth twice. The treatment was conducted once every other day, with five times making up a course of treatment. The method of acupuncture with cupping can improve the blood rheologic indexes of patients with COPD.

Experimental Studies

1. Research on the Efficacy of Single Chinese Medicinals

Ge Xiao-na, et al.[28] established COPD rat models with smoke and repeated intranasal infections with klebsiella pneumoniae. The rats were divided into three groups: the control group, the smoke plus infection group, and the trial group. The rats in the trial group were given Chinese medicinal 814 via gastric lavage for three days before treatment with the smoke and infectious material. The result showed that Chinese medicinal 814 can delay formation and development of COPD induced by smoke plus infection with Klebsiella Pneumoniae.

2. Research on the Efficacy of Herbal Prescriptions

(1) Lowering Pulmonary Arterial Pressure

Sun Zi-kai, et al.[29] created rat models with pulmonary artery hypertension (PAH) that resembles anoxemic PAH under ordinary pressure. The rats were divided into three group: the *Xiè Tíng Hé Jì* (薤葶合剂) group, the nifedipine group, and the ligustrazine group. After treatment, the PAH of the rats in every group decreased, and the effects in the *Xiè Tíng Hé Jì* group were better than those in other groups, with a significant difference (P<0.05). The level of plasma TXB_2 decreased, and the effect in the *Xiè Tíng Hé Jì* group was better than those in ligustrazine group. Xi Zhao-qing, et al.[30] created rat anoxemic models under ordinary pressure, and divided the rats into four groups: the normal group, the nifedipine group, the blank group, and the *Fù Fāng Xiè Bái Jiāo Náng* (复方薤白胶囊) group. The results showed that both nifedipine and *Fù Fāng Xiè Bái Jiāo Náng* can decrease the mean pulmonary artery pressure and the right ventricular pressure in experimental rats, and that there is no significant difference between the two groups. *Fù Fāng Xiè Bái Jiāo Náng* can reduce the thickening of the small arterial wall, pachyhymenia of the tunica media of artery and the right ventricular hypertrophy induced by hypoxia, and the effect is better than that of nifedipine.

(2) Relieving Airway Inflammation

Li Li, et al.[31] created Syrian golden yellow hamster models with COPD by smoking. The hamsters were divided into three groups: the control group, the smoke group and the *Nǎo Fèi Kāng* (脑肺康 , with the main ingredient－ *dān shēn* [Radix et Rhizoma Salviae Miltiorrhizae]) group. *Nǎo Fèi Kāng* (脑肺康) can decrease the level of malonaldehyde and increase the level of SOD that is induced by smoking. Compared with the smoking group, the mean lining interval (MLI) of the lung of hamsters in *Nǎo Fèi Kāng* group was lower, and the mean lung alveolus number (MAN) is higher than those in smoking group. In addition, *Nǎo Fèi Kāng* can relieve bronchial and alveolar inflammation. The bronchial ciliated endothelial cell rank in good order, without obvious lodging and shedding.

(3) Controlling Lung Tissue Matrix Metalloproeinase during the Acute Aggravation Stage of COPD

Li Jiansheng, et al.[32] created rat models with COPD, and divided the rats into five groups: the *Tōng Sè Kē Lì* (通塞颗粒) high-dose group, the middle-dose group, the low-dose group, the Aminofilina group and the *Tíng Bèi Jiāo Náng* (葶贝胶囊) group. *Tōng Sè Kē Lì* (通塞颗粒), which is composed of *tíng lì zǐ* (Semen Lepidii seu Descurainiae), *dì lóng* (Lumbricus), *chì sháo* (Radix Paeoniae Rubra), and *zhì dà huáng* (Radix et Rhizoma Rhei Praeparata), can markedly inhibit the activities of matrix metalloproteinase-2 (MMP-2) and MMP-9 of the lung tissue in the acute aggravation stage of COPD, and the effect is superior to *Tíng Bèi Jiāo Náng* (葶贝胶囊) and Aminofilina.

(4) The Effects of Antioxidants

Li Yuan-qing, et al.[33] created COPD rat models with Lung qi deficiency and used modified *Bǔ Fèi Tāng* (补肺汤) on the experimented rats. This was composed of *huáng qí* (Radix Astragali), *dǎng shēn* (Radix Codonopsis), *sāng bái pí* (Cortex Mori), *bǎi bù* (Radix Stemonae), and *chuān xiōng* (Rhizoma Chuanxiong). modified *Bǔ Fèi Tāng* (补肺汤) can improve signs and symptoms of the experimental rats' respiratory system, and elevate the contents of reduced glutathione hormone (GSH), and the activity of SOD and glutathione peroxidase (GSH-PX) in both the blood and lung tissues. The decoction has an excellent antioxidant effect.

3. Studies on Forms of Chinese Medicinals

(1) Fluid Injections

1) *Tán Rè Qīng Zhù Shè Yè* (痰热清注射液)

Zhang Ying, et al.[34] treated thirty COPD patients with biomedical treatment plus *Tán Rè Qīng Zhù Shè Yè* (痰热清注射液). It was composed of *huáng qín* (Radix Scutellariae), *xióng dǎn fěn* (Pulvis Fellis Suis), *sháng yáng jiáo* (Cornu Naemorhedis), *jīn yín huā* (Flos Lonicerae) and *lián qiào* (Fructus Forsythiae). *Tán Rè Qīng Zhù Shè Yè* (痰热清注射液) had the effects of clearing heat, resolving toxin, and transforming phlegm.

The total effective rate was 96.55%, which was higher than that of the biomedicine group. It was superior to the control group in improving symptoms.

2) *Fù Fāng Dān Shēn Zhù Shè Yè* (复方丹参注射液)

In addition to conventional therapy, Pu Ming-zhi[35] added *Fù Fāng Dān Shēn Zhù Shè Yè* (复方丹参注射液) to treat 20 COPD patients. The result of *Fù Fāng Dān Shēn Zhù Shè Yè* was better that that of only using biomedical therapy in improving lung function and arterial blood gas levels.

3) *Shēng Dì Zhù Shè Yè* (生地注射液)

Zhang Wei, Jiang Chun-juan, et al[36][37] treated COPD patients with *Shēng Dì Zhù Shè Yè* (生地注射液), and found that it can obviously improve lung function and lung capacity, raise the content of tissue plasminogen activator, significantly decrease the content of its inhibitor and the content of plasma D-dimer, improve the patient's pre-thrombotic state, significantly raise the contents of CD_4 and CD_8 in cellular immunity and activity of NK cells, improve the ratio of CD_4/CD_8, and significantly decrease the whole blood viscosity, plasma viscosity and hematocrit.

4) *Mài Luò Níng Zhù Shè Yè* (脉络宁注射液)

Li Hui, et al.[38] added *Mài Luò Níng Zhù Shè Yè* (脉络宁注射液) to conventional therapy. Two weeks made up a course of treatment. Compared with only using biomedical treatment, it could increase the total effective rate, improve the condition of blood gas, and markedly improve whole blood viscosity, blood plasma specific viscosity, hematocrit, platelet aggregation rate and fibrinogen.

(2) Aerosol Inhalation

Lao Wei-guo, et al.[39] used ultrasonic aerosol inhalation of *Yú Xīng Cǎo Zhù Shè Yè* (鱼腥草注射液) combined with conventional biomedical therapy to treat COPD during the acute infection stage. They found it could relieve clinical symptoms of patients with phlegm-heat obstruction in the Lung, increase ventilation function, improve hypoxia state of tissue and organ, and increase patient quality of life. In addition to conventional therapy, Zheng Sheng-jie, et al.[40] added ligustrazine aerosol inhalation to treat patients with complications of pulmonary artery hypertension (PAH) during the acute aggravation stage of COPD. The result revealed that ligustrazine aerosol inhalation could decrease PAH through adjusting the platelet functions.

(3) Bronchoalveolar Lavage

Zhang Wei, et al.[41] carried out bronchoalveolar lavage with *Yú Xīng Cǎo Zhù Shè Yè* (鱼腥草注射液) in the diseased region through a bronchofibroscope. The lavage dose was 20－40ml, two to three times daily; and mechanical ventilation sequential therapy was taken in combination so as to treat COPD patients with the complication of respiratory failure. The results showed that mechanical ventilation combined with bronchoalveolar lavage with *Yú Xīng Cǎo Zhù Shè Yè* (鱼腥草注射液) is superior to mechanical ventilation only in controlling infection, shortening the time of invasive mechanical ventilation, and reducing complications of respirator-dependent pneumonia in tracheal intubation and difficulty in withdrawal of the respirator. In addition it can shorten the duration of hospitalization and improve prognosis.

REFERENCES

[1] Cui Yan, Liang Zhi-ying, Dong Jing-cheng. Clinical Observation on Chronic Obstructive Pulmonary Disease in Acute Aggravation Stage Treated with Activating Blood and Removing Stasis Recipe (活血化瘀方治疗慢性阻塞性肺疾病急性加重期的临床观察). *Chinese Journal of Integrated Traditional and Western Medicine* (中国中西医结合杂志). 2005, 25(4): 327-329.

[2] Shi Ke-hua, Wang Li-xin, Yan Chen, et al. Clinical Research on Therapy of

Clearing the Lung, Dissipating Phlegm and Activating Blood to Treat COPD in the Acute Aggravation Stage · A Report of 33 cases (清肺化湿活血法治疗慢性阻塞肺病急性加重33例临床研究). *Information on Traditional Chinese Medicine* (中医药信息). 2004, 21(4): 56-57.

[3] Li Su-yun, Li Jian-sheng, Ma Li-jun, et al. Effects of *Tōng Sè Kē Lì* on Extracellular Matrix and Adhesion Molecule in Senile COPD Patients in the Acute Aggravation Stage (通塞颗粒对老年慢性阻塞性肺疾病急性加重期患者细胞外基质和粘附分子的影响). *Journal of Traditional Chinese Medicine* (中医杂志). 2003, 44(12): 906-908.

[4] Zhang Li-shan, Wu Wei-ping, Dong An-ming, et al. Clinical Trial of *Fèi Kāng Fāng* for the Treatment of Chronic Obstructive Pulmonary Disease Complicated by Pulmonary Hypertension (肺康方治疗慢性阻塞性肺疾病肺动脉高压的临床研究). *Journal of Beijing University of Traditional Chinese Medicine* (北京中医药大学学报). 2003, 36(3): 70-73.

[5] Lin Jian. Treatment of Chronic Obstructive Pulmonary Disease with *Yáng Hé Tāng* · A Report of 35 Cases (阳和汤为主治疗慢性阻塞性肺病35例). *Zhejiang Journal of Traditional Chinese Medicine* (浙江中医杂志). 2004, 39(4): 151.

[6] Li Su-yun, Li Jian-sheng, Ma Li-jun, et al. Effects of *Bǔ Fèi Yì Shèn Kē Lì* on Extracellular Matrix in Patients with Chronic Obstructive Pulmonary Disease (补肺益肾颗粒对COPD缓解期患者细胞外基质的影响). *Chinese Journal of Information on Traditional Chinese Medicine* (中国中医药信息杂志). 2003, 10(9): 13-15.

[7] Zheng Hong, Tao Jia-ju, Zhao Xue-qun. Clinical Efficacy of a Series of Chinese Medicinals in Treatment of COPD during Remission Stage and Their Effects on Airway Inflammation (系列中药治疗缓解期COPD临床疗效及对气道炎症作用的研究). *Chinese Journal of the Practical Chinese with Modern Medicine* (中华实用中西医杂志). 2005, 18(7): 982-984.

[8] Ji Hong-yan, Hu Guo-jun, Gao Jian, et al. Clinical Observation on the Method of Replenishing Qi and Nourishing Yin for Malnutrition in COPD during Remission Stage (益气养阴对COPD缓解期营养不良患者的临床观察). *Chinese Journal of the Practical Chinese with Modern Medicine* (中华实用中西医杂志). 2003, 16(1): 115-116.

[9] Wu Qi-biao, Li Ju-yun, Ma Li-jun. Effects of Replenishing Qi, Nourishing Yin, Activating Blood and Dissipating Phlegm on Immune Function of Patients with COPD during Stable Stage (益气养阴活血化痰法对COPD稳定期免疫功能的影响). *Academic Periodical of Changchun College of Traditional Chinese Medicine* (长春中医学院学报). 2001, 17(2): 10-11.

[10] Feng Cui-ling, Wu Wei-ping and Wan Xia. Effects of Therapeutic Method of Nourishing Qi, Activating Blood Circulation and Resolving Phlegm on Quality of Life of Patients with Chronic Obstructive Pulmonary Disease (益气活血化痰法对慢性阻塞性肺病

患者生活质量的影响). *Chinese Journal of Integrated Traditional and Western Medicine* (中国中西医结合杂志). 2005, 25(9): 829-831.

[11] Wang Zhi-gang, Liu Hao, Zhang Shu-juan, et al. Therapeutic Effects of Yin-Nourishing, Lung-Cleaning and Stasis-Expelling Method on COPD and Its Influence on Platelet Function (养阴清肺逐瘀法治疗COPD的临床疗效及其对血小板功能的影响). *Acta Universitatis Traditionis Medicalis Sinensis Pharmacologiaeque Shanghai* (上海中医药大学学报). 2002, 16(4): 18-21.

[12] Che Hong-zhu, Pang Jian, Li Chang-jian, et al. Effects of *Zhǐ Ké Qīng Fèi Kǒu Fú Yè* on Interleukin-8 and Tumor Necrosis Factor-α in Sputum of COPD Patients (止咳清肺口服液对25例慢性阻塞性肺疾病患者痰液炎症细胞白细胞介素8、肿瘤坏死因子α的影响). *Journal of Traditional Chinese Medicine* (中医杂志). 2005, 46(10): 759-761.

[13] He Xin, Wu Qing. Clinical Observation on Treatment of Chronic Obstructive Pulmonary Disease with *Shān Ěr Hé Jì* (山耳合剂治疗慢性阻塞性肺病临床观察). *Journal of Emergency in Traditional Chinese Medicine* (中国中医急症). 2003, 12(3): 172-173.

[14] Lin Lin, Fang Hong. Clinical Study on *Jǐ Jiāo Lì Huáng Tāng* with Additions in Treating Pulmonary Hypertension of Chronic Obstructive Pulmonary Disease (加味己椒苈黄汤治疗COPD肺动脉高压的临床研究). *Shanghai Journal of Traditional Chinese Medicine* (上海中医药杂志). 2005, 39(6): 24-25.

[15] Luo Xain-fang, Chai Xiu-juan, Chen Yi-min, et al. Clinical Study on *Bǎo Fèi Dìng Chuǎn Chōng Jì* in Treating Chronic Obstructive Pulmonary Disease · A Report of 36 Cases (保肺定喘冲剂治疗慢性阻塞性肺疾病36例临床研究). *Journal of Traditional Chinese Medicine* (中医杂志). 2002, 43(4): 268-270.

[16] Shi Suo-fang, Cao Shi-hong, Xu Li-hua, et al. Clinical Study of *Qīng Yuán Huà Tán Kē Lì* in Treating COPD in Attack Stage (清源化痰颗粒治疗慢性阻塞性肺疾病[COPD]发作期的临床研究). *Journal of Nanjing University of Traditional Chinese Medicine* (南京中医药大学学报[自然科学版]). 2000, 16(2): 81-83.

[17] Wang Sheng, Ji Hong-yan, Zhang Nian-zhi, et al. Effect of *Yì Fèi Jiàn Pí Fāng* on Count of Inflammatory Cells, Levels of Interleukin-8 and Tumor Necrosis Factor-α in Sputum of Patients with Chronic Obstructive Pulmonary Disease (益肺健脾方对慢性阻塞性肺疾病患者痰液炎症细胞计数和IL-8、TNF-α水平的影响). *Chinese Journal of Integrated Traditional and Western Medicine* (中国中西医结合杂志). 2005, 25(2): 111-113.

[18] Lin Lin, Tang Cui-ying, Xu Yin-ji. Clinical Observation of *Jiàn Pí Yì Fèi Chōng Jì* in Treating Respiratory Muscle Fatigue during Stable Stage of Chronic Obstructive Pulmonary Disease (健脾益肺冲剂治疗慢阻肺稳定期呼吸肌疲劳的临床观察). *Shanghai Journal of Traditional Chinese Medicine* (上海中医药杂志). 2001, 37(11): 10-12.

[19] Zhang Hong-chun, Chao En-xiang. Clinical Trial of *Tiáo Bǔ Fèi Shèn Jiāo Náng* for Treating Chronic Obstructive Pulmonary Disease in Stable Stage (调补肺肾胶囊治疗慢性阻塞性肺疾病稳定期临床研究). *Journal of Beijing University of Traditional Chinese Medicine* (北京中医药大学学报). 2003, 26(2): 53-56.

[20] Yu Xia, Wu Yu-chang, Huang Da-xiang. Treatment of Chronic Obstructive Pulmonary Disease with *Jiā Wèi Yòu Guī Wán* (加味右归丸治疗慢性阻塞性肺病稳定期 35 例). *Chinese Journal of the Practical Chinese with Modern Medicine* (中华实用中西医杂志). 2005, 18(2): 1473-1474.

[21] Ni Wei-min, Shen Jie, Huang Yuan-fang. Transient Therapeutic Effects of Scalp Acupuncture on Anoxia in Patients with Chronic Bronchitis (头针改善慢性支气管炎患者缺氧即时疗效观察). *Chinese Acupuncture & Moxibustion* (中国针灸). 2004, 24(7): 452-454.

[22] Zhang Ling. Treatment of Chronic Obstructive Pulmonary Disease with *Yì Qì Fú Zhèng Tāng* Combining with Acupuncture · A Report of 288 Cases (益气扶正汤加针刺治疗慢性阻塞性肺病288 例). *Shanxi Journal of Traditional Chinese Medicine* (陕西中医). 2003, 24(10): 882-883.

[23] Shi Hong. Therapeutic Effects of Point Injection for Chronic Bronchitis (穴位注射治疗慢性支气管炎疗效观察). *Chinese Journal of the Practical Chinese with Modern Medicine* (中华实用中西医杂志). 2004, 17(6): 834-835.

[24] Xu Xin-yi, Zhou Xun, Liu Wei. Clinical Study of Point Application with *Zhǐ Ké Píng Chuǎn Gāo* Combining with Pharmacotherapy in Treating Chronic Obstructive Pulmonary Disease (止咳平喘膏穴位敷贴配合西药治疗慢性阻塞性肺病36例临床研究). *Journal of Guiyang College of Traditional Chinese Medicine* (贵阳中医学院学报). 2005, 27(2): 38-40.

[25] Sun Shu-qi, Guo Pi-chun. Clinical Observation of Needle-Embedding at Ear Points in Treatment of COPD Complicated by Hemoptysis (耳穴埋针法治疗COPD 并少量咯血临床观察). *Journal of the Practical Chinese with Modern Medicine* (中华实用中西医杂志). 2004, 17(16): 2429.

[26] Chu Wen-hao, Xi Song-mao, Zhang Yan. Prevention and Treatment of Chronic Bronchitis in Old Patients Based on the Principle of "Treating Winter Disease in Summer" ("冬病夏治"防治老年人慢性支气管炎). *Journal of Shanghai University of Traditional Chinese Medicine* (上海中医药杂志). 2001, 20 (3): 8-9.

[27] He Ying-chun, Liu Xiu-mei, Guo Jian-wen. Effects of Acupuncture with Cupping on Patients with Chronic Obstructive Pulmonary Disease in Blood Rheology (针刺配合拔罐疗法改善慢性阻塞性肺病患者血液流变性的影响). *Chinese Journal of Microcirculation* (中国微循环). 2003, 7(6): 387-388.

[28] Ge Xiao-na, Xiong Mi, Hao Chun-rong. Treatment Effect of Chinese Medicinal 814 on Rat of Chronic Obstructive Pulmonary Disease Induced by Smoke in Combination with Klebsiella Pneumoniae. (中药814对吸烟加肺炎克雷白杆菌感染诱发大鼠COPD的防治). *Acta Universitatis Medictnae Tangji* (华中科技大学学报医学版). 2002, 31(4): 359-362.

[29] Sun Zi-kai, Cao Shi-hong, Xi Zhao-qing, et al. Treatment of Chronic Obstructive Pulmonary Disease During the Acute Stage with *Xiè Tíng Hé Jì* and Its Effects on Anoxic Pulmonary Hypertension (薤葶合剂治疗急性发作期COPD及对缺氧性肺动脉高压的影响). *Journal of Nanjing University of Traditional Chinese Medicine* (南京中医药大学学报). 2001, 17(1): 16-19.

[30] Xi Zhang-qing, Jiang Meng, Ju Wen-zheng, et al. Clinical and Empirical Study of *Fù Fāng Xiè Bái Jiāo Náng* in Treatment of Chronic Obstructive Pulmonary Disease (复方薤白胶囊治疗慢性阻塞性肺病36例临床与实验研究). *Journal of Traditional Chinese Medicine* (中医杂志). 2000, 41(4): 218-220.

[31] Li Li, Ruan Ying-mao, Zhang Xu-chen, et al. Establishment of a Hamster COPD Models by Smoking and Preventive and Therapeutic Effect of Chinese Medicine *Nǎo Fèi Kāng* (吸烟导致慢性阻塞性肺疾病地鼠模型的建立及中药脑肺康的防治作用). *Journal of Traditional Chinese Medicine* (中医杂志). 2001, 42(10): 615-618.

[32] Li Jian-sheng, Li Su-yun, Wang You-hong, et al. Changes of Matrix Metalloproteinase of Lung Tissue in Rat Models with Acute Exacerbation of COPD and the Effects of *Tōng Sè Kē Lì* (慢性阻塞性肺疾病急性加重期模型大鼠肺组织基质金属蛋白酶的变化及通塞颗粒的治疗作用). *Chinese Journal of Gerontology* (中国老年学杂志). 2005, 25(2): 174-175.

[33] Li Yuan-qing, Li Ya-guang. Empirical Study of Anti-oxidizing Therapy with modified *Bǔ Fèi Tāng* for Chronic Obstructive Pulmonary Disease (加减补肺汤抗氧化治疗慢性阻塞性肺疾病的实验研究). *Journal of Jiangxi University of Traditional Chinese Medicine* (江西中医学院学报). 2004, 16(4): 61-62.

[34] Zhang Ying, Li Ting-qian, Wang Gang, et al. Randomized Controlled Trial of *Tán Rè Qīng Zhù Shè Yè* in Treatment of Acute Exacerbation of Chronic Obstructive Pulmonary Disease with Pattern of Phlegm-Heat Obstruction in the Lung (痰热清注射液治疗慢性阻塞性肺疾病急性加重期[痰热阻肺证]的随机对照试验). *Chinese Journal of Evidence-Based Medicine* (中国循证医学杂志). 2004, 4(5): 300-305.

[35] Pu Ming-zhi. Effects of *Fù Fāng Dān Shēn Zhù Shè Yè* on Respiratory Function of Chronic Obstructive Pulmonary Disease (复方丹参注射液对COPD患者呼吸功能的影响). *Jilin Journal of Traditional Chinese Medicine* (吉林中医药). 2004, 23(2): 14.

[36] Zhang Wei, Bi Xiao-li. Effects of *Shēng Dì Zhù Shè Yè* on Pre-thrombotic State in

Treating Chronic Obstructive Pulmonary Disease (生地注射液对慢性阻塞性肺病血栓前状态影响的研究). *Journal of Practical Traditional Chinese Medicine* (实用中医药杂志). 2003, 16(3): 3.

[37] Jiang Chun-juan, Bi Xiao-li, Wang Yue. Effects of *Shēng Dì Zhù Shè Yè* on Patients with Chronic Obstructive Pulmonary Disease in Blood Rheology and Pulmonary Function (生地注射液对慢性阻塞性肺疾病患者血流变学及肺功能的影响). *Journal of Practical Traditional Chinese Medicine* (实用中医药杂志). 2002, 18(8): 7-8.

[38] Li Hui, Liu Xiang, Liu Xiao-jun, et al. Clinical Observation of *Mài Luò Níng Zhù Shè Yè* in Treating Chronic Obstructive Pulmonary Disease in Acute Aggravation Stage (脉络宁注射液治疗慢性阻塞性肺疾病急性加重期的临床观察). *Chinese Archives of Traditional Chinese Medicine* (中医药学刊). 2005, 23(8): 1534-1535.

[39] Lao Wei-guo, Li Yan, Zhang Wei. Observation of Curative Effects of *Yú Xīng Cǎo Zhù Shè Yè* Aerosol Inhalation on COPD in Acute Infection Stage with Phlegm-Heat Retention in the Lung (鱼腥草注射液雾化吸入治疗慢性阻塞性肺疾病急性感染期[痰热阻肺型]疗效观察). *Journal of New Chinese Medicine* (新中医). 2005, 37(8): 38-39.

[40] Zheng Sheng-jie, Dai Yong. Effects of Ligustrazine Aerosol Inhalation on Pulmonary Artery Hypertension and the Platelet Function in Patients with COPD in Acute Aggravation Stage (川芎嗪雾化吸入对COPD急性加重期患者肺动脉高压、血小板功能的影响). *Journal of Clinic and Experimental Medicine* (临床与实验医学杂志). 2006, 5(1): 157-158.

[41] Zhang Wei, Sun Zhi-jie, Liu Jian-bo, et al. Effects of Bronchoalveolar Lavage Combining with Mechanical Ventilation Sequential Therapy on COPD Complicated by Respiratory Failure (中药灌洗联合机械通气序贯治疗COPD并发呼吸衰竭23例疗效观察). *Journal of New Chinese Medicine* (新中医). 2006, 38(2): 56-57.

Bronchial Asthma

by **Liu Wei-sheng**, Professor of Chinese Internal Medicine
   Han Yun, M.S. TCM
   Feng Wei-bin, Professor of TCM
   Lin Yan-zhao, M.S. TCM

OVERVIEW 217
CHINESE MEDICAL ETIOLOGY AND PATHOMECHANISM 219
CHINESE MEDICAL TREATMENT 220
Pattern Differentiation and Treatment 220
1. The Treatment During the Attack Stage 221
2. The Treatment During Remission Stage 226

Additional Treatment Modalities 233
1. Chinese Patent Medicine 233
2. Acupuncture and Moxibustion 233
3. Simple Prescriptions and Empirical Formulas 243

PROGNOSIS 247
PREVENTIVE HEALTHCARE 248
Lifestyle Modification 248
1. Pay Attention to Climactic Influences 248
2. Take Precautions against Coming into Contact with Various Asthma Inducing Agents 248
3. Pay Attention to Keeping Warm 248

Dietary Recommendation 249
1. Boiled Chicken with *Dōng Chóng Xià Cǎo* (Cordyceps Sinensis) (冬虫夏草炖鸡) 250
2. Powder of Ginseng and Gecko (*Rén Shēn Gé Jiè Sǎn* 人参蛤蚧散) ... 250
3. Lamb Soup with *Dāng Guī* and Ginger (*Dāng Guī Shēng Jiāng Yáng Ròu Tāng* 当归生姜羊肉汤) 250
4. Pork Tripe Stewed *Hú Jiāo* (Fructus Piperis Nigri) (胡椒煲猪肚) 251
5. Stewed Pork Lung with *Jiàn Huā* (Hylocereus undatus) 251
6. Stewed Lean Pork with *Luó Hàn Guǒ* (Fructus Momordicae) 252
7. Chicken Soup with *Bái Guǒ* (Semen Ginkgo) and *Xìng Rén* (Armeniacae Semen Amarum) 252
8. Lean Meat Soup with *Yú Biāo Jiāo* (Pseudosciaena crocea) and *Dōng Chóng Xià Cǎo* (Cordyceps Sinensis) 252

Regulation of Emotional and Mental Health ·························· 253
CLINICAL EXPERIENCE OF RENOWNED PHYSICIANS ················ 254
Empirical Formulas ·· 254
1. Treating Asthma with Jiàng Qì Dìng Chuǎn Kē Lì Chōng Jì (降气定喘颗粒冲剂) (Liu Wei-sheng) ·· 254
2. Treatment of Cold Asthma with Wēn Fèi Dìng Chuǎn Tāng (温肺定喘汤) (Feng Wei-bin) ·· 255
3. Treatment of Cold Asthma with Wēn Fèi Dìng Chuǎn Tāng (温肺定喘汤) (Yu Shao-yuan) ··· 256
4. Treatment of Wind-Cold Fettering the Lung with Má Xìng Shè Dǎn Tāng (麻杏射胆汤) (Dong Su-liu) ·· 257
5. Treatment of Phlegm-Drool Congestion with Jié Chuǎn Tāng (截喘汤) (Jiang Chun-hua) ·· 260
6. Treatment of Phlegm Obstructing the Lung Collaterals with Píng Chuǎn Fāng (平喘方) (Dong Jian-hua) ·· 261
7. Treatment of Wind Flourishing and Phlegm Blocking with Huáng Lóng Shū Chuǎn Tāng (黄龙舒喘汤) (Chao En-xiang) ·································· 264

Selected Case Studies ··· 265
1. Professor Dong Jian-hua's Case Study: Cold in the Lung and Heat in the Diaphragm ·· 265
2. Professor Chen Shi-an's Case Study: Cold-Phlegm Obstructing the Lung ··· 268
3. Professor Qian Zi-fen's Case: Accumulation of Phlegm-Heat in the Lung ··· 271
4. Professor Zheng Qiao's Case: Phlegm-Fire Assailing the Lung ············ 274
5. Professor Zhu Zhan-yu's Case: Exterior Constraint of Wind-Cold; Accumulation of Turbid-Phlegm in the Lung ·································· 277
6. Professor Zhu Bo-quan's Cases: Failure of the Kidney to Receive Qi ········ 281

Discussions ·· 283
1. Professor Wang Wen-ding: Treating Asthma by Dividing it into the Early, Middle and Late Stages ·· 283

2. Professor Cheng Men-xue: Treating the Lung and Phlegm as the Key to Treating Asthma ·············287
3. Professor Ren Ji-xue: The Treatment of Asthma by Treating Wheezing and Panting as the Same Things ·············290
4. Professor Yu Chang-rong: The Treatment of Asthma Based upon the Condition of the Branch and the Root·············292
5. Professor Guo Zhen-qiu: The Treatment of Senile Asthma by Rectifying the Lung to Treat the Branch, and Consolidating the Kidney to Treat the Root ···295
6. Professor Cen He-ling: The Treatment of Asthma by Treating the Lung and Kidney Simultaneously ·············297
7. Professor Huang Wen-dong: The Treatment of Asthma by the Three Methods of Reliving the Exterior, Attacking and Tonifying ·············299
8. Professor Fu Zai-xi: The Treatment of Asthma Mainly by Opening the Orifices and Dispelling Phlegm ·············302
9. Professor Chao En-xiang: The Treatment of Asthma by Division into Stages, with Emphasis on Dispelling Wind and Resolving Spasms·············305
10. Professor Liu Wei-sheng: Three Steps in the Treatment of Asthma ·············309
11. Professor Feng Wei-bin: Treating Asthma by Paying Attention to the Phase and Variability ·············311
12. Professor Ren Ji-xue: The Treatment of Asthma is Based upon the Recognition that Wheezing and Panting are Similar ·············313

PERSPECTIVES OF INTEGRATIVE MEDICINE ············· 316
Challenges and Solutions ············· 316
Challenge #1: How to Prevent the Occurrence of Asthma ·············316
Challenge #2: How to Reduce the Relapse of Asthma ·············318
Challenge #3: The Treatment of Critical Asthma ·············320
Challenge #4: The Treatment of Hormone-Dependent Asthma·············321
Insight from Empirical Wisdom ············· 323
1. Asthma Outbreaks Occur in Stages ·············323

2. The Complexity of Pattern Types	325
3. The Variability of Pattern Types	326
4. Experience of Using Medicinals in the Treatment of Asthma	327
5. Knowledge from Experience Regarding the Use of *Má Huáng* (Herba Ephedrae)	330
6. If Any of the Below Conditions are Encountered, Treat with Biomedicine or Integrative Medicine as soon as Possible	331

Summary ... 332
SELECTED QUOTES FROM CLASSICAL TEXTS ... 335
MODERN RESEARCH ... 339
Clinical Research ... 339

1. Pattern Differentiation and Corresponding Treatment ... 339
2. Specific Formulas ... 343
3. Additional Treatment Modalities ... 354
4. Acupuncture and Moxibustion ... 356

Experimental Studies ... 363

1. Research on the Efficacy of Single Chinese Medicinals ... 363
2. Research on the Efficacy of Herbal Prescription ... 364
3. Studies on Forms of Chinese Medicinals ... 369

REFERENCES ... 369

OVERVIEW

Bronchial asthma (abbreviated as asthma) is a multi-cellular chronic airway inflammation involving mastocytes, eosinophils and T lymphocytes. Susceptible people can suffer from repeated episodes of wheezing, panting, chest oppression, and coughing, mostly occurring at night or at early dawn. These kinds of symptoms are often accompanied by wide-ranging and variable limitations of ventilation and are characterized by the hyper-reactivity of the airway to different stimulating factors. However, these symptoms can be somewhat alleviated either spontaneously or through treatment.

Clinically, bronchial asthma is usually classified either as extrinsic asthma or intrinsic asthma. Less commonly it can be categorized as drug-induced asthma or exercise-induced asthma.

Biomedicine believes that asthma is frequently induced by either an endogenous or exogenous origin based on heredity. Most patients have a family or personal history of allergies. The pathogenesis of asthma is related to allergic reactions, airway inflammation, airway hyper-reactivity, and neurogenic factors. Clinically, asthma is characterized by recurrent episodes of expiratory dyspnea with wheezing. Symptoms can be alleviated through medication, or may spontaneously disappear. Patients may be completely asymptomatic with no specific physical signs during the remission period. Slight emphysema can be seen in patients with long-term repeated episodes of asthma. During the attack period, there may be thoracic hyperinflation, a decrease of respiratory volume, hyper-resonant sounds upon percussion, prolonged expirations, and wheezing sounds over both lungs heard upon auscultation. If the asthma is complicated by respiratory tract infections, then moist rales can also be heard.

During the attack period, eosinophils may increase by 5%—15%.

Eosinophils and Charcot-Leyden crystals can be found in a sputum smear. The blood serum immunoglobulin E (IgE) is increased in patients with allergies. The arterial PaO_2 (oxygen partial pressure) may decrease, and the $PaCO_2$ (carbon dioxide partial pressure) may not increase, and it might even decrease. A simple bedside pulmonary function test can be helpful so as to confirm the severity of the patient's condition.

A definitive clinical diagnosis of asthma can be made based upon the following factors: a history of asthmatic episodes, typical symptoms and signs, and an alleviative response to bronchial anti-spasmodic agents. For those patients without typical symptoms, bronchiectasis tests or provocation tests should be given, with a positive reaction confirming the diagnosis of asthma.

The purpose of asthma treatment is mainly to inhibit airway inflammation and reduce airway hyper-reactivity. For mild attacks, the following medications can be taken orally aminophylline, theophylline, Bricanyl (terbutaline sulphate solution for nebulization), salbutamol, Volmax (sustained-release salbutamol), or ketotifen. Some medications are given in nebulized aerosol form, such as salbutamol, terbutaline, methylacetic acid beclometasone, or cromolyn sodium. In some cases a clenbuterol hydrochloride suppository may be used. For moderate attacks, aminophylline can be administrated intravenously, corticosteroids can be given intravenously or orally, and an ultrasonic atomizing inhalation of drugs may be given. Anti-infective agents can also be used in cases accompanied by infection. For severe attacks the following treatments can be given oxygen therapy, intravenous transfusion of bronchial anti-spasmodic agents including $β_2$ receptor agitation agents, xanthine bases, anticholinergic agents, inflammation mediator stabilizers (such as corticoid and leukotriene receptor antagonists), antibiotics and anti-phlegmatics. It may also be necessary to correct or maintain the proper acid-base balance. Mechanical ventilation should be applied in cases of respiratory failure, disturbance of consciousness, or respiratory muscle fatigue.

In Chinese medicine, bronchial asthma is referred as *xiào zhèng* (哮证, wheezing pattern).

CHINESE MEDICAL ETIOLOGY AND PATHOMECHANISM

Chinese medicine believes that the etiology of asthma is from the retention of latent phlegm in the Lung. It can be from factors that are hereditary, constitutional, environmental, exogenous, dietary, and related to taxation fatigue. The roots (primary aspect) of asthma are deficiencies of the Lung, Spleen, and Kidney; the branches (secondary aspect) are wind, cold, heat, dampness, phlegm, and stasis. It presents mainly as an excess pattern in the attack stage, and most often as a deficiency pattern in the remission stage.

It is common for the asthma patient to have internal retention of latent phlegm, and deficiency or impairment of yang qi of the Lung, Spleen, and Kidney. The Spleen governs transportation and transformation. If, due to deficiency, the Spleen fails to transform and transport, then turbid phlegm may be engendered and upwardly accumulate in the Lung. The Kidney is the root of yang qi of the body, and is in charge of receiving qi. If the Kidney fails to receive qi because of Kidney essence depletion, there will be panting and dyspnea with little exertion. The Lung governs qi and is in charge of respiration. If the interstices are not secure because of deficiency of Lung qi, then exogenous pathogens can enter the body through the mouth and nose, and the six climatic pathogens can invade the body surface; This results in an adverse rising of Lung qi, leading to unsmooth breathing. Phlegm may ascend following the adverse rising of qi, and qi may also stagnate because of phlegm obstruction. Both the qi and phlegm may act on each other to obstruct the airway, thus there will be a failure of the Lung qi to diffuse and descend, hence the wheezing and panting. If a patient has a yang deficient constitution, and he contracts pathogenic wind-cold which tightens the exterior, then he can have a cold-type asthma. If exogenous pathogens attack the body exteriorly, and the phlegm transforms into heat, then heat-type asthma may occur.

Congenital constitutional insufficiency is a common occurrence in asthmatics. Thus the disease often begins in childhood, but as age increases, the Kidney essence becomes gradually more and more sufficient, thus some child asthmatics may slowly recover. However, if because of repeated attacks or improper treatments, the Kidney qi becomes more and more deficient so that the Kidney fails to receive qi, it is then difficult for asthmatics to be cured as an adult.

If this disease attacks repeatedly for months and years, the Heart and the Kidney may be involved, thus *fèi zhàng* (肺胀, Lung distention) will develop, along with critical signs such as palpitations and edema. During severe asthma attacks, *chuǎn tuō* (喘脱, asthmatic prostration) may occur and the patients may die if first aid is not prompt and effective.

CHINESE MEDICAL TREATMENT

Asthma is a disease that has many complex clinical manifestations. These manifestations are all different, so treatments should be given based on the different clinical manifestations and different stages. In the attack stage, asthma should first be differentiated into cold or heat types. Then treatment should mainly be to eliminate pathogenic factors, downbear qi, resolve phlegm, and relieve asthma. In the remission stage, tonifying the Lung, reinforcing the Spleen, and consolidating the Kidney should be emphasized so as to prevent relapse.

Pattern Differentiation and Treatment

The treatment of asthma during the acute attack stage should focus on the branch (alleviation of symptoms). During the remission stage the focus should be on treating the root. During the attack stage, the main treatments include eliminating pathogenic factors, resolving phlegm, downbearing qi, and calming panting. In the remission stage, suitable treatments include strengthening the right qi so as to secure the root of the body, replenishing the Lung, fortifying the Spleen, and tonifying the Kidney.

1. THE TREATMENT DURING THE ATTACK STAGE

(1) Cold Asthma

【Pattern Characteristics】

Panting, coughing, phlegm wheezing in the throat, difficulty in lying down flat, chest fullness and oppression, breathlessness, and phlegm that is white, clear and watery, accompanied by foam. At the beginning this is accompanied by aversion to cold, fever, headache, clear and profuse urine, and no thirst. The tongue is pale or pink with a white or greasy coating. The pulse is superficial and tight.

【Treatment Principle】

Warm the Lung and dispel cold; resolve phlegm and calm panting.

【Commonly Used Medicinals】

Use *má huáng* (Herba Ephedrae), *sū zǐ* (Fructus Perillae), *xìng rén* (Armeniacae Semen Amarum), *fǎ bàn xià* (Rhizoma Pinelliae Praeparatum), *wǔ wèi zǐ* (Fructus Schisandrae Chinensis), *bái jiè zǐ* (Semen Sinapis Albae), *chén pí* (Pericarpium Citri Reticulatae) and *zhì nán xīng* (Rhizoma Arisaematis Praeparata) to resolve phlegm and calm panting. Use *xì xīn* (Radix et Rhizoma Asari), *bǔ gǔ zhī* (Fructus Psoraleae), *shēng jiāng* (Rhizoma Zingiberis Recens), *zǐ sū* (Folium Perillae), *fáng fēng* (Radix Saposhnikoviae), *jīng jiè* (Herba Schizonepetae), *guì zhī* (Ramulus Cinnamomi) and *gǎo běn* (Rhizoma et Radix Ligustici) to warm the Lung and dispel cold.

【Representative Formula】

Shè Gān Má Huáng Tāng (射干麻黄汤) or *Xiǎo Qīng Lóng Tāng* (小青龙汤) with modifications

【Ingredients】

麻黄	má huáng	9g	Herba Ephedrae
苏子	sū zǐ	12g	Fructus Perillae
杏仁	xìng rén	12g	Armeniacae Semen Amarum
法半夏	fǎ bàn xià	12g	Rhizoma Pinelliae Praeparatum
细辛	xì xīn	6g	Radix et Rhizoma Asari
五味子	wǔ wèi zǐ	9g	Fructus Schisandrae Chinensis
生姜	shēng jiāng	3 pieces	Rhizoma Zingiberis Recens
紫菀	zǐ wǎn	12g	Radix et Rhizoma Asteris
款冬花	kuǎn dōng huā	12g	Flos Farfarae
射干	shè gān	15g	Rhizoma Belamcandae
白芍	bái sháo	15g	Radix Paeoniae Alba
炙甘草	zhì gān cǎo	8g	Radix et Rhizoma Glycyrrhizae Praeparata

Decoct in 800ml of water until 200ml of the decoction is left. Divide into 2 portions. Take warm, 1 dose a day.

【Formula Analysis】

Within this formula, *má huáng* (Herba Ephedrae), *xì xīn* (Radix et Rhizoma Asari) and *shēng jiāng* (Rhizoma Zingiberis Recens) warm the Lung and dispel cold in order to calm panting. *Shè gān* (Rhizoma Belamcandae), *sū zǐ* (Fructus Perillae) and *xìng rén* (Armeniacae Semen Amarum), in combination with with *má huáng* (Herba Ephedrae) and *xì xīn* (Radix et Rhizoma Asari), relive panting. *Fǎ bàn xià* (Rhizoma Pinelliae Praeparatum), *zǐ wǎn* (Radix et Rhizoma Asteris) and *kuǎn dōng huā* (Flos Farfarae) stop cough and resolve phlegm. *Bái sháo* (Radix Paeoniae Alba), *wǔ wèi zǐ* (Fructus Schisandrae Chinensis) and *gān cǎo* (Radix et Rhizoma Glycyrrhizae) are sour and sweet in nature and, used in combination, astringe yin. This prevents *má huáng* (Herba Ephedrae) and *xì xīn* (Radix et Rhizoma Asari), with their acrid flavor, from excessively dispersing, and also restricts the side effects of *má huáng* (Herba Ephedrae) and *xì xīn* (Radix et Rhizoma Asari). Together, all of the medicinals in the formula function to warm the Lung, dispel cold, resolve phlegm, and calm panting.

【Modifications】

➢ For severe wind-cold, chills, headache, and general arthralgia, add *qiāng huó* (Rhizoma et Radix Notopterygii), *guì zhī* (Ramulus Cinnamomi Cassiae) and *wēi líng xiān* (Radix et Rhizoma Clematidis) so as to resolve exterior-tightened wind-cold.

羌活	qiāng huó	15g	Rhizoma et Radix Notopterygii
桂枝	guì zhī	10g	Ramulus Cinnamomi Cassiae
威灵仙	wēi líng xiān	15g	Radix et Rhizoma Clematidis

➢ For profuse phlegm, counterflow of qi and difficult breath, add *jú hóng* (Exocarpium Citri Rubrum), *tíng lì zǐ* (Semen Lepidii seu Descurainiae) and *zhì nán xīng* (Rhizoma Arisaematis Praeparata) to resolve phlegm and stop asthma.

橘红	jú hóng	9g	Exocarpium Citri Rubrum
葶苈子	tíng lì zǐ	12g	Semen Lepidii seu Descurainiae
制南星	zhì nán xīng	10g	Arisaema cum Bile Praeparata

(2) Heat Asthma

【Pattern Characteristics】

Coughing and panting, phlegm wheezing in the throat, difficulty in lying down flat, a dry mouth with a bitter taste, and yellow and sticky sputum that is difficult to expectorate. This is accompanied by fever, headache, a red complexion, sweating, constipation, and yellow urine. There is a red tongue with a yellow and dry, or yellow and greasy coating. The pulse is superficial, slippery and rapid.

【Treatment Principle】

Clear heat and diffuse the Lung; remove phlegm and calm panting.

【Commonly Used Medicinals】

For removing phlegm and calming panting, use *má huáng* (Herba Ephedrae), *xìng rén* (Armeniacae Semen Amarum), *jié gěng* (Radix Platycodonis), *dì lóng* (Lumbricus), *bái guǒ* (Semen Ginkgo), *guā lóu pí* (Pericarpium Trichosanthis) and *shí chāng pú* (Rhizoma Acori Tatarinowii). For clearing heat and diffusing the Lung, select *yú xīng cǎo* (Herba Houttuyniae), *wěi jīng* (Coulis Phragmitis), *huáng qín* (Radix Scutellariae), *pú gōng yīng* (Herba Taraxaci), *zhè bèi mǔ* (Bulbus Fritillariae Thunbergii) and *dǎn nán xīng* (Arisaema cum Bile).

【Representative Formula】

Modified *Dìng Chuǎn Tāng* (定喘汤)

【Ingredients】

白果	bái guǒ	10g	Semen Ginkgo
麻黄	má huáng	9g	Herba Ephedrae
苏子	sū zǐ	10g	Fructus Perillae
甘草	gān cǎo	6g	Radix et Rhizoma Glycyrrhizae
款冬花	kuǎn dōng huā	12g	Flos Farfarae
杏仁	xìng rén	10g	Armeniacae Semen Amarum
桑白皮	sāng bái pí	12g	Cortex Mori
黄芩	huáng qín	12g	Radix Scutellariae
半夏	bàn xià	9g	Rhizoma Pinelliae
鱼腥草	yú xīng cǎo	30g	Herba Houttuyniae

Decoct in 800ml of water until 200ml of the decoction is left. Divide into 2 portions. Take warm, 1 dose a day.

【Formula Analysis】

Within this formula, *má huáng* (Herba Ephedrae) diffuses and lowers Lung qi, it can stop panting and also relieve exterior patterns. *Xìng rén* (Armeniacae Semen Amarum) downbears counterflow in order to relieve panting. In combination, these two herbs have a strong action to diffuse Lung qi, resolve phlegm and stop panting. *Sāng bái pí* (Cortex Mori) and *huáng qín* (Radix Scutellariae) clear Lung heat to stop cough and calm panting. These two herbs are used in combination because one diffuses Lung qi and downbears counterflow, and one clears and resolves heat-phlegm. Therefore the exterior can be resolved, phlegm and heat can be cleared, and the pathogenic factors of disease can be eliminated. *Sū zǐ* (Fructus Perillae), *bàn xià* (Rhizoma Pinelliae) and *kuǎn dōng huā* (Flos Farfarae) downbear counterflow and relieve panting, stop cough and resolve phlegm. In combination with *má huáng* (Herba Ephedrae) and *xìng rén* (Armeniacae Semen Amarum), they strengthen the effect of diffusing the Lung, resolving phlegm and calming panting. *Bái guǒ* (Semen Ginkgo) is sweet in flavor and astringent in nature, it not only resolves phlegm and dispels turbid evil, but also astringes Lung qi and calms panting. It can also restrict the excessively dispersing nature of *má huáng* (Herba Ephedrae). *Gān cǎo* (Radix et Rhizoma Glycyrrhizae) harmonizes all of the herbs in the prescription. Basically, this formula represents the three methods of diffusing, clearing and downbearing. Diffusing and lowering Lung qi, resolving phlegm and calming panting, clearing heat and relieving the exterior can all be achieved, and the wind-cold can be externally scattered, the Lung qi can be diffused and smoothed, the phlegm-heat be removed interiorly, and then panting and cough will calm down.

【Modifications】

➤ For high fever and vexing thirst, and profuse sticky and yellow sputum that is difficult to expectorate, add *lú gēn* (Rhizoma Phragmitis Communis) or *shí gāo* (Gypsum Fibrosum), *qīng tiān kuí* (Nervilia Fordii) and *bò hé* (Herba Menthae Haplocalycis) (to be added at the end) so as to clear Lung heat and resolve both interior and exterior heat.

➤ For constipation, abdominal distention and fullness, a yellowish thick and dry tongue coating, add *dà huáng* (Radix et Rhizoma Rhei) and *zhǐ qiào* (Fructus Aurantii) to clear the interior heat and eliminate the excess of the *fu* organs.

大黄	dà huáng	10g (decocted later)	Radix et Rhizoma Rhei
枳壳	zhǐ qiào	10g	Fructus Aurantii

➤ For serious and protracted panting, add *tíng lì zǐ* (Semen Lepidii seu Descurainiae) and *sū zǐ* (Fructus Perillae) to downbear the Lung qi.

葶苈子	tíng lì zǐ	12g	Semen Lepidii seu Descurainiae
苏子	sū zǐ	10g	Fructus Perillae

2. THE TREATMENT DURING REMISSION STAGE

(1) Deficiency of Lung Qi

【Pattern Characteristics】

There is a cough, expectoration of thin and white sputum, a pale complexion, shortness of breath, a weak voice, spontaneous perspiration and intolerance of wind, susceptibility to catching colds, a pink tongue with a thin and white coating, and a thready and weak pulse.

【Treatment Principle】

Boost qi and consolidate the exterior; tonify the Lung and calm panting.

【Commonly Used Medicinals】

For boosting qi and consolidating the exterior, use *huáng qí* (Radix Astragali), *dōng chóng xià cǎo* (Cordyceps Sinensis), *bái zhú* (Rhizoma Atractylodis Macrocephalae), *fáng fēng* (Radix Saposhnikoviae) and *dǎng shēn* (Radix Codonopsitis). For tonifying the Lung and calming panting, use *qǐ gé* (Solen goudii Conrad), *xìng rén* (Armeniacae Semen Amarum), *wǔ wèi zǐ* (Fructus Schisandrae Chinensis), *chuān bèi mǔ* (Bulbus Fritillariae Cirrhosae), *bǎi hé* (Bulbus Lilii), *hú táo ròu* (Semen Juglandis Regiae), *shā shēn* (Radix Glehniae seu Adenophorae) and *yù zhú* (Rhioma Polygonati Odorati).

【Representative Formula】

Modified *Yù Píng Fēng Sǎn* (玉屏风散)

【Ingredients】

黄芪	huáng qí	30g	Radix Astragali
白术	bái zhú	15g	Rhizoma Atractylodis Macrocephalae
防风	fáng fēng	9g	Radix Saposhnikoviae
桂枝	guì zhī	9g	Ramulus Cinnamomi
白芍	bái sháo	15g	Radix Paeoniae Alba
生姜	shēng jiāng	3pcs	Rhizoma Zingiberis Recens
大枣	dà zǎo	5pcs	Fructus Jujubae
沙参	shā shēn	15g	Radix Glehniae seu Adenophorae
麦冬	mài dōng	15g	Radix Ophiopogonis

Decoct in 800ml of water until 200ml of the decoction is left. Divide into 2 portions. Take warm, 1 dose a day.

【Formula Analysis】

Within this formula, *huáng qí* (Radix Astragali) is sweet in flavor and warm in nature. Interiorly, it can potently tonify the qi of the Spleen and Lung. Exteriorly it can consolidate the exterior to stop perspiration. It is the chief herb in this formula. *Bái zhú* (Rhizoma Atractylodis Macrocephalae) fortifies the Spleen and boosts qi; it can aid *huáng qí* (Radix Astragali) in strengthening the function of boosting qi and consolidating the exterior. It is the deputy herb in this formula. The combination of these two herbs makes the qi flourish and the exterior stable so that the spontaneous perspiration can be stopped and the exterior evils cannot attack the body. Within this formula, *fáng fēng* (Radix Saposhnikoviae) is the assistant herb. It can scatter wind and defend against the exteriors evils, because it functions at the exterior level of the body. *Huáng qí* (Radix Astragali) combined with *fáng fēng* (Radix Saposhnikoviae) can consolidate the exterior while not retaining the exterior evils. *Fáng fēng* (Radix Saposhnikoviae) combined with *huáng qí* (Radix Astragali) can eliminate wind without impairing the right qi. For exterior deficiency with spontaneous perspiration, or general debility with susceptibility to catching colds, this prescription has the effect of boosting qi and consolidating the exterior, as well as supporting the right qi and eliminating the evil qi. *Yù Píng Fēng* is the name of the prescription because the function of the prescription is like a barrier to defend against wind, and its effect is valuable like jade.

【Modifications】

➢ For cough and qi counterflow, add *xìng rén* (Armeniacae Semen Amarum) and *jié gěng* (Radix Platycodonis) to diffuse and lower the Lung qi.

➢ For excessive sweating and non-consolidation of the exterior due to deficiency, use *huáng qí* (Radix Astragali) at a heavier dose, and add *nuò dào gēn* (Radix Oryza Sativa), *má huáng gēn* (Radix et Rhizoma Ephedrae), *wǔ wèi zǐ* (Fructus Schisandrae Chinensis) and *shēng mǔ lì* (Concha Ostreae) in order to consolidate the exterior and astringe sweats

糯稻根	nuò dào gēn		30g	Radix Oryza Sativa
麻黄根	má huáng gēn		10g	Radix et Rhizoma Ephedrae
五味子	wǔ wèi zǐ		6g	Fructus Schisandrae Chinensis
生牡蛎	shēng mǔ lì	30g (decocted first)		Concha Ostreae

(2) Deficiency of Spleen Qi

【Pattern Characteristics】

There is cough and shortness of breath, clear thin sputum, emaciation, a bright pale complexion, loss of appetite with poor digestion, and loose stools. The tongue is pale with teeth-marks on its edges and the coating is white. The pulse is weak.

【Treatment Principle】

Boost qi and fortify the Spleen; reinforce Earth (Spleen) so as to strengthen Metal (Lung).

【Commonly Used Medicinals】

For boosting qi and invigorating the Spleen, use *dǎng shēn*

(Radix Codonopsitis), *fú líng* (Poria), *bái zhú* (Rhizoma Atractylodis Macrocephalae), *jī nèi jīn* (Endothelium Corneum Gigeriae Galli), *mài yá* (Fructus Hordei Germinatus), *gǔ yá* (Fructus Setariae Germinatus), *shā rén* (Fructus Amomi), *huò xiāng* (Herba Agastachis), *dà fù pí* (Pericarpium Arecae), *zhǐ qiào* (Fructus Aurantii), *fǎ bàn xià* (Rhizoma Pinelliae Praeparatum), *chén pí* (Pericarpium Citri Reticulatae), *yí táng* (Saccharum Granorum), *shēng jiāng* (Rhizoma Zingiberis Recens) and *dà zǎo* (Fructus Jujubae).

【Representative Formula】
Modified *Liù Jūn Zǐ Tāng* (六君子汤)

【Ingredients】

党参	dǎng shēn	20g	Radix Codonopsitis
黄芪	huáng qí	20g	Radix Astragali
茯苓	fú líng	12g	Poria
白术	bái zhú	12g	Rhizoma Atractylodis Macrocephalae
炙甘草	zhì gān cǎo	6g	Radix et Rhizoma Glycyrrhizae Praeparata
麦芽	mài yá	15g	Fructus Hordei Germinatus
枳壳	zhǐ qiào	12g	Fructus Citri
法半夏	fǎ bàn xià	12g	Rhizoma Pinelliae Praeparatum
陈皮	chén pí	9g	Pericarpium Citri Reticulatae

Decoct in 800ml of water until 200ml of the decoction is left. Divide into 2 portions. Take warm, 1 dose a day.

【Formula Analysis】
This formula is made up of *Sì Jūn Zǐ Tāng* (四君子汤) plus *chén pí* (Pericarpium Citri Reticulatae) and *bàn xià* (Rhizoma Pinelliae). Within this formula, *rén shēn* (Radix Ginseng) is the chief herb; it is sweet in flavor and warm in nature so that it can boost qi, fortify the Spleen, and nourish the Stomach. *Bái zhú* (Rhizoma Atractylodis Macrocephalae) is the deputy herb. Bitter in flavor and warm in nature, it can fortify the Spleen to dry dampness and enhance the effect of boosting qi to aid transportation. *Fú*

líng (Poria) is the assistant herb. Sweet in flavor and bland in nature, it can fortify the Spleen to discharge dampness. *Fú líng* (Poria) and *bái zhú* (Rhizoma Atractylodis Macrocephalae) work with each other to the effect of enhancing the fortification of the Spleen in order to eliminate dampness. *Zhì gān cǎo* (Radix et Rhizoma Glycyrrhizae Praeparata) is the envoy herb; it can replenish qi and regulate the middle jiao, and harmonize the actions of all of the herbs in the formula. By using these four herbs together, the function of boosting qi and fortifying the Spleen can be achieved. Add *chén pí* (Pericarpium Citri Reticulatae) to rectify qi and scatter counterflow. Add *bàn xià* (Rhizoma Pinelliae) to dry dampness and resolve phlegm. These six herbs are called *Liu Jun (six gentlemen)*, because they are all medicinals with moderate nature, mutual coordinating functions and assistance to the impaired. The ingredients of this prescription are all neutral and warm but not hot and dry. Amongst them some have reinforcing actions, while some others have reducing actions. They tonifying without stagnating, and moderately reinforce without using drastic actions. All of these medicinals function together to make the Spleen qi sufficient so that qi and blood have the source for generation, and thus the turbid phlegm can be removed through sound transportation by the Spleen.

【Modifications】

➢ For cough with excessive sputum, add *qián hú* (Radix Peucedani) and *pí pa yè* (Folium Eriobotryae) to diffuse Lung qi and resolve phlegm.

前胡	qián hú	15g	Radix Peucedani
枇杷叶	pí pá yè	10g	Folium Eriobotryae

➢ For excessive sweats with exterior deficiency, add *má huáng gēn* (Radix et Rhizoma Ephedrae) and *wǔ wèi zǐ* (Fructus Schisandrae Chinensis) to astringe sweating.

麻黄根	má huáng gēn	9g	Radix et Rhizoma Ephedrae
五味子	wǔ wèi zǐ	6g	Fructus Schisandrae Chinensis

➢ For loss of appetite and loose stools, add *shān yào* (Rhizoma Dioscoreae), *shā rén* (Fructus Amomi) (decocted later) and *pèi lán* (Herba Eupatorii) to invigorate the Spleen so as to resolve dampness.

山药	shān yào	20g	Rhizoma Dioscoreae
砂仁	shā rén	6g (decocted later)	Fructus Amomi
佩兰	pèi lán	15g	Herba Eupatorii

(3) Failure of the Kidney to Receive Qi

【Pattern Characteristics】

There is prolonged panting aggravated by exertion, intolerance of cold, spontaneous perspiration or night sweats, emaciation and lassitude, palpitations, and lumbar soreness. There is a pink tongue, and a deep and thready pulse.

【Treatment Principle】

Tonify the Kidney to receive qi.

【Commonly Used Medicinals】

For tonifying the Kidney to receive qi, use *shú dì huáng* (Radix Rehmanniae Praeparata), *shān zhū yú* (Fructus Corni), *dù zhòng* (Cortex Eucommiae), *bā jǐ tiān* (Radix Morindae Officinalis), *ròu cōng róng* (Herba Cistanches), *shú fù zǐ* (Radix Aconiti Lateralis Praeparata), *ròu guì* (Cortex Cinnamomi), *bǔ gǔ zhī* (Fructus Psoraleae), *wǔ wèi zǐ* (Fructus Schisandrae Chinensis), *yì zhì rén* (Fructus Alpiniae Oxyphyllae), *suǒ yáng* (Herba Cynomorii) and *jīn yīng zǐ* (Fructus Rosae Laevigatae).

【Representative Formula】

Modified *Shèn Qì Wán* (肾气丸)

【Ingredients】

熟地黄	shú dì huáng	15g	Radix Rehmanniae Praeparata
山茱萸	shān zhū yú	12g	Fructus Corni
山药	shān yào	15g	Rhizoma Dioscoreae
熟附子	shú fù zǐ	12g	Radix Aconiti Lateralis Praeparata

肉桂	ròu guì	5g (infused before taking)	Cortex Cinnamomi
补骨脂	bǔ gǔ zhī	15g	Fructus Psoraleae
冬虫夏草	dōng chóng xià cǎo	3g (simmered separately)	Cordyceps Sinensis
茯苓	fú líng	12g	Poria
牡丹皮	mǔ dān pí	9g	Cortex Moutan
泽泻	zé xiè	9g	Rhizoma Alismatis
五味子	wǔ wèi zī	6g	Fructus Schisandrae Chinensis

Decoct in 800ml of water until 200ml of the decoction is left. Divide into 2 portions. Take warm, 1 dose a day.

【Formula Analysis】

Within this formula, *fù zǐ* (Radix Aconiti Lateralis Praeparata), *ròu guì* (Cortex Cinnamomi), *shú dì huáng* (Radix Rehmanniae Praeparata), *shān yào* (Rhizoma Dioscoreae) and *shān yú ròu* (Fructus Corni) together can warm the yang qi of the Kidney, tonify the Kidney and replenish the essence to produce Kidney qi so as to promote distribution of water. *Zé xiè* (Rhizoma Alismatis), *dān pí* (Cortex Moutan) and *yún líng* (Poria) can strengthen this tonification through their reducing function. The whole prescription is warm but not hot and dry, and nourishing but not greasy. It tonifies yang with the combination of many yang-invigorating medicinals and a few of yin-nourishing medicinals, thus the deficiency of Kidney yang can be fundamentally cured.

【Modifications】

➢ For severe panting, add the powder of *gé jiè* (Gecko) (infused in hot water before taking) and *bā jǐ tiān* (Radix Morindae Officinalis) to strengthen the function of consolidating the Kidney to receive qi.

蛤蚧末	gé jiè mò	2g (infused in hot water before taking)	Gecko Powder
巴戟天	bā jǐ tiān	15g	Radix Morindae Officinalis

> For a cold body with cold limbs, soreness and weakness of the lower back and knees, add ròu guì (Cortex Cinnamomi) (steamed in air-tight vessel before taking) and yín yáng huò (Herba Epimedii) so as to warm the Kidney and Liver.

| 肉桂 | ròu guì | 5g (steamed in air-tight vessel before taking) | Cortex Cinnamomi |
| 淫羊藿 | yín yáng huò | 15g | Herba Epimedii |

Additional Treatment Modalities

1. Chinese Patent Medicine

(1) *Tán Ké Jìng* (痰咳净)

The dose is one spoonful, four to six times daily. It is suitable for patients with cold asthma.

(2) *Hé Chē Dà Zào Wán* (河车大造丸)

The dose is 10g, 3 times a day. It is suitable for patients in the remission stage with Kidney insufficiency.

(3) *Gé Jiè Dìng Chuǎn Wán* (蛤蚧定喘丸)

The dose is one pill, twice daily. It is suitable for patients with deficiency asthma due to a deficiency of both the Lung and Kidney with the Kidney failing to receive qi.

2. Acupuncture and Moxibustion

(1) Body Acupuncture

【Treatment Principle】
Diffuse Lung qi and calm panting.
【Point Selection】

| EX-B1 | dìng chuǎn | 定喘 |
| BL 12 | fēng mén | 风门 |

BL 13	fèi shù	肺俞
LU 11	shào shāng	少商
LU 7	liè quē	列缺
L 14	hé gǔ	合谷

【Point Modifications】

➢ For excessive phlegm, add ST 36 (*zú sān lǐ*) and ST 40 (*fēng lóng*) to promote qi transformation and move phlegm.

【Manipulation】

Do the acupuncture with an even supplementation and drainage method. Each time chose 3—4 points, using each point 2—3 times. Treat 6 times a week. 24 times is one course of treatment.

(2) Electro-Acupuncture

【Point Selection】

BL 13	fèi shù	肺俞 (both sides)

【Point Modifications】

➢ For cold asthma, add BL 12 (*fēng mén*) (both sides), LI 14 (*hé gǔ*) (both sides) and LU 7 *(liè quē)* (both sides).

➢ For heat asthma, add DU 14 (*dà zhuī*), BL 12 (both sides), and LU 10 (*yú jì*) (both sides).

【Manipulation】

The patient is placed in the prone position. Disinfect BL 13 (*fèi shù*) according to conventional methods. Using a 1.5 *cun* long number 30 filiform needle, insert the needle obliquely with the tip pointed towards the spine. Insert the needle 1.0 to 1.2 *cun* deep according to patient's body build, and then manipulate the needle with a rotating method. After a needling sensation is obtained, connect the Han's electroacupuncture instrument, and use a sparse-dense wave with a frequency of 20Hz. Use a reasonable intensity so that the needle handle vibrates slightly and the patient can tolerate the stimulation. For the rest of the points, needle in a conventional method and retain the needles for 30 minutes. Acupuncture treatment is conducted once a day, with two weeks of treatments making up a course. The cautions are the same as those for body acupuncture.

(3) Moxibustion

1) Point Combination 1

【Treatment Principle】

Boost the Lung, dispel cold, and calm panting.

【Point Selection】

DU 14	dà zhuī	大椎
BL 13	fèi shù	肺俞
BL 43	gāo huāng	膏肓
EX-B1	dìng chuǎn	定喘

【Manipulation】

Do suspended moxibustion for 20 minutes every time, once or twice a day.

2) Point Combination 2

【Treatment Principle】

Tonify the Kidney to receive qi; warm and supplement the Ren and Du vessels; return yang, stem desertion, and stem counterflow.

【Point Selection】

RN 4	guān yuán	关元
DU 20	bǎi huì	百会
KI 1	yǒng quán	涌泉

【Manipulation】

Use ginger moxibustion for 3—5 *zhuang* and suspended moxibustion for 15—20 minutes, once or twice a day.

3) Point Combination 3

【Treatment Principle】

Warm and tonify the Lung, Spleen and Kidney; greatly tonify the gathering qi and original qi.

【Point Selection】

DU 14	dà zhuī	大椎
BL 13	fèi shù	肺俞
BL 17	gé shù	膈俞
BL 23	shèn shù	肾俞
LU 1	zhōng fǔ	中府
RN 22	tiān tū	天突
RN 17	dàn zhōng	膻中
RN 6	qì hǎi	气海
RN 4	guān yuán	关元
ST 36	zú sān lǐ	足三里

【Manipulation】

Use suspended moxibustion or ginger moxibustion, once a day. Alternate using 3 to 5 points every time. 7 days makes up one course of treatment.

(4) External Application at Points

1) Approach 1

【Treatment Principle】

Acridly warm to expel phlegm, dispel and resolve cold evil.

【Point Selection】

BL 13	fèi shù	肺俞
BL 15	xīn shù	心俞
BL 17	gé shù	膈俞

【Manipulation】

Application of *Xīn Jiè Gāo* 辛芥膏 (Asarum and Brassicae Albae Semen Plaster) on acupuncture points: Use *bái jiè zǐ* (Semen Sinapis Albae), *gān suí* (Radix Kansui) 1.2 portions, respectively, *xì xīn* (Radix et Rhizoma Asari) 1.5 portions and *shè xiāng* (Secretio Moschi) 0.05 portion. Grind them together into a powder, mix with ginger juice to prepare as a plaster, and use as an external compress. Do this once every 5 days, with 3 times making up a course of treatment.

2) Approach 2

【Treatment Principle】

Dispel phlegm, calm panting, invigorate blood, and transform stasis.

【Point Selection】

DU 14	dà zhuī	大椎
EX-B1	dìng chuǎn	定喘 (both sides)
BL 13	fèi shù	肺俞 (both sides)
BL 43	gāo huāng	膏肓 (both sides)
BL 15	xīn shù	心俞 (both sides)

【Manipulation】

Use *bái jiè zǐ* (Semen Sinapis Albae), *xì xīn* (Radix et Rhizoma Asari), *gān suí* (Radix Kansui), *é zhú* (Rhizoma Curcumae), *yán hú suǒ* (Rhizoma Corydalis) and *liú huáng* (Sulphur) in the ratios of 6:5:4:3:2:1. Grind these together into a powder. Add *shè xiāng* (Secretio Moschi) 0.9g to every 100g of powder. Gently mix together with fresh ginger juice. Dissolve *bīng piàn* (Borneolum Syntheticum) in a 75% alcohol saturated solution. Mix together the ginger juice and *bīng piàn* (Borneolum Syntheticum) alcohol solution in a 5:1 ratio. After this process, form the medicine into a cake with the size and thickness of a 5 *fen* coin. Stick the medicinal cake on the above-mentioned points for 4 to 6 hours at a time (2 hours for children). Stop the treatment if erythema or blisters appear locally on the skin. The application should be done on the first days of the initial, middle and last periods of the greatest heat days in summer. 3 times makes up a course of treatment.

3) Approach 3

【Treatment Principle】

Warm the Lung and dispel cold to calm panting.

【Point Selection】

BL 13	fèi shù	肺俞
RN 20	huá gài	华盖
RN 17	dàn zhōng	膻中
RN 8	shén què	神阙

【Manipulation】

Use *Qīng Lóng Tiē* (青龙贴). There are 11 ingredients: *má huáng* (Herba Ephedrae), *dì lóng* (Lumbricus), *guì zhī* (Ramulus Cinnamomi), *bái sháo* (Radix Paeoniae Alba), *gān jiāng* (Rhizoma Zingiberis), *xì xīn* (Radix et Rhizoma Asari), *wǔ wèi zǐ* (Fructus Schisandrae Chinensis), *chuān wū tóu* (Radix Aconiti Carmichaeli), *bàn xià* (Rhizoma Pinelliae), *tíng lì zǐ* (Semen Lepidii seu Descurainiae) and *gān cǎo* (Radix et Rhizoma Glycyrrhizae).

麻黄	má huáng	Herba Ephedrae
地龙	dì lóng	Lumbricus
桂枝	guì zhī	Ramulus Cinnamomi
白芍药	bái sháo yào	Radix Paeoniae Alba
干姜	gān jiāng	Rhizoma Zingiberis
细辛	xì xīn	Radix et Rhizoma Asari
五味子	wǔ wèi zǐ	Fructus Schisandrae Chinensis
川乌头	chuān wū tóu	Radix Aconiti Carmichaeli
半夏	bàn xià	Rhizoma Pinelliae
亭苈子	tíng lì zǐ	Semen Lepidii seu Descurainiae
甘草	gān cǎo	Radix et Rhizoma Glycyrrhizae

After processing this mixture, compress the plaster onto the above-mentioned points. Use 1 plaster per day. 14 days makes up a course of treatment.

4) Approach 4

【Treatment Principle】

Transform phlegm, resolve spasms, and calm panting.

【Points Selection】

| KI 1 | yǒng quán | 涌泉 (both sides) |

【Manipulation】

Use *Mǎ Xìng Zhǐ Xiào Sǎn* (马杏止哮散). The ingredients are *mǎ qián zǐ* (Semen Strychni) 20g, *dì biē chóng* (Eupolyphaga seu steleophaga) 15g and *běi xìng rén* (Armeniacae Semen Amarum) 15g.

马钱子	mǎ qián zǐ	20g	Semen Strychni
地鳖虫	dì biē chóng	15g	Eupolyphaga seu steleophaga
北杏仁	běi xìng rén	15g	Armeniacae Semen Amarum

Break them into pieces, add water and mix them into a paste. The patient is asked to lie in bed, and externally apply the paste on both KI 1 (*yǒng quán*) points for 24 hours. This is done once a week.

5) Approach 5

【Treatment Principle】

Tonify the Lung and resolve phlegm to arrest panting.

【Point Selection】

BL 13	fèi shù	肺俞
BL 43	gāo huāng shù	膏肓俞
EX-HN15	bǎi láo	百劳

【Manipulation】

Use appropriate qualities of *bái jiè zǐ* (Semen Sinapis Albae), *bàn xià* (Rhizoma Pinelliae), *xì xīn* (Radix et Rhizoma Asari) and *yán hú suǒ* (Rhizoma Corydalis), and grind them into a powder. Make this powder into a paste by using fresh ginger juice, and then make this mixture into medicinal cakes to apply on the above-mentioned points. The application is usually used during the three periods of the greatest heat days in summer, once during each period, 2 hours for each time.

(5) Ear Acupuncture
【Treatment Principle】
Boost the Kidney and calm panting.
【Point Selection】

anti-asthmatic		píng chuǎn	平喘
adrenal gland	TG2p	shèn shàng xiàn	肾上腺
sympathetic	AH6a	jiāo gǎn	交感

【Manipulation】
Disinfect using conventional methods. Insert the needles with moderate or light stimulation, and retain the needles for 15 to 30 minutes. Do once every other day, with 12 times making up a course of treatment. There should be a 3 to 5 day interval between two courses. The cautions are the same as those for body acupuncture.

Auricular Points Pellet-Pressing Therapy: Disinfect the auricular area of the ear. Adhere *wáng bù liú xíng zǐ* (Semen Vaccariae) to the center of an adhesive plaster that is 0.5cm×0.5cm in size. Then apply the seeds on the auricular points with appropriate pressure in order to induce a feeling of heat and distending pain in the auricle of ear. It is common that for each treatment with *wáng bù liú xíng zǐ* (Semen Vaccariae) that only points in one ear are used. The treatment uses alternate sides each time, though both ears can be treated at once. During this treatment, the patient can press the seeds himself, for 1 to 2 minutes for each point every time. The pellets are retained for 3 to 5 days each time. Seven times makes up a course of treatment.

(6) Eye Acupuncture
【Treatment Principle】
Transform phlegm and calm panting.

【Point Selection】.

| Lung | CO14 | fèi qū | 肺区 (both sides) |
| Upper Jiao | | shàng jiāo qū | 上焦区 (both sides) |

【Manipulation】

Select a needle with a length of 5 *fen*. Insert the needle obliquely with an angle of 45° to reach the eye bone until there is a needling sensation. Pay attention not to injury the eyeball. Retain the needle for 15 minutes, manipulating the needle every 5 minutes. The symptoms can be relieved after 10 minutes.

(7) Miscellaneous Modalities

1) Cupping

Use a three-edged needle to prick DU 14 (*dà zhuī*) and *dìng chuǎn* in order to cause some bleeding; then apply cups. Afterwards, insert needles at RN 17 (*dàn zhōng*), LI 11 (*qū chí*) and SP 6 (*sān yīn jiāo*). For cases of qi deficiency of the Spleen and Lung, add BL 20 (*pí shù*) and BL 13 (*fèi shù*). For cases of yin deficiency of the Lung and Kidney, add BL 23 (*shèn shù*), KI 3 (*tài xī*) and KI 7 (*fù liū*). This treatment is suitable during an acute episode of asthma.

2) Three-Edged Needle Acupuncture

Use *dìng chuǎn* and BL 13 (*fèi shù*) as the main acupuncture points, and use BL 20 (*pí shù*), BL 23 and LI 11 (*shào shāng*) as subsidiary points. Chose one main point and one subsidiary point each time, and using a three-edged needle, insert into the points until it reaches the muscular layer. Then withdraw and insert the needle up and down 5 to 10 times until a needling sensation is induced. Treat this way 2 to 3 times each week. 6 to 8 times makes up a course of treatment. 2 to 3 successive courses of treatment are needed.

3) Three-Acupuncture Points, Five Needles, One Cup" Therapy

Insert needles at BL 13 (*fèi shù*) (bilaterally), BL 12 (*fēng mēn*) (bilaterally), and DU 14 (*dà zhuī*). Other acupuncture points can be chosen according to symptoms. Retain the needles for 30 minutes after a needling sensation is induced. Use an even supplementation and drainage method for the needling, and then use cupping therapy after acupuncture. Treat once every other day. 15 times makes up a course of treatment.

4) Needle-Pricking Therapy

Select DU 14 (*dà zhuī*), *dìng chuǎn*, BL 13 (*fèi shù*), RN 15 (*jiū wěi*), and RN 12 (*zhōng wǎn*). Use a hook-shaped pricking needle and insert at the points to a depth of 1 *fen*. Prick out white fiber-like subcutaneous tissue. Treat once a week. 7 times makes up a course of treatment. 1 to 3 courses of treatment are needed.

5) Implantation Therapy

Decoct the suture thread and *xī xiān cǎo* (Herba Siegesbeckiae) together for 30 minutes. Then cut the suture thread to 0.5cm long and implant it subcutaneously at RN 17 (*dàn zhōng*). Repeat once a month, for 3 months in a row. 3 times makes up a course of treatment.

Use medicated thread implanted subcutaneously at BL 13 (*fèi shù*), BL 12 (*fēng mēn*), ST 40 (*fēng lōng*), *dìng chuǎn*, BL 20 (*pí shù*) and BL 23 (*shèn shù*).

6) Needle-Implantation Therapy

For excess patterns, use BL 13 (*fèi shù*), *dìng chuǎn*, and tender points on the back. For deficiency patterns, use BL 17 (*gé shù*), BL 23 (*shèn shù*) and tender points on the back. Implant needles subcutaneously and retain them for 3 to 5 days. Treat 1 to 2 times a week. A course of treatment is 4 weeks.

7) Acupuncture Point Taping Therapy

Use BL 13 (*fèi shù*) and *dìng chuǎn* as the primary points. In cases of wind and cold, add LU 7 (*liè quē*) and BL 12 (*fēng mēn*). In cases with profuse expectoration, add RN 17 (*dàn zhōng*) and ST 40 (*fēng lōng*). For deficiency patterns, add LU 9 (*tài yuān*), KI 3 *(tài xī)*, RN 6 (*qì hǎi*) and BL 23 *(shèn shù)*. Use a magnetic round needle to tap the points with a bird-pecking technique. Tap each point for 3 minutes, once a day. 10 times makes up a course of treatment.

8) Plum-Blossom Needling

Tap lightly up and down the Bladder channel along the thoracic spine 3 times. Then tap the skin of the Ren Vessel from RN 22 (*tiān tū*) to RN 17 (*dàn zhōng*) until the skin is flushed. Add moxibustion therapy at DU 14 (*dà zhuī*), BL 12 (*fēng mén*), BL 13 (*fèi shù*), RN 22 (*tiān tū*), and RN 17 (*dàn zhōng*). Treat for 15 minutes each time, once every four days. 3 times makes up a course of treamtent.

9) Lipid Cutting Therapy

Chose RN 17 (*dàn zhōng*) and anesthetize locally. Cut into the fat layer of the skin and remove local fatty tissue. Then clean and suture the cut. Take out the stitches a week later. 3 times makes up a course of treatment.

3. Simple Prescriptions and Empirical Formulas

(1) *Zào Jiá Wán* (皂荚丸)
【Ingredients】

红枣	hóng zǎo	500g	Fructus Jujubae
炙皂荚	zhì zào jiá	90g	Fructus Forsythiae

Take the *hóng zǎo* (Fructus Jujubae) 500g, peel it and pound it into a paste. Add *zhì zào jiá* (Fructus Gleditsiae Sinensis Praeparata) 90g, and mix with water. Form the mixture into 3g pills. Take one pill orally, 3 times a day. This is suitable for patients with bronchial asthma and profuse sputum.

(2) *Gé Jiè* (Gecko) and *Jí Lín Shēn* (Radix Ginseng Indici)
【Ingredients】

| 蛤蚧 | gé jiè | Gecko |
| 吉林参 | jí lín shēn | Radix Ginseng Indici |

Use a mixture of half *gé jiè* (Gecko) and half *jí lín shēn* (Radix Ginseng Indici) and grind them together into a fine powder. Take 2g orally in the morning and evening. This is suitable for patients in the remission stage of bronchial asthma, with deficiency of the Lung and Kidney.

(3) *Má Huáng* (Herba Ephedrae), *Shēng Bái Guǒ* (Semen Ginkgo Raw) and *Wǔ Wèi Zǐ* (Fructus Schisandrae Chinensis)
【Ingredients】

麻黄	má huáng	3g	Herba Ephedrae
生白果	shēng bái guǒ	5 pieces	Semen Ginkgo (raw)
五味子	wǔ wèi zǐ	2g	Fructus Schisandrae Chinensis

Take *má huáng* (Herba Ephedrae) 3g, *shēng bái guǒ* (Semen Ginkgo Raw) 5 pieces and *wǔ wèi zǐ* (Fructus Schisandrae Chinensis) 2g, and decoct them with water. Take orally, 3 to 4 times a day. Add 9g of Yinde black tea into the boiling water, and drink to strengthen the therapeutic effects. This is suitable for bronchial asthma with wheezing sounds, panting and cough.

(4) *Guǎng Dì Lóng* (Lumbricus) Powder
【Ingredients】

| 广地龙 | guǎng dì lóng | 3g | Lumbricus |

Take 3g of *guǎng dì lóng* (Lumbricus) per dose, 3 times a day. This can be swallowed in capsules.

(5) *Yáng Jīn Huā* (Flos Daturae)
【Ingredients】

| 洋金花 | yáng jīn huā | Flos Daturae |

Dry *yáng jīn huā* (Flos Daturae) in the sun and cut into filaments, then roll them into cigarette-like forms. When the patient experiences an asthma attack, he should light the roll and smoke it like a cigarette. The symptoms can be relieved after 3 or 4 inhalations.

(6) Placenta Therapy

Rinse the fresh placenta until it is clean. Place it on a new earthenware tile and bake it over a slow fire. Afterwards, grind it into a fine powder and sieve the powder, and then pack them up and seal with cera. The dosage is 2g each time, twice a day. 2 weeks makes up a course of treatment. The therapeutic effects using this method are a potent invigoration of the original qi, and a tonification of the Lung and Kidney. This is outstanding for asthmatic children and old men.

(7) *Lái Fú Zǐ Sǎn* (莱菔子散)

【Ingredients】

莱菔子	lái fú zǐ	500g	Semen Raphani
猪牙皂角	zhū yá zào jiǎo	15g	Spina Gleditsiae Abnormalis

Take *lái fú zǐ* (Semen Raphani) 500g (steamed, and dried in the sun), and *zhū yá zào jiǎo* (Spina Gleditsiae Abnormalis) 15g (with the peel and back spine removed), and grind them together into a fine powder. Put the mixture into bottles in order to prevent off-gassing. The dosage is 3g, taken after mixing the liquid.

(8) *Xìng Bèi Chōng Jì* (杏贝冲剂)

【Ingredients】

麻黄	má huáng	Herba Ephedrae
杏仁	xìng rén	Armeniacae Semen Amarum
金银花	jīn yín huā	Flos Lonicerae Japonicae
桑白皮	sāng bái pí	Cortex Mori
牛蒡子	niú bàng zǐ	Fructus Arctii

川贝母	chuān bèi mǔ	Bulbus Fritillariae Cirrhosae
前胡	qián hú	Radix Peucedani
丹参	dān shēn	Radix et Rhizoma Salviae Miltiorrhizae
地龙	dì lóng	Lumbricus

The ingredients are *má huáng* (Herba Ephedrae), *xìng rén* (Armeniacae Semen Amarum), *jīn yín huā* (Flos Lonicerae Japonicae), *sāng bái pí* (Cortex Mori), *niú bàng zǐ* (Fructus Arctii), *chuān bèi mǔ* (Bulbus Fritillariae Cirrhosae), *qián hú* (Radix Peucedani), *dān shēn* (Radix et Rhizoma Salviae Miltiorrhizae) and *dì lóng* (Lumbricus). There should be 50g of crude medicinals per bag. The dosage is one bag, taken twice a day orally as a draft. 20 days makes up a course of treatment.

(9) *Tíng Lì Píng Chuǎn Shuān* (葶苈平喘栓)

【Ingredients】

葶苈子	tíng lì zǐ	24g	Semen Lepidii seu Descurainiae
皂荚	zào jiá	10g	Fructus Gleditsiae Sinensis
麻黄	má huáng	12g	Herba Ephedrae
杏仁	xìng rén	6g	Armeniacae Semen Amarum
大黄	dà huáng	12g	Radix et Rhizoma Rhei
芒硝	máng xiāo	3g	Natrii Sulfas
大枣	dà zǎo	3g	Fructus Jujubae

The ingredients are *tíng lì zǐ* (Semen Lepidii seu Descurainiae) 24g, *zào jiá* (Fructus Gleditsiae Sinensis) 10g, *má huáng* (Herba Ephedrae) 12g, *xìng rén* (Armeniacae Semen Amarum) 6g, *dà huáng* (Radix et Rhizoma Rhei) 12g, *máng xiāo* (Natrii Sulfas) 3g and *dà zǎo* (Fructus Jujubae) 3g. Form these herbs into suppositories, with 10g crude medicinals in each one. Use 3 a day. 7 days makes up a course of treatment.

(10) *Má Bái Hé Jì* (麻白合剂)

【Ingredients】

| 麻黄 | má huáng | Herba Ephedrae |

白果	bái guǒ	Semen Bilobae
杏仁	xìng rén	Armeniacae Semen Amarum
枳实	zhǐ shí	Fructus Aurantii Immaturus
辛夷	xīn yí	Flos Magnoliae
细辛	xì xīn	Radix et Rhizoma Asari
丹参	dān shēn	Radix et Rhizoma Salviae Miltiorrhizae
川芎	chuān xiōng	Rhizoma Chuanxiong
黄芩	huáng qín	Radix Scutellariae
甘草	gān cǎo	Radix et Rhizoma Glycyrrhizae

The ingredients are *má huáng* (Herba Ephedrae), *bái guǒ* (Semen Bilobae), *xìng rén* (Armeniacae Semen Amarum), *zhǐ shí* (Fructus Aurantii Immaturus), *xīn yí* (Flos Magnoliae), *xì xīn* (Radix et Rhizoma Asari), *dān shēn* (Radix et Rhizoma Salviae Miltiorrhizae), *chuān xiōng* (Rhizoma Chuanxiong), *huáng qín* (Radix Scutellariae) and *gān cǎo* (Radix et Rhizoma Glycyrrhizae), for a total of 10 ingredients. Add water and decoct 3 times in a row, and then filter into a concentrated preparation. Use 20ml as an atomized inhalation, twice a day, for 20 minutes each time.

PROGNOSIS

In general, the symptoms and signs of an asthma attack can be quickly relieved through prompt treatment. However, improper treatments, repeated attacks, or prolonged illnesses can impair pulmonary function, induce emphysema, or even lead to pulmonary heart disease. This can cause the patient to lose his capacity for work, and affect his quality of life.

Status asthmaticus is a critical emergency condition of asthma, which can seriously endanger the patient's life. Therefore the treatment of this condition needs to be given sufficient and ample attention. A combination of Chinese medicine and biomedicine should be given, such as oxygen therapy, ample amounts of sensitive antibiotics to fight infection, large amounts of steroids for anti-inflammatory purposes, prompt monitoring of patient blood gas levels, and timely and efficacious treatment of respiratory failure, so as to save the patient's life.

PREVENTIVE HEALTHCARE

Because asthma attacks are related to allergies, we should pay attention to avoid sensitizing agents, emphasize the regulation of diet, strengthen the disease resistance of the body, and avoid flare ups. For these reasons, attention should be paid to the following aspects.

Lifestyle Modification

1. Pay Attention to Climactic Influences

Particularly in the autumn and winter seasons, when there may be violent changes in temperature, one should promptly add clothing and blankets so as to avoid from catching colds. This prevents against episodes induced by exogenous evils.

2. Take Precautions against Coming into Contact with Various Asthma Inducing agents

For example, avoid allergens such as coal gas, nitro diluent, insecticide aerosols, pesticides, gasoline, paints, indoor dust, cockroaches, and pollen. One must also absolutely stop smoking.

3. Pay Attention to Keeping Warm

During asthma attacks, because of coughing, panting and dyspnea, patients frequently sweat all over the body. The sweats can be so profuse that the clothes become wet. Therefore, in order to avoid catching colds, patients should change underwear promptly and pay attention to keeping warm.

Dietary Recommendation

A bland diet is suitable. One should avoid rich and heavy food, raw and cold food, and acrid and hot food, so as to eliminate the source of phlegm. Foods that in the past induced allergic reactions and episodes of asthma, such as fish, shrimp and crab, should be absolutely avoided. Clinically, during the remission stage of asthma, tonification is the major method of Chinese dietary therapy. This includes tonifying the Lung, Spleen, and Kidney. In general, it is not suitable to eat raw and cold food such as fish, shrimp, crab, raw chicken, carp, and *fā wù* (发物 , stimulating and illness-inducing foods). For cases of bronchial asthma complicated by infection one should not eat dry and hot food, or phlegm-condensing food. This is because there are symptoms like difficult expectoration, a dry mouth and a bitter taste in the mouth.

Medicinals and foods for dietary therapy include *xìng rén* (Armeniacae Semen Amarum), *zǐ sū* (Folium Perillae), *shēng jiāng* (Rhizoma Zingiberis Recens), *luó hàn guǒ* (Fructus Momordicae), *bǎi hé* (Bulbus Lilii), *bái guǒ* (Semen Ginkgo), *chuān bèi mǔ* (Bulbus Fritillariae Cirrhosae), *pí pa guǒ* (Fructus Eriobotryae), *hé táo* (Semen Juglandis), *qīng pí* (Pericarpium Citri Reticulatae Viride), *chén pí* (Pericarpium Citri Reticulatae), *fó shǒu* (Fructus Citri Sarcodactylis), *dīng xiāng* (Flos Caryophylli), *hú jiāo* (Fructus Piperis Nigri), *jiāo mù* (Semen Zanthoxyli Bungeani), *rén shēn* (Radix Ginseng), *fú líng* (Poria), *shān yào* (Rhizoma Dioscoreae), *lián zǐ* (Semen Nelumbinis), *qiàn shí* (Semen Euryales), *dāng guī* (Radix Angelicae Sinensis), *huáng qí* (Radix Astragali), *chuān xiōng* (Rhizoma Chuanxiong), *dōng chóng xià cǎo* (Cordyceps Sinensis), *gé jiè* (Gecko), *zǐ hé chē* (Placenta Hominis), *yín yáng huò* (Herba Epimedii), as well as Silkies (black chicken), quail, squab, sparrow, Chinese partridge, turtledove, mutton, pig lung, cat meat, crocodile meat, and jerboa .

1. Boiled Chicken with Dōng Chóng Xià Cǎo (Cordyceps Sinensis) (冬虫夏草炖鸡)

冬虫夏草	dōng chóng xià cǎo	5g	Cordyceps Sinensis
竹丝鸡 (乌鸡)	zhú sī jī	75g	Silkies (black chicken)
生姜	shēng jiāng	3 pieces	Rhizoma Zingiberis Recens
蜜枣	mì zǎo	1 piece	preserved date

Add 180ml of water, as well as salt and oil to taste, and cook over a slow fire for 2 hours. Drink the soup and eat the meat. This is suitable for patients in the remission stage of asthma, with Lung yin deficiency. The manifestations are dyspnea, shortness of breath and occasional cough with no expectoration, and a red tongue with little coating.

2. Powder of Ginseng and Gecko (Rén Shēn Gé Jiè Sǎn 人参蛤蚧散)

吉林参	jí lín shēn	0.25g	Radix Ginseng Indici
蛤蚧	gé jiè	1 pair	Gecko
紫河车	zǐ hé chē	1.75g	Placenta Hominis

Prepare these herbs and grind them into a fine powder, then preserve them in a bottle. The oral dose is 1.5 to 3g, 1 to 3 times a day. This is suitable for patients in the remission stage of asthma with yin deficiency of the Lung and Kidney. This manifests with dyspnea that is aggravated by exertion, spontaneous perspiration and night sweats, a low and weak voice due to insufficieny of the gathering qi. This is accompanied by soreness and weakness of the waist and knees.

3. Lamb Soup with Dāng Guī and Ginger (Dāng Guī Shēng Jiāng Yáng Ròu Tāng 当归生姜羊肉汤)

当归	dāng guī	15g	Radix Angelicae Sinensis
生姜	shēng jiāng	3 pieces	Rhizoma Zingiberis Recens
羊肉	yáng ròu	120g	mutton

Using an appropriate amount of water, decoct the above ingredients with salt and oil to taste. Drink the soup and eat the meat. This is suitable for patients in the remission stage of asthma, and a deficiency of qi and blood due to prolonged disease. This manifests as dyspnea, a reluctance to talk, a pale complexion, pale lips, poor appetite, and a thin body.

4. Pork Tripe Stewed Hú Jiāo (Fructus Piperis Nigri) (胡椒煲猪肚)

胡椒	hú jiāo	10 grains	Fructus Piperis Nigri
猪肚(猪胃)	zhū dù	120g	Pork tripe

Decoct with an appropriate amount of water, adding salt and oil to taste. Drink the soup and eat the meat. This is suitable for patients in the remission stage of asthma, with cold due to Stomach qi deficiency. This manifests as eating only a small amount, constant acid regurgitation, belching, and a dull pain in the epigastrium.

According to the above-mentioned recipes, patients can select one kind of medicinal herb and one kind of meat to make various stewed soups. These are suitable for weak patients in the remission stage of asthma.

5. Stewed Pork Lung with Jiàn Huā (Hylocereus undatus)

剑花	jiàn huā	20g	Hylocereus undatus
猪肺	zhū fèi	120g	Pig lung

Decoct with an appropriate amount of water, adding add salt and oil to taste. Drink the soup and eat the meat. This is suitable for patients in the remission stage of asthma, with heat in the Lung. This manifests as cough, a dry mouth, a bitter taste in the mouth, and a white and sticky sputum that difficult to expectorate. This therapy has the effect of clearing heat and tonifying the Lung.

6. Stewed Lean Pork with *Luó Hàn Guǒ* (Fructus Momordicae)

| 罗汉果 | luó hàn guǒ | 1/6 of a piece | Fructus Momordicae |
| 瘦肉 | shòu ròu | 120g | Lean meat |

Decoct with an appropriate amount of water, adding salt and oil to taste. Drink the soup and eat the meat. This is suitable for patients in the remission stage of asthma, with yin deficiency of the Lung. This manifests as a dry mouth and tongue, cough without expectoration, and itching and pain in the throat. This decoction has the effect of moistening the Lung and nourishing yin.

7. Chicken Soup with *Bái Guǒ* (Semen Ginkgo) and *Xìng Rén* (Armeniacae Semen Amarum)

白果	bái guǒ	15 pieces	Semen Ginkgo
杏仁	xìng rén	10g	Armeniacae Semen Amarum
陈皮	chén pí	3g	Pericarpium Citri Reticulatae

Take one chicken with the internal organs and skin removed, and stuff the above ingredients into the cavity, then stitch it shut with thread, stew it in water. Do not add salt. This therapy is suitable for patients whose panting has been relieved, but who still have a cough with little sputum.

8. Lean Meat Soup with *Yú Biāo Jiāo* (Pseudosciaena crocea) and *Dōng Chóng Xià Cǎo* (Cordyceps Sinensis)

鱼膘胶	yú biāo jiāo	15g	Pseudosciaena crocea
冬虫夏草	dōng chóng xià cǎo	10g	Cordyceps Sinensis
瘦猪肉	shòu zhū ròu	100g	Lean pork meat

Decoct the above in water until it is well done. Eat with a little salt. This therapy is suitable for those patients whose panting has been relieved, in order to strengthen the physique of the body and increase resistance to disease.

[Note: *Fā wù* (发物) refers to certain foods which can easily induce some diseases (especially chronic diseases) or aggravate already existing illness. *Fā wù* contraindications are important for dietary health care and dietary therapy. In general, *fā wù* are foods that most people can eat moderately without suffering from side effects or uncomfortable feelings. Only for those with special constitutions and related diseases can *fā wù* induce illness. According to their nature, *fā wù* can be classified into six types. First, foods that induce heat, such as Chinese onion, ginger, *huā jiāo* (Pericarpium Zanthoxyli), mutton and dog meat. Second, foods that induce wind, such as shrimp, crab and ailanthus sprout. Third, foods that induce dampness, such as *yí táng* (Saccharum Granorum), polished glutinous rice, glutinous wine and rice wine. Fourth, foods that induce cold accumulation, such as pear, persimmon and various raw and cold foods. Fifth, foods that induce bleeding, such as cayenne and *hú jiāo* (Fructus Piperis Nigri). Sixth, foods that induce qi stagnation, such as potato, *lián mǐ* (Stamen Nelumbinis Nuciferae), *qiàn shí* (Semen Euryales) and various foods made with beans.]

Regulation of Emotional and Mental Health

Asthma patients should avoid emotional and mental irritations and excessive overwork because these things can result in asthma attacks and are detrimental to physical recovery. During the remission stage of asthma, young patients should take part in appropriate physical exercise to promote the growth and development of the mind and body. Older patients with lower resistance may take part in physical fitness activities such as *Taiji* and *Qi Gong* to nourish the body through movement, increase lung capacity, reduce asthma attacks, improve pulmonary function and strengthen the resistance of body against disease.

CLINICAL EXPERIENCE OF RENOWNED PHYSICIANS

Empirical Formulas

1. TREATING ASTHMA WITH JIÀNG QÌ DÌNG CHUǍN KĒ LÌ CHŌNG JÌ (降气定喘颗粒冲剂) (LIU WEI-SHENG)

【Ingredients】

炙麻黄	zhì má huáng	12g	Herba Ephedrae Praeparata
白芥子	bái jiè zǐ	9g	Semen Sinapis Albae
苏子	sū zǐ	12g	Fructus Perillae
葶苈子	tíng lì zǐ	15g	Semen Lepidii
桑白皮	sāng bái pí	15g	Cortex Mori
陈皮	chén pí	3g	Pericarpium Citri Reticulatae

【Indications】

Bronchial asthma or asthmatic bronchitis presenting with panting and dyspnea as the main symptoms, accompanied with cough and expectoration.

【Formula Analysis】

Zhì má huáng (Herba Ephedrae Praeparata) is warm in nature. It is the main medicinal for eliminating phlegm and calming panting. *Sū zǐ* (Fructus Perillae) and *bái jiè zǐ* (Semen Sinapis Albae) descend qi and relieve qi stagnation so as to assist *zhì má huáng* (Herba Ephedrae Praeparata) to diffuse the Lung and calm panting. *Chén pí* (Pericarpium Citri Reticulatae) regulates qi and invigorates the Spleen, dries dampness and resolves phlegm. *Tíng lì zǐ* (Semen Lepidii) and *sāng bái pí* (Cortex Mori) eliminate heat from the Lung and promote the circulation of water so as to treat cough, panting and dyspnea, and remove phlegm. Together, all of the medicinals in the formula work to diffuse the Lung, descend qi, calm panting, eliminate phlegm, and promote qi flow.

【Modifications】

➤ For cases without obvious heat, remove *sāng bái pí* (Cortex Mori) to avoid excessive cold. This called "dependence on warm-natured medicinals in treating asthma". Never excessively use cold and cool natured medicinals in treating the attack stage of asthma.

➤ For cases with yellow sputum, add *yú xīng cǎo* (Herba Houttuyniae) 30g to clear heat from the Lung and resolve phlegm.

(Guangdong Provincial Hospital of Traditional Chinese Medicine)

2. Treatment of Cold Asthma with Wēn Fèi Dìng Chuǎn Tāng (温肺定喘汤) (Feng Wei-bin)

【Ingredients】

麻黄	má huáng	10g	Herba Ephedrae
白芥子	bái jiè zǐ	9g	Semen Sinapis Albae
干姜	gān jiāng	9g	Rhizoma Zingiberis Officinalis
苏子	sū zǐ	12g	Fructus Perillae
法半夏	fǎ bàn xià	12g	Rhizoma Pinelliae Praeparatum
杏仁	xìng rén	12g	Armeniacae Semen Amarum
陈皮	chén pí	6g	Pericarpium Citri Reticulatae
补骨脂	bǔ gǔ zhī	15g	Fructus Psoraleae
莱菔子	lái fú zǐ	12g	Semen Raphani
甘草	gān cǎo	9g	Radix et Rhizoma Glycyrrhizae

【Indications】

The beginning of cold asthma manifests as aversion to cold, headache, itching in the throat, and cough. This is followed by dyspnea, panting, stridor in the throat like the sound of a frog, fullness and oppression in the chest and diaphragm, difficulty in lying flat, a pale complexion, no thirst, and a preference for hot drinks. There is a pink tongue with a white and glossy coating, and a floating and tight pulse.

【Formula Analysis】

Within this formula, *má huáng* (Herba Ephedrae), *bǔ gǔ zhī* (Fructus Psoraleae) and *gān jiāng* (Rhizoma Zingiberis Officinalis) are the main medicinals. They warm the Lung and expel cold. *Bái jiè zǐ* (Semen Sinapis Albae), *sū zǐ* (Fructus Perillae) and *lái fú zǐ* (Semen Raphani) descend qi and eliminate phlegm. *Chén pí* (Pericarpium Citri Reticulatae), *fǎ bàn xià* (Rhizoma Pinelliae Praeparatum) and *xìng rén* (Armeniacae Semen Amarum) diffuse the Lung and resolve phlegm. Taken together, all of the medicinals warm the Lung and expel cold, resolve phlegm and calm panting.

【Modifications】

➢ For cases with severe chills and a headache due to invasion by severe wind-cold, add *zǐ sū* (Folium Perillae) 6g (decocted at the end) and *xì xīn* (Radix et Rhizoma Asari) 6g to relieve the exterior, diffuse the Lung, and eliminate the exogenous evils.

➢ For cases with profuse sputum and dyspnea, add *shè gān* (Rhizoma Belamcandae) 12g, *dǎn nán xīng* (Arisaema cum Bile) 12g and *jié gěng* (Radix Platycodonis) 12g to help *má huáng* (Herba Ephedrae) eliminate phlegm, stop asthma, and diffuse the Lung qi.

(Liu Wei-sheng, Feng Wei-bin. *Pattern Differentiation and Treatment of Tumors and Respiratory Diseases in Chinese Medicine* 中医肿瘤、呼吸病临证证治. Guangzhou: The People's Publishing House of Guangdong, 1999. 268)

3. Treatment of Cold Asthma with *Wēn Fèi Dìng Chuǎn Tāng* (温肺定喘汤) (Yu Shao-yuan)

【Ingredients】

麻黄	má huáng	10g	Herba Ephedrae
白芥子	bái jiè zǐ	9g	Semen Sinapis Albae
干姜	gān jiāng	9g	Rhizoma Zingiberis
苏子	sū zǐ	12g	Fructus Perillae

法半夏	fǎ bàn xià	12g	Rhizoma Pinelliae Praeparatum
杏仁	xìng rén	12g	Armeniacae Semen Amarum
陈皮	chén pí	6g	Pericarpium Citri Reticulatae
补骨脂	bǔ gǔ zhī	15g	Fructus Psoraleae
莱菔子	lái fú zǐ	12g	Semen Raphani
甘草	gān cǎo	9g	Radix et Rhizoma Glycyrrhizae

【Indications】

The beginning of cold asthma manifests as aversion to cold, headache, itching in the throat and cough. Then there is dyspnea, panting, throat stridor that sounds like a frog, fullness and oppression in the chest and diaphragm, difficulty in laying flat, a pale complexion, no thirst, and a preference for hot drinks. There is a pink tongue with a white and glossy coating, and a floating and tight pulse.

【Modifications】

➢ For cases with severe aversion to cold and a headache due to invasion by severe wind-cold, add *zǐ sū* (Folium Perillae) and *xì xīn* (Radix et Rhizoma Asari).

➢ For cases with profuse sputum and dyspnea, add *shè gān* (Rhizoma Belamcandae), *dǎn nán xīng* (Arisaema cum Bile) and *jié gěng* (Radix Platycodonis) to aid *má huáng* (Herba Ephedrae) in eliminating phlegm, stopping asthma, and diffusing the Lung qi.

(Yu Shao-yuan. *Treatment of Common Internal Diseases with Combination of Chinese Medicine and Biomedicine* 中西医结合治疗常见内科病. Guangzhou: The People's Publishing House of Guangdong, 1996. 130)

4. Treatment of Wind-Cold Fettering the Lung with *Má Xìng Shè Dǎn Tāng* (麻杏射胆汤) (Dong Su-liu)

【Ingredients】

| 麻黄 | má huáng | 5g | Herba Ephedrae |
| 杏仁 | xìng rén | 10g | Armeniacae Semen Amarum |

射干	shè gān	9g	Rhizoma Belamcandae
桔梗	jié gěng	6g	Radix Platycodonis
苏子	sū zǐ	9g	Fructus Perillae
蝉蜕	chán tuì	4.5g	Periostracum Cicadae
炒僵蚕	chǎo jiāng cán	9g	Bombyx Batryticatus Tostum
法半夏	fǎ bàn xià	9g	Rhizoma Pinelliae Praeparatum
陈皮	chén pí	4.5g	Pericarpium Citri Reticulatae
生甘草	shēng gān cǎo	4.5g	Radix et Rhizoma Glycyrrhizae
鹅管石	é guǎn shí	12g	Balanophyllia (calcinined, crushed)
枳实	zhǐ shí	6g	Fructus Aurantii Immaturus
制胆星	zhì dǎn xīng	6g	Arisaema cum Bile Praeparata

【Indications】

Bronchial asthma with acute episodes of chronic bronchitis, manifesting as cough with profuse sputum, difficulty with expectoration, oppression in the chest, shortness of breath, itching and stridor in the throat, difficulty in laying flat at night, and tonsillitis with swelling. There is a thin, white and greasy tongue coating, and a slippery pulse. The Chinese medical pattern differentiation is wind-cold settling in the Lung, with interior obstruction of turbid phlegm, and a failure of the Lung qi to diffuse.

【Modifications】

➢ For cases with thirst and restlessness, sticky sputum, and a red tongue with a yellow coating, remove *fǎ bàn xià* (Rhizoma Pinelliae Praeparatum) and *chén pí* (Pericarpium Citri Reticulatae); add *shí gāo* (Gypsum Fibrosum), *zhī mǔ* (Rhizoma Anemarrhenae) and *zhè bèi mǔ* (Bulbus Fritillariae Thunbergii).

➢ For cases that appear cold, with cold limbs, no sweating, white frothy sputum, and a white and glossy tongue coating, remove *chán tuì* (Periostracum Cicadae), *bái jiāng cán* (Bombyx Batryticatus) and *jié gěng* (Radix Platycodonis); add *guì zhī* (Ramulus Cinnamomi), *xì xīn* (Radix et Rhizoma Asari) and *gān jiāng* (Rhizoma Zingiberis).

➢ For cases with congested throat, tonsillitis with swelling and pain, sticky sputum, a red tongue, and a rapid pulse, remove *fǎ bàn xià* (Rhizoma Pinelliae Praeparatum) and *chén pí* (Pericarpium Citri Reticulatae); add *jīn yín huā* (Flos Lonicerae Japonicae), *lián qiào* (Fructus Forsythiae), *chǎo niú bàng zǐ* (Fructus Arctii Tostum), and replace *shēng má huáng* (Herba Ephedrae Recens) with *shuǐ zhì má huáng* (Herba Ephedrae Praeparata).

➢ For cases with yellow urine, constipation, and a red tongue, remove *jié gěng* (Radix Platycodonis) and *gān cǎo* (Radix et Rhizoma Glycyrrhizae); add *huáng qín* (Radix Scutellariae) and *sāng bái pí* (Cortex Mori), replace *shēng má huáng* (Herba Ephedrae Recens) with *mì zhì má huáng* (Herba Ephedrae Praeparata), replace *zhì fǎ bàn xià* (Rhizoma Pinelliae Preparata) with *zhú lì fǎ bàn xià* (Rhizoma Pinelliae, Prepared by *zhú lì* [Succus Bambusae]), and replace *chén pí* (Pericarpium Citri Reticulatae) with *jú luò* (Retinervs Citri Reticulatae Fructus).

➢ For cases with cough, panting, counterflow of qi, abdominal distention and hypochondriac pain, remove *jié gěng* (Radix Platycodonis) and *gān cǎo* (Radix et Rhizoma Glycyrrhizae); add *lái fú zǐ* (Semen Raphani) and *bái jiè zǐ* (Semen Sinapis Albae).

➢ For cases with fullness and distention of epigastrium, a sticky feeling in the mouth, and poor appetite, remove *chán tuì* (Periostracum Cicadae) and *bái jiāng chán* (Bombyx Batryticatus); add *hòu pò* (Cortex Magnoliae Officinalis) and *jiāo liù qū* (Massa Medicata Fermentata).

➢ For cases with pain and distention of the head, and stuffy nose with profuse nasal discharge, remove *fǎ bàn xià* (Rhizoma Pinelliae Praeparatum) and *chén pí* (Pericarpium Citri Reticulatae); add *xīn yí* (Flos Magnoliae) and *cāng ěr zǐ* (Fructus Xanthii).

(Zhang Feng-qiang, et al. *Essentials of Effective and Proved Secret Prescriptions of the First Group of Famous Veteran Doctors in State Level* 首批国家级名老中医效验秘方精选. Beijing: China Press of Traditional Chinese Medicine, 1996. 119-121)

5. Treatment of Phlegm-Drool Congestion with *Jié Chuǎn Tāng* (截喘汤) (Jiang Chun-hua)

【Ingredients】

佛耳草	fó ěr cǎo	15g	Gnaphalium Affine D.Don
碧桃干	bì táo gān	15g	Fructus Persicae Viride
老鹳草	lǎo guàn cǎo	15g	Herba Geranii
旋覆花	xuán fù huā	10g	Flos Inulae
全瓜蒌	quán guā lóu	10g	Fructus Trichosanthis
姜法半夏	jiāng fǎ bàn xià	10g	Rhizoma Pinelliae Praeparatum
防风	fáng fēng	10g	Radix Saposhnikoviae
五味子	wǔ wèi zǐ	6g	Fructus Schisandrae Chinensis

【Indications】

Cough with profuse expectoration, dyspnea, and panting.

【Modifications】

➢ For qi deficiency, add *bái shēn* (Radix Ginseng Alba) and *huáng qí* (Radix Astragali).

➢ For Kidney deficiency, add *ròu cōng róng* (Herba Cistanches) 15g, *bā jǐ tiān* (Radix Morindae Officinalis) 15g, *bǔ gǔ zhī* (Fructus Psoraleae) 15g, and *gé jiè* (Gecko) 3—6g.

➢ For yin deficiency with heat, add *huáng bǎi* (Cortex Phellodendri), *zhī mǔ* (Rhizoma Anemarrhenae), *xuán shēn* (Radix Scrophulariae) and *shēng dì huáng* (Radix Rehmanniae Recens), 9g for each.

➢ For severe cough, and panting with no expectoration or just a little sputum, add *nán tiān zhú zǐ* (Fructus Nandinae Domesticae) 6g, *mǎ bó* (Lasiosphaerae seu Calvatia) 6g and *tiān jiāng ké* (Rhizoma Metaplexis Japonicae) 3 pieces.

➢ For heat panting, add *shí gāo* (Gypsum Fibrosum) 15g, *zhī mǔ* (Rhizoma Anemarrhenae) 10g and *huáng qín* (Radix Scutellariae) 10g.

➢ For profuse sputum that is difficult to expectorate, add *sū zǐ* (Fructus Perillae), *bái jiè zǐ* (Semen Sinapis Albae) and *lái fú zǐ* (Semen Raphani), 9g each.

➤ For gastrointestinal excess pattern with constipation, add one dose of *Tiáo Wèi Chéng Qì Tāng* (调胃承气汤), taken orally.

➤ After the panting has stopped, it is customary to take *Hé Chē Dà Zào Wán* (河车大造丸), *Zuǒ Guī Wán* (左归丸) or *Yòu Guī Wán* (右归丸), orally, 3g, twice a day.

(Zhang Feng-qiang, et al. *Essentials of Effective and Proved Secret Prescriptions of the First Group of Famous Veteran Doctors in State Level* 首批国家级名老中医效验秘方精选 . Beijing: China Press of Traditional Chinese Medicine, 1996. 116-117)

6. Treatment of Phlegm Obstructing the Lung Collaterals with *Píng Chuǎn Fāng* (平喘方) (Dong Jian-hua)

【Ingredients】

麻黄	má huáng	5g	Herba Ephedrae
杏仁	xìng rén	10g	Armeniacae Semen Amarum
地龙*	dì lóng	10g	Lumbricus
全蝎**	quán xiē	3g (ground and dissolved in water before taking)	Scorpio
川芎	chuān xiōng	10g	Rhizoma Chuanxiong

【Indications】

This treats asthma attack, presenting with mild aversion to cold, cough and panting, dyspnea, and white sputum that is difficult to expectorate. There is also a white and glossy tongue coating, and a floating and tight pulse.

【Modifications】

1) Excess pattern (attack stage of asthma)

a. Internal accumulation of phlegm-heat: This manifests as fever,

---

* *Dì lóng* is a medicinal substance from animal body parts and can easily cause allergic reactions. If inappropriate measures are taken in the preparation or storage of this substance, it may cause mildew to build up making it smell. Therefore, it is not recommended for independent use or any use in further reference to this medicinal substance here after in this book.
** *Quán xiē* is a medicinal substance from animal body parts. Since it contains foreign proteins and can easily cause allergic reactions, it is not recommended for a medicinal substance from an animal use.

yellow and sticky sputum that is difficult to expectorate, and a yellow and greasy tongue coating. Prescribe *Píng Chuǎn Fāng* (平喘方) plus *huáng qín* (Radix Scutellariae), *chuān bèi mǔ* (Bulbus Fritillariae Cirrhosae) and *tíng lì zǐ* (Semen Lepidii).

➤ For excessive heat, add *shēng shí gāo* (Gypsum Fibrosum).

➤ For profuse sputum, add *lái fú zǐ* (Semen Raphani), *sū zǐ* (Fructus Perillae) and *quán guā lóu* (Fructus Trichosanthis).

➤ For sticky and turbid sputum that is difficult to expectorate, add *hǎi fú shí* (Os Costaziae) and *shēng gé qiào* (Concha Meretricis seu Cyclinae).

b. Dry heat in the Lung: This manifests as a dry throat and dry tongue, itching in the throat, a hacking cough with little sputum that is difficult to expectorate, and a red tongue with little moisture. Prescribe *Píng Chuǎn Fāng* (平喘方) plus *běi shā shēn* (Radix Glehniae), *mài mén dōng* (Radix Ophiopogonis), *yù zhú* (Rhioma Polygonati Odorati) and *sāng bái pí* (Cortex Mori).

c. Interior retention of cold fluids and repeated contraction of cold evil: This manifests as profuse thin sputum and aversion to cold. Use *Píng Chuǎn Fāng* (平喘方) plus *guì zhī* (Ramulus Cinnamomi), *gān jiāng* (Rhizoma Zingiberis), *xì xīn* (Radix et Rhizoma Asari) and *wǔ wèi zǐ* (Fructus Schisandrae Chinensis).

2) Deficiency pattern (remission stage of asthma)

For these patterns, *má huáng* (Herba Ephedrae) is not used. Herbs are used according to the principles of pattern differentiation.

a. Qi deficiency of the Lung and Spleen: This manifests as shortness of breath, a low weak voice, a reluctance to talk, loss of appetite, and a pale tongue with a yellow coating. Prescribe *Píng Chuǎn Fāng* (平喘方) plus *huáng qí* (Radix Astragali), *dǎng shēn* (Radix Codonopsis), *bái zhú* (Rhizoma Atractylodis Macrocephalae) and *gōng láo yè* (Folium Ilex).

b. Deficiency of both qi and yin: This manifests as shortness of breath with a reluctance to talk, palpitations, and a pink tongue with little coating. Prescribe *Píng Chuǎn Fāng* (平喘方) plus *huáng qí* (Radix Astragali), *dǎng shēn* (Radix Codonopsitis), *shā shēn* (Radix Glehniae seu Adenophorae), *mài mén dōng* (Radix Ophiopogonis), *dōng chóng xià cǎo* (Cordyceps) and *xiān hè cǎo* (Herba Agrimoniae).

c. Deficiency of Kidney yang: This manifests as intolerance of cold, cold limbs, and a deep pulse that is weak at *chi* portion. Prescribe *Píng Chuǎn Fāng* (平喘方) plus *shú fù zǐ* (Radix Aconiti Lateralis Praeparata), *zǐ hé chē* (Placenta Hominis), *ròu guì* (Cortex Cinnamomi), *zǐ shí yīng* (Fluoritum) and *chén xiāng* (Lignum Aquilariae Resinatum).

d. Deficiency of Kidney yin: This manifests as a feverish sensation in the chest, palms and soles, emaciation, shortness of breath, and a red tongue with little coating. Prescribe *Píng Chuǎn Fāng* (平喘方) plus *shēng shú dì huáng* (Radix Rehmanniae Recens and Radix Rehmanniae Praeparata), *nǚ zhēn zǐ* (Fructus Ligustri Lucidi), *hé táo ròu* (Semen Juglandis Regiae), *wǔ wèi zǐ* (Fructus Schisandrae Chinensis) and *chén xiāng* (Lignum Aquilariae Resinatum).

3) Concurrent deficiency and excess pattern (status asthmaticus)

a. Deficiency of the Lung and excess of the Stomach: This is a pattern of Lung and Spleen qi deficiency combined with gastric distention or pain, and unsmooth defecation. Based on the formula for qi deficiency of the Lung and Spleen, add *sū zǐ* (Fructus Perillae), *sū gěng* (Caulis Perillae), *guā lóu* (Fructus Trichosanthis), *fǎ bàn xià* (Rhizoma Pinelliae Praeparatum), *zhǐ qiào* (Fructus Aurantii) and *jiāo sān xiān* (Stir-fried Combination of Fructus Crataegi, Massa Fermentata and Fructus Hordei Vulgaris Germinatus).

b. Kidney deficiency and exterior excess pattern: For this pattern of Kidney deficiency combined with an exogenous contraction, use as a basis the formula for Kidney deficiency. For Lung-heat, add *má huáng* (Herba Ephedrae), *huáng qín* (Radix Scutellariae) and *tíng lì zǐ* (Semen Lepidii seu Descurainiae). For Lung-dryness, add *shēng dì huáng* (Radix Rehmanniae Recens), *shā shēn* (Radix Glehniae seu Adenophorae), *mài mén dōng* (Radix Ophiopogonis) and *yù zhú*

(Rhizoma Polygonati Odorati). For fluid retention in the Lung, add *gān jiāng* (Rhizoma Zingiberis), *xì xīn* (Radix et Rhizoma Asari), *wǔ wèi zǐ* (Fructus Schisandrae Chinensis) and *má huáng* (Herba Ephedrae).

(Shi Yu-guang, Shan Shujian. *The Clinical Essence of Contemporary Famous Physicians: Special Monograph of Asthma* 当代名医临证精华·咳喘专辑. Beijing: China Ancient Writings Publishing House, 1991. 108)

7. Treatment of Wind Flourishing and Phlegm Blocking with *Huáng Lóng Shū Chuǎn Tāng* (黄龙舒喘汤) (Chao En-xiang)

【Ingredients】

炙麻黄	zhì má huáng	10g	Herba Ephedrae Praeparata
蝉蜕	chán tuì	10g	Periostracum Cicadae
苏叶	sū yè	10g	Folium Perillae
苏子	sū zǐ	10g	Fructus Perillae
地龙*	dì lóng	10g	Lumbricus
石菖蒲	shí chāng pú	10g	Rhizoma Acori Tatarinowii
白芍	bái sháo	15g	Radix Paeoniae Alba
白果	bái guǒ	10g	Semen Ginkgo
五味子	wǔ wèi zǐ	10g	Fructus Schisandrae Chinensis

【Indications】

Dyspnea and a wheezing sound due to wind flourishing and phlegm blocking.

【Modifications】

➢ For heat panting, add *shēng shí gāo* (Gypsum Fibrosum), *huáng qín* (Radix Scutellariae) and *sāng bái pí* (Cortex Mori).

➢ For obvious cold manifestations, add *guì zhī* (Ramulus Cinnamomi) and *xì xīn* (Radix et Rhizoma Asari).

➢ For cases with no obvious cold or heat manifestations, use the above-mentioned formula with no changes.

---

* see above.

[Zhang Hongchun, Chao En-xiang. Clinical Study of Allergic Bronchial Asthma Treated with Method of Scattering Wind and Relieving Spasm. *Journal of Emergency in Traditional Chinese Medicine* 中国中医急症. 1998, (2): 54]

Selected Case Studies

1. Professor Dong Jian-hua's Case Study: Cold in the Lung and Heat in the Diaphragm

Chen, female, age 15.

【Initial Visit】

The initial visit was on July 12th, 1976. The patient had suffered from asthma since she was 3 years old. Attacks were mild at the beginning, then frequent and severe in the spring and summer. In the attack phase the manifestations were shortness of breath, panting and wheezing sounds, difficulty in laying flat, and loss of appetite. The symptoms were usually be relieved by antitussives and anti-asthmatics such as aminophylline and ephedrine, and antibiotics such as penicillin and streptomycin. Recently, because of an exogenous contraction of wind-cold, she had another asthma attack. The manifestations were, gasping with the shoulders raised, panting, wheezing sounds over both lungs, scattered dry and moist rales heard upon auscultation, profuse thick sputum, and a pale complexion. She also had a red tongue with a yellow and greasy coating, and a thready and wiry pulse.

【Pattern Differentiation】

Retained phlegm lies deep in the interior, becomes depressed over the long run, and turns into heat. This and exterior coldness are mutually creative, with the result that asthma occurs repeatedly. The pattern belongs to cold in the Lung and heat in the diaphragm. The root is deficiency and the branch is excess.

【Treatment Principle】

"In an emergency, treat the branch". Thus first diffuse the Lung and clear heat; stop cough and calm panting.

【Formulas and Medicinals】

Modified *Dìng Chuǎn Tāng* (定喘汤)

麻黄	má huáng	10g	Herba Ephedrae
白果	bái guǒ	3 pieces	Semen Ginkgo (crushed)
黄芩	huáng qín	10g	Radix Scutellariae
苏子	sū zǐ	10g	Fructus Perillae
地龙*	dì lóng	15g	Lumbricus
杏仁	xìng rén	12g	Armeniacae Semen Amarum
款冬花	kuǎn dōng huā	10g	Flos Farfarae
川芎	chuān xiōng	10g	Rhizoma Chuanxiong
全蝎**	quán xiē	5g	Scorpio

Decocted in water. Taken orally, one dose daily, 6 doses in total.

【Second Visit】

August 13th. The asthma was relieved after taking the decoction. Only one or two episodes occurred in the past month, and the patient's condition was milder than before. When an asthma attack did occur, taking above-mentioned decoction provided relief. The patient's remaining manifestations were panting upon slight exertion, hyperhidrosis (excessive sweating), and loss of appetite. "For chronic cases, treat the root". Therefore the treatment should be to tonify the Kidney so as to receive qi, and reinforce the Lung and removing phlegm so as to stop asthma.

熟地黄	shú dì huáng	20g	Radix Rehmanniae Praeparata
五味子	wǔ wèi zǐ	5g	Fructus Schisandrae Chinensis
冬虫夏草	dōng chóng xià cǎo	10g	Cordyceps
紫河车***	zǐ hé chē	5g	Placenta Hominis
甘草	gān cǎo	5g	Radix et Rhizoma Glycyrrhizae

*,** see above.

*** *Zǐ hé chē* is human placenta. It is not recommended for use, because it may carry the hepatitis B virus if the preparation is not done appropriately.

沉香末	chén xiāng mò	1g (dissolved in hot water before taking)	Lignum Aquilariae Resinatum
苏子	sū zǐ	5g	Fructus Perillae
川贝母	chuān bèi mǔ	3g	Bulbus Fritillariae Cirrhosae
党参	dǎng shēn	5g	Radix Codonopsis
麦门冬	mài mén dōng	3g	Radix Ophiopogonis
煅牡蛎	duàn mǔ lì	12g	Concha Ostreae Calcinatun

Decocted in water. Taken orally, one dose daily, 6 doses in total.

【Third Visit】

September 6th. The account from the patient was the following: For asthma attacks, the formula given during the initial visit was used. For the remission stage, the formula given during the second visit was used. These were taken alternately for about one year (sometimes there were breaks or a dose was taken every other day). The asthma was basically controlled. The present symptoms are slight expectoration, mild wheezing and panting upon exertion. There were no severe attacks for a long time. The patient was told she could do ordinary movements (exercises) The patient was advised to double the dosage of the formula given during the second visit, and to prepare them into pills to take orally, so as to consolidate the treatment.

【Comments】

In terms of clinical treatment, the attack stage should be divided according to whether it is a cold pattern or a heat pattern. There is difference between warmly transforming and diffusing the Lung, and clearing, transforming and depurating the Lung. Normally, the main treatment is to fortify the Spleen, boost the Kidney and tonify the Lung. During the attack stage of asthma, if the pattern is cold in the Lung and heat in the diaphragm, the priority is to treat the branch. This involves diffusing the Lung, clearing heat from the Lung, stopping cough, and calming asthma. The prescription is *Dìng Chuǎn Tāng* (定喘汤), with modifications, which has the function of diffusing the Lung and relieving asthma, clearing heat and resolving phlegm. Subtract *gān cǎo* (Radix et Rhizoma Glycyrrhizae), *sāng bái pí* (Cortex Mori) and *fǎ bàn xià* (Rhizoma Pinelliae Praeparatum), and add *dì lóng* (Lumbricus), *chuān xiōng* (Rhizoma Chuanxiong) and *quán xiē* (Scorpio) so as to relieve asthma and alleviate spasms. Taken together, the medicinals in the formula can not only clear heat from the Lung, descend qi and resolve phlegm, but can also eliminate retained liquid. In the remission stage, use *shú dì huáng* (Radix Rehmanniae Praeparata), *wǔ wèi zǐ* (Fructus Schisandrae Chinensis), *zǐ hé chē* (Placenta Hominis) and *dōng chóng xià cǎo* (Cordyceps) to tonify the Kidney so it can receive qi. Use *dǎng shēn* (Radix Codonopsis), *mài mén dōng* (Radix Ophiopogonis), *chuān bèi mǔ* (Bulbus Fritillariae Cirrhosae), *sū zǐ* (Fructus Perillae), *chén xiāng* (Lignum Aquilariae Resinatum) and *gān cǎo* (Radix et Rhizoma Glycyrrhizae) to reinforce the Lung, promote qi movement and resolve phlegm. Use a small amount of *mǔ lì* (Concha Ostreae) to stop sweats. This is a treatment based on the condition of the root Thus one should alternate treating the branch in urgent situations, and treating the root in chronic situations. Thereby the functions of the Lung and Kidney can be recovered quickly.

(Dong Jian-hua. *Clinical Experience of Diagnosis and Treatment* 临证治验. The Friendship Publishing Company of China, 1986. 289)

2. Professor Chen Shi-an's Case Study: Cold-Phlegm Obstructing the Lung

Xu, female, age 29.

【Initial Visit】

The patient had suffered from asthma from childhood for about 20 years. The asthma episodes often occurred whenever she caught cold, and manifested as panting, difficulty lying down, and extraordinary anguish. She went to the veteran physician Chen in the winter of 1959.

Examination: Panting with the shoulders raised, difficultly in lying down at night, rapid breathing, wheezing in the throat, lumbar soreness, abdominal distention, panting aggravated by exertion, and chest pain with oppression. She had a pale tongue with a white and greasy coating, and a deep, wiry and thready pulse that at the same time seemed slippery.

【Pattern Differentiation】

Cold-phlegm obstructing the Lung, insufficiency of both the Lung and Kidney.

【Treatment Principle】

Diffuse the Lung and transform phlegm to relieve panting; boost the Lung to receive qi and return to the origin.

【Formulas and Medicinals】

麻黄	má huáng	6g	Herba Ephedrae
桂枝	guì zhī	10g	Ramulus Cinnamomi
细辛	xì xīn	3g	Radix et Rhizoma Asari
杏仁	xìng rén	10g	Armeniacae Semen Amarum
法半夏	fǎ bàn xià	10g	Rhizoma Pinelliae Praeparatum
陈皮	chén pí	10g	Pericarpium Citri Reticulatae
参蛤散	shēn gé sǎn (1.5g each)	3g	Ginseng and Gecko Powder

【Second Visit】

The asthma was relieved after taking the above decoction, and the patient could lie flat at night a little bit, but the chest pain still worried the patient. She had a pale tongue with a white and greasy coating, and a deep, wiry and thready pulse that at the same time seemed slippery. She continued the treatment with the above formula, with some modifications.

麻黄	má huáng	10g	Herba Ephedrae
桂枝	guì zhī	10g	Ramulus Cinnamomi
细辛	xì xīn	3g	Radix et Rhizoma Asari
川贝	chuān bèi	6g	Bulbus Fritillariae Cirrhosae
杏仁	xìng rén	10g	Armeniacae Semen Amarum
桃仁	táo rén	6g	Semen Persicae
法半夏	fǎ bàn xià	10g	Rhizoma Pinelliae Praeparatum
陈皮	chén pí	10g	Pericarpium Citri Reticulatae
参蛤散	Shēn gé sǎn (1.5g each)	3g	Ginseng and Gecko Powder

【Third Visit】

The patient took several doses of the above decoction and the asthma was gradually relieved. The chest pain had been alleviated; and the tongue was pale with a thin white coating. The pulse was wiry and thready. In order to consolidate the therapeutic effect, the patient was given the powder to take orally over a long time, so as to avoid relapses. The formula was as follows:

野人参	yě rén shēn	10g	Radix Ginseng Indici
藏红花	zàng hóng huā	10g	Flos Carthami Tinctorii
大蛤蚧	dà gé jiè	1 pair	Gecko (remove the head and feet)
川贝母	chuān bèi mǔ	10g	Bulbus Fritillariae Cirrhosae
杏仁	xìng rén	10g	Armeniacae Semen Amarum
桃仁	táo rén	10g	Semen Persicae

The medicinals were ground into a fine powder, and taken twice a day, 1g to 2g each time.

After the patient took the powder for half a month, the asthma was relieved, and her mental status became much better. In addition, the symptoms such as sore low back and chest pain had also been relieved. After this, there were no relapses for nearly 20 years.

【Comments】

If there are repeated asthma attacks for several years, it is usually due to deficiency of the Lung, Spleen and Kidney. Therefore the treatment is not only to diffuse the Lung and relieve asthma to treat the branch, but also to tonify the Lung, fortify the Spleen, and benefit the Kidney to treat the root. In addition, attention should be given to the obstruction of Lung qi caused by prolonged asthma; this inevitably leads to stagnation and obstruction of the Lung collaterals. Therefore auxiliary medicinals that activate the blood and remove stasis, like *táo rén* (Semen Persicae) and *hóng huā* (Flos Carthami), should be added to promote the circulation of qi and blood. This can not only alleviate symptoms but also enhance the treatment effect of diffusing the Lung and relieving asthma.

(Editorial committee. *Collection of Experience of Renowned and Veterane Physicians of Chinese Medicine* 名老中医经验选编. Beijing: Beijing Publishing House, 1994. 283)

3. Professor Qian Zi-fen's Case: Accumulation of Phlegm-Heat in the Lung

Gao, female, age 29.

【Initial Visit】

The initial visit was on August 5th, 1987. The asthma attacks started three years ago, with episodes occurring many times every year. The patient has taken many pharmacological therapies (both Chinese medicine and biomedicine), but without satisfactory effect. A week ago, she caught a cold, manifesting with headache, muscle soreness, low fever, intolerance of cold, cough, and panting. When the patient saw the doctor, some symptoms had disappeared, like headache, muscle soreness, low fever, and intolerance of cold. However, the cough and panting were worse. At the same time, the patient was expectorating a moderate amount of yellow and thick phlegm. Her appetite and stool were normal. Wheezing sounds over both lungs were heard upon auscultation, but no abnormalities were found in chest fluoroscopy. The number of leukocytes was 13500/mm³. She had a red tongue with a thin yellow coating, and a thready and slippery pulse.

【Pattern Differentiation】

Accumulation of phlegm-heat in the Lung.

【Treatment Principle】

Clear heat from the Lung and resolve phlegm; stop cough and calm panting.

【Formulas and Medicinals】

Modified *Má Xìng Shí Gān Tāng* (麻杏石甘汤)

麻黄	má huáng	3g	Herba Ephedrae
杏仁	xìng rén	10g	Armeniacae Semem Amarum
甘草	gān cǎo	6g	Radix et Rhizoma Glycyrrhizae
地龙	dì lóng	10g	Lumbricus
黄芩	huáng qín	10g	Radix Scutellariae
鱼腥草	yú xīng cǎo	30g	Herba Houttuyniae
款冬花	kuǎn dōng huā	10g	Flos Farfarae
紫菀	zǐ wǎn	10g	Radix et Rhizoma Asteris
瓜蒌	guā lóu	30g	Fructus Trichosanthis
葶苈子	tíng lì zǐ	20g	Semen Lepidii seu Descurainiae
苏子	sū zǐ	10g	Fructus Perillae
莱菔子	lái fú zǐ	30g	Semen Raphani

Decocted in water. One dose taken daily, divided into two portions.

【Second Visit】

August 12th, 1987. After taking 6 doses of the above decoction, the cough and panting had been relieved, the expectoration had been reduced, and the wheezing sounds had decreased. However, diarrhea occurred, with the passage of loose stools 3 or 4 times a day. The tongue picture and the pulse condition were almost the same as before.

From the above formula, *lái fú zǐ* (Semen Raphani) was removed, the quantity of *guā lóu* (Fructus Trichosanthis) was reduced from 30g to 15g, and *wǔ wèi zǐ* (Fructus Schisandrae Chinensis) 10g was added. Six doses were prescribed, with the same preparation and dosage as the previous formula.

【Third Visit】

August 19th, 1987. After taking the above decoction for 6 doses, the cough and panting had disappeared, and patient felt only some chest oppression. Her stools were normal. The tongue picture and the pulse condition were normal. The wheezing sounds over both lungs had disappeared. The formula from the second visit was prescribed with the addition of *hòu pò* (Cortex Magnoliae Officinalis) 10g. The preparation and dosage was the same as the previous formulas. 6 doses were given.

After a month and a half, a follow-up exam revealed that the general condition of the patient was normal, with only slight coughing and panting occurring on occasion.

【Comments】

In this case, the patient's signs and symptoms such as yellow and sticky sputum and yellow coating on a red tongue, belong to the Chinese medical pattern of "accumulation of phlegm-heat in the Lung". This pattern is usually caused by wind-heat or heat transformed from wind-cold. It is obvious that this case was caused by wind-cold transforming into heat. This patient's asthma attack was induced by a typical exogenous contraction of wind-cold, manifesting as intolerance of cold, fever, headache, and muscle soreness. The heat combined with phlegm in the body to accumulate in the Lung, obstructing the airway and resulting in a failure of the Lung qi to diffuse and descend. Thus there were symptoms of coughing and panting. Heat can burn the body fluids, so there was yellow and sticky phlegm. The key points of treatment, in addition to stopping cough and calming panting, were clearing heat and resolving phlegm. Within the first formula, *má huáng* (Herba Ephedrae), *dì lóng* (Lumbricus), *tíng lì zǐ* (Semen Lepidii seu Descurainiae), *sū zǐ* (Fructus

Perillae) and *lái fú zǐ* (Semen Raphani) calm panting. *Xìng rén* (Armeniacae Semen Amarum), *kuǎn dōng huā* (Flos Farfarae) and *gān cǎo* (Radix et Rhizoma Glycyrrhizae) stop cough. *Huáng qín* (Radix Scutellariae) and *yú xīng cǎo* (Herba Houttuyniae) clear heat and detoxify. *Guā lóu* (Fructus Trichosanthis) and *zǐ wǎn* (Radix et Rhizoma Asteris) resolve phlegm. The second formula was based on the first formula, with a subtraction of *lái fú zǐ* (Semen Raphani), a reduced quantity of *guā lóu* (Fructus Trichosanthis), and an addition of *wǔ wèi zǐ* (Fructus Schisandrae Chinensis) in order to alleviate diarrhea. The third formula was a modification of the second formula, with the addition of *hòu pò* (Cortex Magnoliae Officinalis) to alleviate chest oppression.

In terms of biomedicine, the presentation of panting, wheezing sounds over both lungs, leukocytosis, and sticky yellow phlegm can be diagnosed as bronchial asthma with an accompanying respiratory tract infection. The pharmacological research shows that *má huáng* (Herba Ephedrae) and *dì lóng* (Lumbricus) have anti-asthmatic functions. *Huáng qín* (Radix Scutellariae) and *yú xīng cǎo* (Herba Houttuyniae) have obvious anti-inflammatory functions, and usually are used to treat bacteria and viral infections. *Guā lóu* (Fructus Trichosanthis), *xìng rén* (Armeniacae Semen Amarum), *zǐ wǎn* (Radix et Rhizoma Asteris), *kuǎn dōng huā* (Flos Farfarae) and *gān cǎo* (Radix et Rhizoma Glycyrrhizae) have the functions of relieving cough and resolving phlegm.

(Chen Ke-ji. *Clinical Proved Cases in Point of Chinese Medicine* 中医药学临床验案范例. Beijing: New World Publishing House, 1994. 66)

4. Professor Zheng Qiao's Case: Phlegm-Fire Assailing the Lung

Kang, female, age 26.

【Initial Visit】

The initial visit was on March 5th, 1970. The patient had been ill for several months, and was given a biomedical diagnosis of bronchial asthma. The manifestations were cough and panting, stridor in the throat, dyspnea, expectoration of yellow and sticky phlegm, chest oppression and pain, thirst and vexation, flushed face and red lips, a red tongue with a yellow coating, and a powerful slippery and rapid pulse.

【Pattern Differentiation】

Phlegm-fire assailing the Lung and stagnating and blocking the Lung orifice, Lungs unable to depurate and downbear, airways inhibited.

【Treatment Principle】

Clear heat and transform phlegm; diffuse the Lung and disinhibit qi.

【Formulas and Medicinals】

Personally created *Qián Hú Tāng* (前胡汤) with modifications.

前胡	qián hú	12g	Radix Peucedani
杏仁	xìng rén	9g	Armeniacae Semen Amarum
桑叶	sāng yè	12g	Folium Mori
知母	zhī mǔ	12g	Rhizoma Anemarrhenae
麦门冬	mài mén dōng	9g	Radix Ophiopogonis
黄芩	huáng qín	9g	Radix Scutellariae
金银花	jīn yín huā	15g	Flos Lonicerae Japonicae
款冬花	kuǎn dōng huā	15g	Flos Farfarae
枇杷叶	pí pa yè	12g	Folium Eriobotryae
桔梗	jié gěng	9g	Radix Platycodonis
甘草	gān cǎo	6g	Radix et Rhizoma Glycyrrhizae

【Second Visit】

After the patient had taken four doses continuously, the pulse condition became moderate and slippery, the yellow tongue coating had mostly lessened, expectoration was easier, the phlegm was slightly yellow and not sticky, the chest oppression and pain had been relieved, respiration was even, and the asthma had stopped. These changes showed that the phlegm-fire had disappeared, and the airways were disinhibited. Still, the above formula was used with the subtraction of *kuǎn dōng huā* (Flos Farfarae) and the addition of *tiān huā fěn* (Radix Trichosanthis) 12g. After five successive doses of this formula, the asthma was relieved.

【Comments】

Zhu Dan-xi first put forth the name of *xiào chuǎn* (asthma), and clarified its pathomechanism as "particularly caused by phlegm (专主于痰)". It is due mainly to qi and phlegm joining and obstructing, blocking the airways and causing a failure of the Lung to depurate and descend. According to the theory that "all disorders of the five emotions and vexation are ascribed to fire", the pathomechanism in the case of this patient is that the seven emotions stagnated and transformed into fire. This fire consumed the fluids and became phlegm which damaged the Lung, and lead to the obstruction of the Lung orifice and an inhibition of the airway. As a result there was coughing and panting, stridor in the throat, dyspnea, fullness, and oppression and pain in the chest. The vexation and thirst were caused by the accumulation of phlegm-fire and consumption of the fluids by the scorching heat. The red tongue, yellow coating, and slippery rapid pulse were the indicators of excessive phlegm-fire. "Heat patterns should be treated with cold-natured remedies." In terms of treatment, use *Qián Hú Tāng* (前胡汤), which is bitter-cold and mildly acrid-sweet in order to clear heat and resolve phlegm. Add *jié gěng* (Radix Platycodonis) as the assistant so as to be a guide to the Lung. *Kuǎn dōng huā* (Flos Farfarae) purges heat and moistens the Lung, eliminates phlegm, relieves restlessness, and alleviates cough, dyspnea, panting and oppression in the chest. *Pí pa yè* (Folium Eriobotryae) purges the fire that is accumulated in the Lung. After four doses of the medication, the fire was expelled, the phlegm was eliminated, and the asthma was stopped. From the above formula, remove *kuǎn dōng huā* (Flos Farfarae); and add *tiān huā fěn* (Radix Trichosanthis). Its sour, sweet and mildly bitter flavor and cold nature can promote the production of body fluids, moisturize the Lung, and recover the Lung yin that was damaged by phlegm-fire. Five successive doses cured the disease.

(Anonymous. *Collection of Experience of Distinguished Veteran Doctors of Chinese Medicine · Volume One* 老中医经验汇编 · 第一集. Beijing: People's Medical Publishing House, 1978. 2)

5. Professor Zhu Zhan-yu's Case: Exterior Constraint of Wind-Cold; Accumulation of Turbid-Phlegm in the Lung

Wang, female, age 34.

【Initial Visit】

The initial visit was on December 9th, 1991. The chief complaint was episodic asthma for 4 years that was aggravated for the past three months. In the autumn of 1987, the patient had coughing and asthma after catching colds. After that the asthma occurred every autumn, and lasted to the spring of next year. Stridor usually appeared in the morning, the wheezing sounds were like a drawing saw, and the patient could not lie flat. The attack could be temporarily alleviated by taking oral antibiotics and anti-asthmatics, but it would relapse with the withdrawal of medication. The asthma had lasted for the past 3 months. In the allergy department of our hospital, the results of the skin test (inhaling group) for the patient revealed many kinds of prophylactic substances such as indoor dust, spring, summer and autumn pollens, ragweed pollen, fungus, dust mites, fluffed cotton, cigarette fumes, animal, fur, and feathers. The patient was diagnosed as having bronchial asthma. She had been given complex desensitization therapies, and oral compounded Clorprenaline and Ketotifen for two months. However, there were no obvious effects. The current manifestations were asthma attack occurring whenever the patient caught colds, with symptoms of runny nose, frequent sneezing, white and sticky phlegm, chest oppression, an obstructed feeling in the throat, lassitude, unsmooth defecation, lying flat at night, a dark tongue with a white, thick and greasy coating, and a wiry and thready pulse.

【Pattern Differentiation】

Accumulation of turbid-phlegm in the Lung, with an exterior constraint of wind-cold.

【Treatment Principle】

Eliminate phlegm and descend qi; scatter cold and calm panting.

【Formulas and Medicinals】

Personally-created *Wǔ Zǐ Dìng Chuǎn Tāng* (五子定喘汤) with additions.

炙苏子	zhì sū zǐ	10g	Fructus Perillae Praeparata
莱菔子	lái fú zǐ	10g	Semen Raphani
白芥子	bái jiè zǐ	3g	Semen Sinapis Albae
葶苈子	tíng lì zǐ	15g	Semen Lepidii seu Descurainiae
杏仁	xìng rén	10g	Armeniacae Semen Amarum
前胡	qián hú	10g	Radix Peucedani
白前	bái qián	10g	Radix et Rhizoma Cynanchi Stauntonii
桔梗	jié gěng	10g	Radix Platycodonis
炙紫菀	zhì zǐ wǎn	10g	Radix et Rhizoma Asteris Praeparata
款冬花	kuǎn dōng huā	10g	Flos Farfarae
桑白皮	sāng bái pí	10g	Cortex Mori
荆芥	jīng jiè	10g	Herba Schizonepetae
防风	fáng fēng	10g	Radix Saposhnikoviae
炙甘草	zhì gān cǎo	6g	Radix et Rhizoma Glycyrrhizae Praeparata

【Second Visit】

December 16th. After treatment with 7 doses of the above decoction, the asthma attacks did not appear in the morning, and runny nose and sneezing were markedly alleviated, but there was still an obstructed feeling in the throat and an expectoration of white phlegm. This is a case in which wind-cold has been eliminated, but the turbid-phlegm was still excessive. The original formula was prescribed, with subtractions of *jīng jiè* (Herba Schizonepetae), *fáng fēng* (Radix Saposhnikoviae), *jié gěng* (Radix Platycodonis) and *qián hú* (Radix Peucedani), and with additions of *zhì pa yè* (Folium Eriobotryae Praeparata) 10g, *wǔ wèi zǐ* (Fructus Schisandrae Chinensis) 10g, *fǎ bàn xià* (Rhizoma Pinelliae Praeparatum) 10g and *chén pí* (Pericarpium Citri Reticulatae) 10g. A total of 14 doses were taken.

【Third Visit】

January 3rd, 1992: The asthma attacks didn't occur for a long time, coughing was relieved, and expectoration had been reduced. The prescription was not changed because it was effective, and another 14 doses were given. At the same time, a pill form was prepared and given to consolidate the effect.

炙苏子	zhì sū zǐ	30g	Fructus Perillae Praeparata
莱菔子	lái fú zǐ	30g	Semen Raphani
白芥子	bái jiè zǐ	10g	Semen Sinapis Albae
葶苈子	tíng lì zǐ	50g	Semen Lepidii seu Descurainiae
杏仁	xìng rén	30g	Armeniacae Semen Amarum
赤小豆	chì xiāo dòu	50g	Semen Phaseoli
炙杷叶	zhì pa yè	30g	Folium Eriobotryae Praeparata
炙紫菀	zhì zǐ wǎn	30g	Radix et Rhizoma Asteris Praeparata
款冬花	kuǎn dōng huā	30g	Flos Farfarae
生甘草	shēng gān cǎo	30g	Radix et Rhizoma Glycyrrhizae

The medicinals were ground together into a fine powder, and prepared into pills with honey. Each one weighed 10g. One pill was taken, 3 times a day.

The follow-up in August 1992 found that the asthma did not relapse again.

【Comments】

Asthma is a disease that is difficult to permanently cure. Like the saying of Zhang Jing-yue, "*Chuǎn* (panting) has an latent cause, and it will occur as the patient is exposed to cold; it is also called *xiào chuǎn* (asthma)." Master Zhu believes that the retention of phlegm and fluids in the Lung is the potential pathologic factor for inducing repeated asthma attacks, and this is the so-called "latent cause". He emphasizes "resolving phlegm first to treat asthma, and regulating qi to resolve phlegm". He prescribes *Wǔ Zǐ Dìng Chuǎn Tāng* (五子定喘汤) with additions to treat this disease. In this case, the disease had been prolonged for four years, turbid phlegm had accumulated in the Lung, and asthma attacks were induced when exogenous cold invaded the body. Because the airways were obstructed by a combination of phlegm and stagnated qi, there was stridor. In terms of treatment, *Sān Zǐ Yǎng Qīn Tāng* (三子养亲汤) was given. It has the basic function of resolving phlegm and lowering qi. *Xìng rén* (Armeniacae Semen Amarum) was added to diffuse the Lung and relieve panting, and *tíng lì zǐ* (Semen Lepidii seu Descurainiae) was added to purge heat in the Lung and promote water circulation. Thus one diffuses and one purges, smoothing the qi dynamic. Hence the asthma will be relieved. In the initial visit, there was a pattern of exterior constrainr of wind-cold, manifesting as nasal obstruction, runny nose, and frequent sneezing, so *jīng jiè* (Herba Schizonepetae) and *fáng fēng* (Radix Saposhnikoviae) were added to dispel wind and expel cold, *qián hú* (Radix Peucedani), *bái qián* (Radix et Rhizoma Cynanchi Stauntonii), *zǐ wǎn* (Radix et Rhizoma Asteris) and *kuǎn dōng huā* (Flos Farfarae) were added to arrest cough, resolve phlegm and calm panting. Although the patient was found, (through allergic reaction examinations), to be hypersensitive to many kinds of substances, the key was to eliminate phlegm. This was understood by looking at the pattern differentiation, and thus a therapeutic effect was naturally achieved.

(Dong Zhen-hua, et al. *Essentials of Zhu Shen-yu's Clinical Proved Cases* 祝谌予临证验案精选. Beijing: Learning Center Press, 1996. 7)

6. Professor Zhu Bo-quan's Cases: Failure of the Kidney to Receive Qi

Gao, female, aged 57.

【Initial Visit】

The patient had suffered on and off from asthma for many years. With the asthma attacks, the manifestations were shortness of breath, panting with the shoulders raised, difficulty in lying flat, symptoms aggravated with exertion, palpitations, loss of appetite, dark yellow urine and constipation, emaciation with a pale complexion, a dry tongue with a white coating, and a thready weak pulse.

【Pattern Differentiation】

Insecurity of the lower origin, failure of the Kidney to receive qi.

【Treatment Principle】

Supplement the Kidney to receive qi; settle counterflow panting.

【Formulas and Medicinals】

熟地黄	shú dì huáng	10g	Radix Rehmanniae Praeparata
山茱萸	shān zhū yú	6g	Fructus Corni Officinalis
山药	shān yào	10g	Rhizoma Dioscoreae
茯苓	fú líng	10g	Poria
五味子	wǔ wèi zǐ	3g	Fructus Schisandrae Chinensis
知母	zhī mǔ	10g	Rhizoma Anemarrhenae
杏仁	xìng rén	6g	Armeniacae Semen Amarum
川贝母	chuān bèi mǔ	10g	Bulbus Fritillariae Cirrhosae
麦门冬	mài mén dōng	10g	Radix Ophiopogonis
沙参	shā shēn	10g	Radix Glehniae seu Adenophorae
阿胶珠	ē jiāo zhū	10g	Colla Corii Asini
生甘草	shēng gān cǎo	6g	Radix et Rhizoma Glycyrrhizae

The patient took the above formula when she had an asthma attack, and after treatment of three to six doses, the symptoms were relieved. She had taken the formula successively for four to five years, and up to now, there had been no asthma attacks. The patient is nearly seventy years old and alive and well.

【Comments】

Plain questions: On Cough (素问·咳论篇, *Sù Wèn · Ké Lùn Piān*) says: "Both the five *zang* organs and the six *fu* organs can cause cough, not alone the Lung … ". *Classic of Difficulties: The Fourth Problem* (难经·四难, *Nàn Jīng · Sì Nàn*) points out that "Expiration is related to the Heart and Lung, inspiration is related to the Kidney and Liver." Therefore asthma is not only a disease of the Lung, but also related to the other *zang* organs. The causative factors are the retention of damp-heat in the interior of the Lung, Spleen and Heart meridians, or yin deficiency of the Liver and Kidney. The exogenous contraction of evils is the inducing factor. In clinic, deficient patterns and excess patterns should be differentiated. In treating excess patterns of asthma I use *Má Xìng Shí Gān Tāng* (麻杏石甘汤), *Tíng Lì Dà Zǎo Xiè Fèi Tāng* (葶苈大枣泻肺汤) and *Èr Chén Tāng* (二陈汤) with modifications. For deficient patterns I use *Liù Wèi Dì Huáng Tāng* (六味地黄汤), *Èr Mǔ Níng Sòu Wán* (二母宁嗽丸) and *Sì Jūn Zǐ Tāng* (四君子汤) with modifications. Usually a better effect can be achieved.

In this case, the patient had suffered from asthma for a long time, and the disease involved the Kidney. The Kidney is the root of qi; if the Kidney is insecure and fails to receive qi, the pattern belongs to deficiency asthma. Treatment should be to tonify the Kidney to receive qi, descend qi, and calm panting. Within the formula, *shú dì huáng* (Radix Rehmanniae Praeparata) and *shān zhū yú* (Fructus Corni Officinalis) nourish yin and tonify the Kidney; *shān yào* (Rhizoma Dioscoreae) fortifies the Spleen and tonifies the Lung, *fú líng* (Poria) transforms dampness, resolves phlegm, calms the mind, and replenishes qi. *Wǔ wèi zǐ* (Fructus Schisandrae Chinensis) astringes the Lung and assists the Kidney to receive qi; *zhī mǔ* (Rhizoma Anemarrhenae) and *chuān bèi mǔ* (Bulbus Fritillariae Cirrhosae) clear heat from the Lung and moisturize the Lung, resolve phlegm and arrest cough. *Xìng rén* (Armeniacae Semen Amarum) descends qi and calms panting, *mài mén dōng* (Radix Ophiopogonis) and *shā shēn* (Radix Glehniae seu Adenophorae) moisturize the Lung, promote the production of body fluids and stops cough. *Gān cǎo* (Radix et Rhizoma Glycyrrhizae) fortifies the Spleen and harmonizes the qi of the middle jiao, In addition, *ē jiāo zhū* (Colla Corii Asini) nourishes yin and moisturizes the Lung, and is good at treating prolonged cough.

(Editorial committee. *Collection of Experience of Renowned and Veteran Physicians of Chinese Medicine in Beijing · Book Two* 北京市名老中医经验选编·第二集. Beijing: Beijing Publishing House, 1986. 287)

Discussions

1. Professor Wang Wen-ding: Treating Asthma by Dividing it into the Early, Middle and Late Stages

Asthma is generally divided into new, prolonged, excess and deficiency types. New and excess types of asthma are ascribed to the Lung; an excess means that there are evils. The prolonged and deficiency types of asthma are ascribed to the Kidney; a deficiency means that there is no evil. Initially asthma is caused by contraction of cold, and the branch (emergent symptoms) should be treated as an emergency. For panting with a rapid and hasty pulse, *Fǎ Bàn Xià Hòu Pò Tāng* (法半夏厚朴汤) with modifications should be prescribed when the presentation is mild. *Yuè Bì Zhú Xià Tāng* (越婢术夏汤) with modifications should be prescribed when the presentation is severe. The herbs are *má huáng* (Herba Ephedrae), *shēng shí gāo* (Gypsum Fibrosum), *fǎ bàn xià* (Rhizoma Pinelliae Praeparatum), *zhì gān cǎo* (Radix et Rhizoma Glycyrrhizae Praeparata), *bái zhú* (Rhizoma Atractylodis Macrocephalae), *shēng jiāng* (Rhizoma Zingiberis Recens), *dà zǎo* (Fructus Jujubae), *hòu pò* (Cortex Magnoliae Officinalis), *xì xīn* (Radix et Rhizoma Asari), and *wǔ wèi zǐ* (Fructus Schisandrae Chinensis) . For distention and fullness in the chest and abdomen, *Hòu Pò Má Huáng Tāng* (厚朴麻黄汤) is appropriate. For cases with serious phlegm and fluid retention, with stridor in the throat like the sound of a frog, *Shè Gān Má Huáng Tāng* (射干麻黄汤) is a very good remedy. For cases of cold enveloping fire, *Má Xìng Shí Gān Tāng* (麻杏甘石汤) or *Bái Guǒ Dìng Chuǎn Tāng* (白果定喘汤) can be used directly. For cases with a complication of vexation, *Dà Qīng Lóng Tāng* (大青龙汤) with an increased amount of *shí gāo* (Gypsum Fibrosum) can be selected. For cases of exterior cold with interior fluids and productive expectoration of white frothy sputum, *Xiǎo Qīng Lóng Tāng* (小青龙汤) is most suitable. In the above prescriptions, when *gān jiāng* (Rhizoma Zingiberis Officinalis) or *shēng jiāng* (Rhizoma Zingiberis Recens), *xì xīn* (Radix et Rhizoma Asari), and *wǔ wèi zǐ* (Fructus Schisandrae Chinensis) are used together, the three herbs must be in the same quantity. If one is worried about a large quantity of *xì xīn* (Radix et Rhizoma Asari), and just a small quantity of it is used, then the effect will be immediately reduced. The saying "*xì xīn* (Radix et Rhizoma Asari) should not be taken more than one *qian* [about 3 grams]" refers to the dosage of *xì xīn* (Radix et Rhizoma Asari) used in powder. As it is used in a compound in each prescription, its dose could be 6-9g decocted and divided into 2—3 portions for oral use. This administration is of no harm, but does have a special effect to quickly relieve the condition. In treating a disease, one must take into consideration the disease mechanism, as well as the actions of the medicinals to upbear, downbear, open, and close. The compatibility of the *gān jiāng* (Rhizoma Zingiberis Officinalis) or *shēng jiāng* (Rhizoma Zingiberis Recens), *xì xīn* (Radix et Rhizoma Asari), and *wǔ wèi zǐ* (Fructus Schisandrae Chinensis) in Zhong-jing' prescriptions have provided a good example of these principles.

As for the middle stage of asthma, there can be deficiency and there can be excess or there can be a deficiency of the root and an excess of the branch. At this time, *Sān Niù Tāng* (三拗汤), *Dà Qīng Lóng Tāng* (大青龙汤), *Xiǎo Qīng Lóng Tāng* (小青龙汤) and *Shè Gān Má Huáng Tāng* (射干麻黄汤)

are not appropriate. *Rén Shēn Dìng Chuǎn Tāng* (人参定喘汤) and *Rén Shēn Má Huáng Tāng* (人参麻黄汤) used by later generations both are formulas that treat the branch as well as the root, but predominantly used in the treatment of qi deficiency patterns. An asthma attack during the course of a prolonged illness is not affected by seasonal climatic influences. If the pulse is floating and rapid in the *cun* positions, and deep and thready in the *chi* positions, it is a case of excess in the upper and deficiency in the lower with the lower deficiency being primary. The treatment should be to greatly reinforce the Lung and promote the Kidney to receive qi. The prescription is modified *Quán Zhēn Yī Qì Tāng* (全真一气汤):

人参	rén shēn	30~60g	Radix Ginseng
熟地黄	shú dì huáng	30g	Radix Rehmanniae Praeparata
山萸肉	shān yú ròu	12g	Fructus Corni Officinalis
麦门冬	mài mén dōng	15g	Radix Ophiopogonis
五味子	wǔ wèi zǐ	3g	Fructus Schisandrae Chinensis
怀牛膝	huái niú xī	10g	Radix Achyranthis Bidentatae
白芥子	bái jiè zǐ	6g	Semen Sinapis Albae
生姜	shēng jiāng	5 pieces	Rhizoma Zingiberis Recens

Professor Wang used this prescription to cure or control asthma is several patients who had this type of prolonged asthma. For example, a 20 year old female patient with bronchial asthma for 17 years was treated with this formula for about a month. A good short term treatment effect of controlling the asthma was achieved unexpectedly. Professor Wang believes that when it is used in a small quantity, the nature of *rén shēn* (Radix Ginseng) is ascending; however, when used in a large quantity its nature is descending. *Rén Shēn Dìng Chuǎn Tāng* (人参定喘汤) is used for cases of half deficiency and half excess. The idea is to use *rén shēn* (Radix Ginseng) and *má huáng* (Herba Ephedrae) at the same time. *Rén shēn* (Radix Ginseng) was once used in a high quantity of 90g by our predecessors, but I use it in doses of 30—60g according to the condition; the result is also good. In

Collected Treatises of Jing-yue (景岳全书, *Jǐng Yuè Quán Shū*) *Zhēn Yuán Yǐn* (贞元饮) is used. The herbs are *shú dì huáng* (Radix Rehmanniae Praeparata) 120g, *dāng guī* (Radix Angelicae Sinensis) 21g, and *gān cǎo* (Radix et Rhizoma Glycyrrhizae) 12g. Xu Ling-tai even advocates using pieces of *rén shēn* (Radix Ginseng). However, if this is used for an excess pattern, it will be a violation of the taboo of reducing the deficiency and tonifying the excess.

For asthma in the late stage, with phlegm like a gushing spring, *Guì Fù Dì Huáng Tāng* (桂附地黄汤) can be used in order to warm and transform phlegm and fluids, and replenish and supplement the lower origin. A patient with a prolonged deficiency often has a failure of the Spleen to transform and transport, thus phlegm will be constantly produced. If no measures are taken, in time it will gradually cause a serious qi deficiency. Then Kidney water will affect the upper jiao, fire of the Kidney and Liver will become hyperactive, and the patient might eventually die. In late stage asthma, there are deficiencies of the Lung, Spleen and Kidney. *Rén shēn* (Radix Ginseng) and *shú dì huáng* (Radix Rehmanniae Praeparata) can treat the root; at the same time they are also very good medicinals to resolve phlegm. For a sudden episode of asthma during a prolonged illness, *gé jiè wěi* (Exremitas Gecko) 0.2g can be ground into a fine powder, and taken at a draught after mixing with water. It is very effective to stop asthma. It is quite helpful in cases of deficiency asthma to take 3—5 pieces of honey-prepared *hé táo* (Semen Juglandis Regiae Praeparata) every day as an auxiliary food. According to theories of Chinese medicine, after the condition is controlled (static stage) *Shèn Qì Wán* (肾气丸) plus *chén xiāng* (Lignum Aquilariae Resinatum) and *wǔ wèi zǐ* (Fructus Schisandrae Chinensis) can be prescribed to improve the Kidney's function in receiving qi and returning it to the root Continue to simultaneously treat the Spleen and Kidney. That is to say, lay equal priority upon both organs. Take *Wǔ Wèi Yì Gōng Sǎn* (五味异功散) or *Liù Jūn Zǐ Wán* (六君子丸) in the early morning and *Shèn Qì Wán* (肾气

丸) in the evening in order to strengthen the right qi so as to reinforce the root and consolidate the curative effect.

"Three tenths is medication, seven tenths is taking care of oneself", and asthma is no exception. First, one must know what is appropriate and what to avoid. Prevent common colds in order to avoid triggering internal fluid retention by exogenous contraction. Patients with asthma that induced by salt and sugar should avoid consuming sugar and salt. Second, one must work and rest appropriately. Overstrain or prolonged lying down can both damage qi, therefore both work and rest must be done in moderation. Patients with enduring asthma in particular should avoid sexual intercourse in order to protect the origin. Third, one must have a moderate diet. Mild foods are good; but greasy and rich foods can result in damp-heat, and thus should be limited.

(Liu Qiang, et al. *Medical Talks of Famous Veteran Physicians of Chinese Medicine* 名老中医医话. Scientific and Technical Documents Publishing House, 1985. 43)

2. Professor Cheng Men-xue: Treating the Lung and Phlegm as the Key to Treating Asthma

One of the features of asthma is repeated and stubborn episodes. The most appropriate way to describe this feature of asthma is "a sound in the throat like a frog". The original formula for asthma is *Shè Gān Má Huáng Tāng* (射干麻黄汤) from the *Essentials of the Golden Cabinet* (金匮, *Jīn Guì*). *Shè Gān Má Huáng Tāng* is different from *Xiǎo Qīng Lóng Tāng* (小青龙汤). In both formulae *má huáng* (Herba Ephedrae) serves as the chief medicinal, but in *Shè Gān Má Huáng Tāng*, *Guì Zhī Tāng* (桂枝汤), with its actions of relieving the exterior with pungency and warmth, is not used. However, *shè gān* (Rhizoma Belamcandae), with its bitter-cold nature that clears heat from the throat, is taken in combination with *má huáng* (Herba Ephedrae), *kuǎn dōng* (Flos Tussilaginis Farfarae) and *zǐ wǎn* (Radix et Rhizoma Asteris). These assistant herbs are pungent, moistening, and descend qi. Thus the actions of pungent-opening, bitter-purging and the acid-astringing are contained in a formula, which obviously treats the Lung. It should be the special formula for treating asthma.

Asthma is a disease that may develop into fluid retention in the diaphragm. Asthma has stubborn phlegm, so an attacking method must be used during episodes, but during its remission the treatment must be to fortify the Spleen and tonifying the Kidney in order to support the right qi and aid recuperation. Wang Xu-gao treats childhood asthma with *Liù Jūn Zǐ Tāng* (六君子汤) and *Píng Wèi Sǎn* (平胃散), with additions of *chuān bèi* (Bulbus Fritillariae Cirrhosae) and *fěi zǐ* (Semen Torreyae), which are ground into a fine powder. This powder is put into the *dà zǎo* (Fructus Jujubae), and *tíng lì* (Semen Lepidii seu Descurainiae); the medicinals are decocted together and taken orally. The creativity is quite ingenious, and it is a model to follow. Previously, an external medicine, *Yáng Hé Tāng* (阳和汤), was used to treat a child with a pale complexion and weak constitution. He had suffered from asthma of yang deficiency pattern for several years, and a good treatment effect was achieved. The formula is:

熟地黄	shú dì huáng	30g	Radix Rehmanniae Praeparata
白芥子	bái jiè zǐ	3g	Semen Sinapis Albae (toasted and pulverized)
鹿角胶	lù jiǎo jiāo	9g	Colla Cornus Cervi
姜炭	jiāng tàn	1.5g	Rhizoma Zingiberis Praeparatum Carbonisata
麻黄	má huáng	1.5g	Herba Ephedrae
肉桂	ròu guì	3g	Cortex Cinnamomi
生甘草	shēng gān cǎo	3g	Radix et Rhizoma Glycyrrhizae (raw)
五味子	wǔ wèi zǐ	1.5g	Fructus Schisandrae Chinensis

Lěng Xiào Wán (冷哮丸) is composed of *má huáng* (Herba Ephedrae), *chuān wū* (Radix Aconiti), *xì xīn* (Radix et Rhizoma Asari), *shǔ jiāo* (Pericarpium Zanthoxyli Bungeani), *bái fán* (Alumen), *yá zào* (Fructus Gleditsiae Abnormalis), *fǎ bàn xià qū* (Rhizoma Pinelliae Fermentata), *chén dǎn xīng* (Arisaema cum Bile), *xìng rén* (Armeniacae Semen Amarum), *gān căo* (Radix et Rhizoma Glycyrrhizae), *zĭ wăn* (Radix et Rhizoma Asteris), *kuăn dōng huā* (Flos Farfarae).

麻黄	má huáng	Herba Ephedrae
川乌	chuān wū	Radix Aconiti
细辛	xì xīn	Radix et Rhizoma Asari
蜀椒	shŭ jiāo	Pericarpium Zanthoxyli Bungeani
白矾	bái fán	Alumen
牙皂	yá zào	Fructus Gleditsiae Abnormalis
法半夏曲	fă bàn xià qū	Rhizoma Pinelliae Fermentata
陈胆星	chén dăn xīng	Arisaema cum Bile
杏仁	xìng rén	Armeniacae Semen Amarum
甘草	gān căo	Radix et Rhizoma Glycyrrhizae
紫菀	zĭ wăn	Radix et Rhizoma Asteris
款冬花	kuăn dōng huā	Flos Farfarae

It is from *Comprehensive Medicine According to Master Zhang* (张氏医通, *Zhāng Shì Yī Tōng*). Along with *Sān Jīn Gāo* (三津膏), it is applied on BL 13 (*fèi shù*). This is also a very effective treatment.

Dìng Chuăn Tāng (定喘汤) is not suitable for treating asthma of a yin deficiency and phlegm-heat pattern. A formula for asthma recorded in Cheng Xing Xuan's book (Qing Dynasty) *Medical Essays* (医述, *Yī Shù*) can consulted as a reference. The composition of the formula is:

熟地黄	shú dì huáng	15g	Radix Rehmanniae Praeparata
当归	dāng guī	3g	Radix Angelicae Sinensis
茯苓	fú líng	4.5g	Poria
法半夏	fă bàn xià	4.5g	Rhizoma Pinelliae Praeparatum
橘红	jú hóng	4.5g	Exocarpium Citri Rubrum
金沸草	jīn fèi căo	4.5g	Herba Inulae
麦门冬	mài mén dōng	4.5g	Radix Ophiopogonis
甘草	gān căo	1.5g	Radix et Rhizoma Glycyrrhizae
淡豆豉	dàn dòu chĭ	3g	Semen Sojae Praeparatum
黑山栀	hēi shān zhī	3g	Fructus Gardeniae Praeparatus
海浮石	hăi fú shí	6g	Os Costaziae

Jīn Shuǐ Liù Jūn (金水六君) is the main element of the above formula. It enriches yin and nourishes blood in order to treat phlegm. *Shān zhī zhǐ* (Fructus Gardeniae) and *dàn dòu chǐ* (Semen Sojae Praeparatum) clear fire; *jīn fèi cǎo* (Herba Inulae), with its salty flavor, can eliminate phlegm, and *hǎi fú shí* (Os Costaziae), with its salty flavor, can reduce fire. If *Dài Gé Sǎn* (黛蛤散) is added the result will be much better.

(Shi Yu-guang, Shan Shu-jian. *The Clinical Essence of Contemporary Famous Physicians: Special Monograph of Asthma* 当代名医临证精华 · 咳喘专辑 . Beijing: China Ancient Writings Publishing House, 1988. 19)

3. Professor Ren Ji-xue: The Treatment of Asthma by Treating Wheezing and Panting as the Same Things

Some ancient doctors considered wheezing and panting to be two patterns. Professor Ren, through clinical observations for 40 years, believes that there is no strict difference between wheezing and panting, and that they are not easy to distinguish. The *Orthodox Medical Records* (医学正传 , *Yī Xué Zhèng Zhuàn*) simply proposed that "panting is the name of the breath, wheezing is the name of the sound". But Wang Ken-tang of the Ming dynasty did not agree with this theory and proposed that "wheezing and panting are the same as each other". This opinion is in accordance with clinical actuality, and the name *xiào chuǎn* (哮喘 , wheezing and panting, or asthma) should be used.

This disease often originates from an exogenous contraction of one of the six climatic pathogens or pestilent evils, and a delayed or mistaken treatment that causes a failure of the body in expelling evil qi. This then obstructs the Lung. It can also result because a residual measles toxin invades and lodges in the Lung. As it becomes entrenched in the Lung, the breath cannot be vent outward. In addition, there can be a cough that lingers for several years which damages the Lung membranes and invades the Lung collaterals. It can, further affects the trachea and impair the Lung body. Then a prolonged illness will cause an obstruction of blood circulation in the collaterals, and the bronchi may enter a pathological state of spasms. As a result, water can not be normally distributed, and the defensive and nutritive qi are in disharmony. The result is an insecurity of the defensive qi and a failure of the Lung qi to diffuse. After a long time, the disease mechanism is congested qi in the chest, stubborn phlegm in the diaphragm, and contraction of exterior evils at the improper times; thus the disease appears. Therefore the treatment must place emphasis on diffusing the Lung, opening phlegm, regulating qi, and resolving spasms. The medicinals needed are *quán xiē* (Scorpio), *bái jiè zǐ* (Semen Sinapis Albae), *tán xiāng* (Lignum Santali Albi), *qīng pí* (Pericarpium Citri Reticulatae Viride), *chuān xiōng* (Rhizoma Chuanxiong), *jiāo mù* (Semen Zanthoxyli Bungeani), *wū méi* (Fructus Mume), *hē zǐ ròu* (Fructus Terminaliae Chebulae), *bái guǒ rén* (Semen Ginkgo), *xìng rén* (Armeniacae Semen Amarum), *hǎi fú shí* (Os Costaziae).

全蝎	quán xiē	Scorpio
白芥子	bái jiè zǐ	Semen Sinapis Albae
檀香	tán xiāng	Lignum Santali Albi
青皮	qīng pí	Pericarpium Citri Reticulatae Viride
川芎	chuān xiōng	Rhizoma Chuanxiong
椒目	jiāo mù	Semen Zanthoxyli Bungeani
乌梅	wū méi	Fructus Pruni Mume
诃子肉	hē zǐ ròu	Fructus Terminaliae Chebulae
白果仁	bái guǒ rén	Semen Ginkgo
杏仁	xìng rén	Armeniacae Semen Amarum
海浮石	hǎi fú shí	Os Costaziae

Decoct with water and take orally. For cold phlegm, add *xiān máo* (Rhizoma Curculiginis), *ròu guì* (Cortex Cinnamomi), and *yín yáng huò* (Herba Epimedii). For heat phlegm, add medicinals like *shēng shí gāo*

(Gypsum Fibrosum) and *huáng qín* (Radix Scutellariae). After the panting is calmed, use *tāi pán* (Placenta Hominis), *dōng chóng xià cǎo* (Cordyceps Sinensis), *hē zǐ ròu* (Fructus Terminaliae Chebulae), *bái guǒ* (Semen Ginkgo), *hǎi mǎ* (Hippocampus), *gé jiè* (Gecko), *chén xiāng* (Lignum Aquilariae Resinatum), and *shān zhū yú* (Fructus Corni Officinalis) to support the right qi.

胎盘	tāi pán	Placenta Hominis
冬虫夏草	dōng chóng xià cǎo	Cordyceps Sinensis
诃子肉	hē zǐ ròu	Fructus Terminaliae Chebulae
白果	bái guǒ	Semen Ginkgo
海马	hǎi mǎ	Hippocampus
蛤蚧	gé jiè	Gecko
沉香	chén xiāng	Lignum Aquilariae Resinatum
山茱萸	shān zhū yú	Fructus Corni Officinalis

Or use *bái fán* (Alumen) and *shēng fǎ bàn xià* (Rhizoma Pinelliae Praeparatum) put into pig's feet, and place into an earthenware jar and calcine. Then add a little bit of *shè xiāng* (Secretio Moschi). Grind them all together into a fine powder. Take 5–10g each time, with boiled water, twice a day. Thus there is a cure.

(Ren Ji-xue. *Experience Collection of China Famous Veteran Physicians of Traditional Chinese Medicine* 中国名老中医经验集萃. Beijing Science and Technology Publishing House, 1993. 190)

4. Professor Yu Chang-rong: The Treatment of Asthma Based upon the Condition of the Branch and the Root

Professor Yu treats bronchial asthma basically according to these principles: "its branch is the Lung, and its root is the Kidney" and "for new asthma treat the Lung, and for prolonged asthma treat the Kidney". Initially, the symptoms (the branch) of asthma are often caused by an invasion of cold-pathogen exogenously leading to a restraint of Lung qi.

So the treatment should mainly be to diffuse Lung qi and dispel cold. The most commonly used formula is *Xiǎo Qīng Lóng Tāng* (小青龙汤):

桂枝	guì zhī	10g	Ramulus Cinnamomi
白芍	bái sháo	10g	Radix Paeoniae Alba
法半夏	fǎ bàn xià	10g	Rhizoma Pinelliae Praeparatum
麻黄	má huáng	6g	Herba Ephedrae
五味子	wǔ wèi zǐ	6g	Fructus Schisandrae Chinensis
干姜	gān jiāng	5g	Rhizoma Zingiberis Officinalis
炙甘草	zhì gān cǎo	5g	Radix et Rhizoma Glycyrrhizae Praeparata
细辛	xì xīn	3g	Radix et Rhizoma Asari
红枣	hóng zǎo	3 pieces	Fructus Jujubae

The above formula has the function of dispelling cold, resolving fluid retention, diffusing the Lung, and calming panting. If the patient ordinarily has a deficiency of Lung qi, or cold complicated by heat, it is not suitable to warm and disperse. Then the formula *Dìng Chuǎn Tāng* (定喘汤) can be used instead. In the prescription there are not only warming and downbearing medicinals such as *má huáng* (Herba Ephedrae), *xìng rén* (Armeniacae Semen Amarum) and *sū zǐ* (Fructus Perillae), but also cooling and draining herbs such as *huáng qín* (Radix Scutellariae) and *sāng bái pí* (Cortex Mori). *Bái guǒ* (Semen Ginkgo) and *kuǎn dōng* (Flos Farfarae) have astringing and moistening effects. This is suitable for cases of excess mixed with deficiency and cold accompanied by heat. According to my own view from clinical practice, patients who suffer from new asthma seldom go to the hospital, but those who suffer from prolonged asthma often do. New asthma can be treated easily, but prolonged asthma is hard to cure. So-called prolonged asthma refers to the repeated episodes of asthma for long period (more than 1 year), on and off, or several episodes a day, or one episode from several days up to 10 days. During asthma attacks there is suffocation and rapid breathing with the shoulders raised. While in the remission phase, the patient seems like a normal person. Prolonged asthma is either due to damage to the Lung qi first and then involvement of the Kidney, or an original deficiency of the Kidney. Either case can lead to failure of the Kidney to receive qi, resulting in asthma. Therefore the main treatment should be to boost the Kidney so as to consolidate qi. There are many formulas for this, but. I prefer to use *Jīn Guì Shèn Qì Wán* (金匮肾气丸) (changed into a decoction).

熟地黄	shú dì huáng	15g	Radix Rehmanniae Praeparata
山药	shān yào	15g	Rhizoma Dioscoreae
茯苓	fú líng	15g	Poria
枸杞子	gǒu qí zǐ	10g	Fructus Lycii
牡丹皮	mǔ dān pí	10g	Cortex Moutan
泽泻	zé xiè	10g	Rhizoma Alismatis
熟附子	shú fù zǐ	10g	Radix Aconiti Lateralis Praeparata
肉桂心	ròu guì xīn	3g (ground into fine power, and taken separately by infusing)	Olumula Cinnamomi
地龙干*	dì lóng gān	10g	Lumbricus
胆南星	dǎn nán xīng	6~10g	Arisaema cum Bile

Most patients can have some relief or a cure after this treatment. Also, some patients who had suffered asthma for 10 or 20 years do not have relapses after being cured. In cases of failure of the Kidney to receive qi, there is usually a deficiency of both Kidney yin and Kidney yang. In the prescription, the first 6 medicinals are responsible for replenishing Kidney yin. For non-serious case of yang deficiency, remove *shú fù zǐ* (Radix Aconiti Lateralis Praeparata) and *ròu guì xīn* (Olumula Cinnamomi), and add *wǔ wèi zǐ* (Fructus Schisandrae Chinensis). For severe yang deficiency, remove *zé xiè* (Rhizoma Alismatis), and add *tù sī zǐ* (Semen Cuscutae) and *hú lú bā* (Semen Trigonellae). In both cases *dì lóng* (Lumbricus), *dǎn nán xīng* (Arisaema cum Bile) should be added as adjuvant herbs. The treatment

---

* see above.

of prolonged asthma by adding *dì lóng* (Lumbricus) and *dǎn nán xīng* (Arisaema cum Bile) is based on my own experience in clinical practice, and is from theoretical deduction. According to biomedical theory, asthma is due to allergies causing the spasms of the bronchial smooth muscle. According to records of the traditional Chinese pharmacy, *dì lóng gān* (Lumbricus) can act to dredge the collaterals and stop spasms, and *dǎn nán xīng* (Arisaema cum Bile) can resolve phlegm, extinguish wind, and stop spasms. This shows that both medicinals can stop spasms. I had once used the two medicinals to treat whooping cough, with a better effect on alleviating the spasmodic cough. Consequently, I inferred that they would be useful for bronchial asthma and probably have an effect; in practice this proved to be correct.

(Song Zu-jing. *Essential Collection of Diagnosis and Treatment by Contemporary Famous Doctors* 当代名医证治汇粹. Shijiazhuang: Hebei Science and Technology Publishing House, 1990. 31)

5. Professor Guo Zhen-qiu: The Treatment of Senile Asthma by Rectifying the Lung to Treat the Branch, and Consolidating the Kidney to Treat the Root

Guo Zhen-qiu believes that senile asthma is usually due to lingering phlegm panting (asthma) leading to wheezing. Clinically, it is characterized by the sound resulting from phlegm-qi in the throat. There is much phlegm in the chest, and it congeals and blocks the throat, then the phlegm and breath mingle together to make a sound. The pathogenesis may be due to eating acidic and salty foods in excess, or an invasion of pathogenic wind, cold, dampness, or heat. As qi depresses and phlegm obstructs an attack occurs. Asthma attacks may be divided into cold asthma, heat asthma, and phlegm asthma; thus the treatment should be to rectify the Lung to treat the branch. After the asthma attack has stopped, the treatment should be to consolidate the Kidney to treat the root.

Cold asthma: It is usually due to contraction of wind-cold. The evil invades the Lung, cold fluids settle in the interior, and turbid phlegm accumulates; the airway is obstructed. The symptoms are gasping for breath, stridor in the throat, expectoration of sticky or thin sputum, oppression and stuffiness in the chest and hypochondrium, a dark complexion, a white tongue coating, and a tight pulse. The treatment should be to warm the Lung, scatter cold, clear phlegm, and disinhibit the orifices. The formulas are *Shè Gān Má Huáng Tāng* (射干麻黄汤), *Sān Zǐ Yǎng Qīn Tāng* (三子养亲汤), and *Wēn Fèi Tāng* (温肺汤), with modifications. For coagulation of cold phlegm, *Lěng Xiào Wán* (冷哮丸) may be prescribed accordingly.

Heat asthma: It is usually due to stubborn phlegm-heat resulting in Lung qi obstruction and counterflow. The clinical manifestations are stridor in the throat, chest hyperinflation, hoarse breathing and dyspnea, expectoration of thick yellow phlegm, vexing oppression in the chest and hypochondrium, a red face, spontaneous perspiration, thirst with a desire to drinks, a red tongue with a yellow coating, and a slippery and rapid pulse. The treatment should be to diffuse the Lung and clear heat. The formulas are *Dìng Chuǎn Tāng* (定喘汤) and *Sāng Bái Pí Tāng* (桑白皮汤). If a case arises from invasion of cold, it belongs to cold enveloping fire. Then the treatment should be to dispel the stagnated cold by taking *Sān Niù Tāng* (三拗汤) or *Yuè Bì Jiā Fǎ Bàn Xià Tāng* (越婢加法半夏汤) in order to dispel cold evil and relieve exterior depression.

Phlegm asthma: It is usually due to wind-cold fettering the exterior and phlegm-turbidity obstruction. The clinical manifestations are dyspnea and wheezing, and stridor in the throat like the sound of sawing. The treatment should be to diffuse the Lung and downbear qi, eliminate phlegm and clear fire. Use *Wǔ Hǔ Tāng* (五虎汤), *Bái Guǒ Tāng* (白果汤) with modifications.

Kidney asthma: It is usually due to the depletion of Kidney essence (*jing*) and Kidney qi, failure of the Kidney to receive qi, and deficiency below and exuberance above. The clinical manifestations are dyspnea, panting, shortness of breath, expectoration of frothy phlegm, palpitations induced by exertion, lumbar soreness, knee weakness, dizziness, and tinnitus. The treatment should be to tonify the Kidney to receiving qi. Use *Shèn Qì Wán* (肾气丸) or *zǐ hé chē* (Placenta Hominis) powder.

(Shi Yu-guang, Shan Shu-jian. *The Clinical Essence of Contemporary Famous Physicians: Special Monograph of Asthma* 当代名医临证精华·咳喘专辑 . Beijing: China Ancient Writings Publishing House, 1988. 203)

6. Professor Cen He-ling: The Treatment of Asthma by Treating the Lung and Kidney Simultaneously

Chinese medicine believes that asthma "has its branch in the Lung, and its root in the Kidney". The treatment should be "at the branch in acute [cases], and at the root in chronic [cases]". That means treating the Lung when an asthma attack occurs, and tonifying the Kidney when it remits. This standard is quite inflexible, and impractical. If the asthma is serious, of course the Lung must be treated first to stop the panting. However, the medicinals treating the Lung usually only alleviate the asthma, and cannot be a total cure. If the medications are withdrawn for several days, panting will recur. It is possible that the asthma will not totally disappear even during the period of medication. Therefore it is unreasonable to apply the remedy of tonifying the Kidney only when the asthma has alleviated and ceased.

Professor Cen advocates treating the Lung and Kidney concurrently when an asthma attack occurs. After the asthma remits slightly, tonifying the Kidney will be the main treatment. Only in this way can a total cure of asthma be affected. Although bronchial asthma and asthmatic bronchitis are different, they both belong to *xiào chuǎn* (哮喘 , asthma) in the pattern differentiation of Chinese medicine.

Ma, 28 years old. He visited in the spring of this year because he was suffering from asthmatic bronchitis. The main complaint was asthma lasting for a year; it came following a cold with a cough. The clinical manifestations were a tight feeling in the throat and stridor. Before an asthma attack, there was chest discomfort. The attacks were always at night, in any season, and they could occur every day. Occasionally a cough appeared. The patient had a healthy body in his childhood, without a history of asthma. At the beginning, I thought it was a case of invasion of the Lung by a water pathogen, so I prescribed *Xiǎo Qīng Lóng Tāng* (小青龙汤) for him for a week. It only reduced the severity of asthma attack and decreased the frequency, but it could not effect a cure. For a change, I then used the method of tonifying the Kidney. The formula was *Liù Wèi Dì Huáng Tāng* (六味地黄汤) with additions.

熟地黄	shú dì huáng	24g	Radix Rehmanniae Praeparata
山药	shān yào	24g	Rhizoma Dioscoreae
泽泻	zé xiè	18g	Rhizoma Alismatis Orientalis
牡丹皮	mǔ dān pí	12g	Cortex Moutan
茯苓	fú líng	18g	Poria
山茱萸	shān zhū yú	15g	Fructus Corni Officinalis
淫羊藿	yín yáng huò	18g	Herba Epimedii
丹参	dān shēn	15g	Radix et Rhizoma Salviae Miltiorrhizae

He took one pack a day, with an additional *gé jiè* (Gecko) powder 6 *fen* taken with boiled water, twice a day. The patient was also advised to eat 10 pieces of *hé táo ròu* (Semen Juglandis Regiae), several times, everyday.

Mr. Ma took the prescription for ten days, and his asthma did not relapse. In the past whenever he ate shrimp, it would induce an asthma attack. This time he ate shrimp again, but the asthma did not recur. I told him to take the remedy for 3 successive months in order to consolidate the effect.

(Cen He-ling. *Medical Essays of He's House* 鹤庐医话. Hong Kong: Xingdao Publishing House, 1994. 9)

7. PROFESSOR HUANG WEN-DONG: THE TREATMENT OF ASTHMA BY THE THREE METHODS OF RELIVING THE EXTERIOR, ATTACKING AND TONIFYING

Patients with asthma since childhood mostly have "insufficiency of earlier heaven" and Kidney qi deficiency. Cold asthma with abiding phlegm is often due to a sudden invasion of cold or heavy rain. Cold evil invades the body through BL 13 (*fèi shù*), obstructing the yang qi and leading to cold fluid retention in the interior. The Lung qi fails to diffuse, the phlegm cannot to be expectorated, and qi fails to descend. This results in cough and panting. Heat asthma is usually due to a preference for acidic and salty foods, and an indulgence in eating rich, fatty, and sweet foods. This may cause an accumulation of phlegm and a production of heat. Then wind-cold invades the Lung, leading to a depression of qi and accumulation of phlegm; this results in heat asthma that has exterior cold and interior heat.

The two principles of deficiency and excess must be grasped in order to treat asthma. Generally speaking, if asthma is of the Lung it is excess, and if it is of the Kidney it is deficient. New cases are mostly excess, and long-standing cases are mostly deficient. Frequent attacks are mainly excess, and infrequent attacks are mainly deficient. Cases with invasion of evils belong mostly to excess, and cases with no evils belong mostly to deficiency. Cases that are exogenously contracted mostly pertain to excess, and cases induced by endogenous injury mostly pertain to deficiency. In principle, the treatment of excess cases should stress the elimination of pathogens, using such methods as dispersing wind and expelling cold, clearing heat and purging phlegm, promoting digestion and downbearing qi. The treatment of deficient cases should focus mainly on strengthening the right qi, using such methods as fortifying the Spleen to boost qi, and tonifying the Kidney to grasp qi.

Patients with asthma usually have deficiency as the root and excess as the branch. The deficiency of the root refers to deficiency of both the Spleen and Kidney, while the excess of the branch refers to internal smoldering phlegm-fluids or phlegm-heat. Exogenous contraction of wind-cold or wind-heat can cause a failure of the Lung qi to diffuse, thus inducing asthma or aggravating asthma. Therefore, for an asthma attack, the treatment of the branch is the key; use methods of relieving the exterior or attacking. During the remission period between episodes, treatment of the root is the key; use methods of tonifying the Spleen and Kidney. That is to say "during remission, give precedence to supporting the right qi; during episodes urgently attack the evil qi".

An exterior method is to scatter the wind and cold from the surface. Because most asthma patients have a deficient physique and their exterior *wèi* (卫 , defense) is not consolidated, they are susceptible to sneak-attack invasions by wind-cold and wind-heat evils. During these times, it is most important to dispel evils. Use *Xiǎo Qīng Lóng Tāng* (小青龙汤) for cases of wind-cold. The prescription can not only dispel wind-cold from the exterior, but can also resolve fluid retention and stopping panting. In the prescription, *gān jiāng* (Rhizoma Zingiberis Officinalis) is good at dispelling cold and resolving phlegm. *Gān jiāng* (Rhizoma Zingiberis Officinalis) and *wǔ wèi zǐ* (Fructus Schisandrae Chinensis) are compatible with each other, as one dispels and one astringes. For cases of wind-heat, use *Xiǎo Qīng Lóng Tāng* (小青龙汤) plus *shí gāo* (Gypsum Fibrosum) and *huáng qín* (Radix Scutellariae). However, *gān jiāng* (Rhizoma Zingiberis Officinalis) should be replaced by *shēng jiāng* (Rhizoma Zingiberis Recens). For cases accompanied by sore throat, add *shè gān* (Rhizoma Belamcandae); or prescribe *Shè Gān Má Huáng Tāng* (射干麻黄汤) minus *dà zǎo* (Fructus Ziziphi Jujubae), for an equally obvious effect.

An attacking method is used to warm and transform phlegm-fluids, or to clear and transform phlegm-heat. Asthmatics usually have an abiding ailment of phlegm-fluids, or an exogenous contraction of wind-cold leading to the production of phlegm-fluids internally. There are also patients who have an accumulation of phlegm-heat internally and are repeatedly invaded by exogenous evils, resulting in a depression of qi and blockage of phlegm. Therefore, in treatment, besides exterior-relieving medicinals, those that remove visible phlegm are also needed. For cases belonging to phlegm-fluid [retention], in accordance with the saying from *Essentials of the Golden Cabinet* (金匮要略 , *Jīn Guì Yào Luè*): "The patient that suffers from phlegm-fluid retention should be given warming medicine for harmonization (病痰饮者，当以温药和之)", use *Xiǎo Qīng Lóng Tāng* (小青龙汤). One can also consider using *Líng Guì Zhú Gān Tāng* (苓桂术甘汤) as the basic formula, plus *sū zǐ* (Fructus Perillae), *xìng rén* (Armeniacae Semen Amarum), *chén pí* (Pericarpium Citri Reticulatae), *fǎ bàn xià* (Rhizoma Pinelliae Praeparatum), *zǐ wǎn* (Radix et Rhizoma Asteris), and *dāng guī* (Radix Angelicae Sinensis). Grind these into a fine powder, then prepare them with water, as pills to take orally. For cases belonging to accumulation of phlegm–heat internally, prescribe *Dìng Chuǎn Tāng* (定喘汤) to clear and resolve phlegm-heat. For cases of severe asthma with accumulation of turbid phlegm in the Lung, when prescriptions do not seem effective, use *Dǎo Tán Tāng* (导痰汤) plus *Sān Zǐ Yǎng Qīn Tāng* (三子养亲汤) to achieve a definite effect.

A tonifying method is used to warm and tonify the Spleen and Kidney in order to build up the root. Asthma can have a tendency to be yang deficient or yin deficient. Clinically these are not the same circumstances, therefore they should be treated accordingly. For a predominance of yang deficiency, use *Líng Guì Zhú Gān Tāng* (苓桂术甘汤), or *Shèn Qì Wán* (肾气丸). For a predominance of yin deficiency, use

Shēng Mài Sǎn (生脉散), or *Qī Wèi Dū Qì Wán* (七味都气丸). In addition, agents that can downbear qi and resolve phlegm such as *zǐ wǎn* (Radix et Rhizoma Asteris), *kuǎn dōng huā* (Flos Farfarae), *yuǎn zhì* (Radix Polygalae), *jīn fèi cǎo* (Herba Inulae), *é guǎn shí* (Balanophyllia), and *gé ké* (Concha Meretricis seu Cyclinae) may be employed in the formulas so as to treat deficiency.

After calming asthma, treatment of the root should be paid attention to in order to prevent relapse. This is usually more important than treating the branch to stop panting. The Spleen and Stomach need also to be considered at the same time that the Kidney is tonified. Fortifying the Spleen and harmonizing the Stomach have the same significance as tonifying the Kidney. Because the Spleen is the root of acquired constitution, it is the source of qi and blood generation and transformation. When the Spleen and Stomach are both fortified, then the right qi flourishes, and evils cannot attack.

(Shi Yu-guang, Shan Shu-jian. *The Clinical Essence of Contemporary Famous Physicians: Special Monograph of Asthma* 当代名医临证精华·咳喘专辑. Beijing: China Ancient Writings Publishing House, 1988. 5)

8. Professor Fu Zai-xi: The Treatment of Asthma Mainly by Opening the Orifices and Dispelling Phlegm

Asthma with episodes induced by cold is called cold asthma, and asthma with episodes induced by heat is called heat asthma. From clinical experience, cold asthma is more common. Regardless of whether it is cold asthma or heat asthma, the cause is internal. Both are caused by enduring latent abiding phlegm. Thus Dan-xi has a saying "particularly caused by phlegm (专主于痰)". Because there is stubborn phlegm accumulated within the Lung orifices, in normal times it lies latent and does not move. In the cases of it not moving, the patient is no different from an ordinary person. If the patient contracts wind, cold, summer-heat, or dampness, or overeats greasy, raw, cold, sour, or salty foods, this will trigger the latent phlegm and lead to a sudden episode of asthma. This manifests as wheezing with dyspnea, stridor in the throat, difficulty in coughing, heavy sweating on the head, fullness and stuffiness in the chest, and inability to lie flat. At this time, the treatment should primarily use methods of opening the orifices and removing phlegm. The following formulas may be taken: *Zào Jiá Wán* (皂荚丸), *Qiān Mín Tāng* (千缗汤), *Xiǎo Qīng Lóng Tāng* (小青龙汤), and *Shè Gān Má Huáng Tāng* (射干麻黄汤). Such medicinals as *má huáng* (Herba Ephedrae), *xì xīn* (Radix et Rhizoma Asari), *yá zào* (Fructus Gleditsiae Abnormalis), *bái jiè zǐ* (Semen Sinapis Albae) may be used. Since all asthma episodes are caused by a blockage of stubborn phlegm, medicinals like *má huáng* (Herba Ephedrae) and *xì xīn* (Radix et Rhizoma Asari) can be used to open the Lung orifice. For phlegm-drool that is sticky, stubborn and hard to cough up, such medicinals as *xiǎo yá zào* (Fructus Gleditsiae Abnormalis), and *bái jiè zǐ* (Semen Sinapis Albae) can be used. After medication, if patients expectorate tough yellowish green thick sputum, the asthma will stop at once. If only common herbs that resolve phlegm and calm panting are used, such as *sū zǐ* (Fructus Perillae), *zǐ wǎn* (Radix et Rhizoma Asteris), *kuǎn dōng huā* (Flos Farfarae), and *fǎ bàn xià* (Rhizoma Pinelliae Praeparatum), no effect will be achieved. Clinically for this condition, I usually apply the above prescriptions as the base, and make additions or subtractions to make my own formula. A good effect can usually be achieved. The medicinals are:

麻黄	má huáng	6g	Herba Ephedrae
小牙皂	xiǎo yá zào	6g	Fructus Gleditsiae Abnormalis (roasted, skin peeled)
厚朴	hòu pò	6g	Cortex Magnoliae Officinalis
陈皮	chén pí	6g	Pericarpium Citri Reticulatae
白芥子	bái jiè zǐ	9g	Semen Sinapis Albae (fried, ground)

姜法半夏	jiāng fǎ bàn xià	9g	Rhizoma Pinelliae Praeparatum
茯苓	fú líng	9g	Poria
细辛	xì xīn	3g	Radix et Rhizoma Asari
甘草	gān cǎo	3g	Radix et Rhizoma Glycyrrhizae
生姜	shēng jiāng	3 pieces	Rhizoma Zingiberis Recens
红枣	hóng zǎo	3 pieces	Fructus Jujubae

If asthma is induced by heat evils, and accompanied by thirst and a red complexion, then *má huáng* (Herba Ephedrae), *xì xīn* (Radix et Rhizoma Asari), *yá zào* (Fructus Gleditsiae Abnormalis), and *bái jiè zǐ* (Semen Sinapis Albae) may also be used (in the same quantities). Within the formula, combine only *shí gāo* (Gypsum Fibrosum) 24g and *huáng qín* (Radix Scutellariae Baicalensis) 9g; be sure not to use only cold medicinals in a formula. The treatment of asthma by Chinese medicine, although difficult to affect a permanent cure, can guarantee a short-term effect if the treatment is appropriate and the patient earnestly follows a set diet.

During acute episodes of asthma, it is not suitable to use such medicinals as *rén shēn* (Radix Ginseng), or *huáng qí* (Radix Astragali) to tonify and lift qi. It is also not appropriate to use yin–natured medicinals as they can congeal and consolidate phlegm. Commonly, some practitioners fail to understand the principles of medicine, and when they see urgent panting they fear for qi collapse and absurdly use such medicinals as *rén shēn* (Radix Ginseng), *huáng qí* (Radix Astragali), *gǒu qí* (Fructus Lycii), and *shú dì huáng* (Radix Rehmanniae Praeparata). This can occur to such an extent that death or accidents can occur very often, and one must learn lessons from these experiences. Also, it is common that asthma and panting result from a failure of the Kidney to receive qi, and this is quite different, so *Hēi Xī Dān* (黑锡丹) cannot be used for descending qi.

(Lu Xiang-zhi. *The Unique Skills in Treatment of Diseases by Famous Doctors of Chinese Medicine* 名中医治病绝招 . China Medical Science and Technology Publishing House, 1998. 202)

9. Professor Chao En-xiang: The Treatment of Asthma by Division into Stages, with Emphasis on Dispelling Wind and Resolving Spasms

(1) Dispelling Wind and Resolving Spasms during the Attack Stage of Asthma

The main factor of an asthmatic episode is "wind flourishing". Phlegm, as a secondary pathogenic factor resulting from invasion of wind evil, can exacerbate the disturbance of the Lung's ability to diffuse and descend. The whole pathological process can be generalized as "excess of wind and blockage of phlegm leading to spasms of airway". Wind evil, as the initial factor to cause asthma, invades the Lung and causes a failure of diffusing and descending. Thus, the essential substances cannot be distributed above, and the water passages cannot be dredged and regulated below. Finally, body fluids accumulate to form phlegm. This is like the saying in *Symptom, Cause, Pulse and Treatment* (症因脉治 , *Zhèng Yīn Mài Zhì*): "The etiology of wind-phlegm is that exogenous wind evil invades the body surface, binds up the interiorly stagnated fire and makes it fail to go out, then the exterior evil goes into the interior, and an enhance wind–phlegm disorder develops (风痰之因，外感风邪，袭人肌表，束其内郁之火，不得发泄，外邪传内，内外熏蒸，则风痰之证作矣)." "Excessive wind leads to spasms (风盛则挛急)."Wind and phlegm combine to obstruct the Lung and airway, resulting in a contraction of the airway and disturbance of the Lung "tube", hence wheezing occurs. Furthermore, the narrow airway and disturbance of the Lung tube may inhibit the expectoration of phlegm, thus deteriorating the condition of illness.

Dispelling wind and resolving spasms are the most important methods in the treatment of asthma. In prescription and medication the stress should be upon the wind evil. As for dispelling wind and resolving spasms, dispelling wind treats the root (being the primary aspect), while resolving spasms treats the branch (being the secondary aspect). Through dispelling wind, the exterior evil can be outthrust, the Lung qi can be cleared and depurated, the respiratory tract can be disinhibited, the phlegm can be expelled through opening the collaterals, and thus asthma can be calmed. For asthmatic episodes, dispelling wind is the most pressing matter of the moment. Nevertheless, when choosing wind-dispelling medicinals, it must be in accord with the physiological characteristics of the Lung. This means that it is suitable to diffuse and downbear, open and close, and ascend and descend.

Qū Fēng Jiě Jìng Píng Chuǎn Tāng (祛风解痉平喘汤) may be used. The ingredients are:

麻黄	má huáng	10g	Herba Ephedrae
蝉衣	chán yī	10g	Periostracum Cicadae
僵蚕	jiāng cán	10g	Bombyx Batryticatus
苏叶	sū yè	10g	Folium Perillae
苏子	sū zǐ	10g	Fructus Perillae
地龙	dì lóng	10g	Lumbricus
石菖蒲	shí chāng pú	10g	Rhizoma Acori Tatarinowii
白芍	bái sháo	15g	Radix Paeoniae Alba
白果	bái guǒ	10g	Semen Ginkgo
五味子	wǔ wèi zǐ	10g	Fructus Schisandrae Chinensis

In the prescription, *má huáng* (Herba Ephedrae) dispels wind and expels cold, diffuses the Lung and stops panting. There is dispersing within the diffusing, and it works well with *dì lóng* (Lumbricus), for one is warm and the other is cold, one is diffusing and the other is descending. *Sū yè* (Folium Perillae) and *sū zǐ* (Fructus Perillae) combine with *má huáng* (Herba Ephedrae) not only to enhance the effect of dispelling wind, but also to promote harmony between ascending and descending. As a result the diffusing and descending functions of the Lung will recover.

Chán yī (Periostracum Cicadae) and *jiāng cán* (Bombyx Batryticatus) can both expel wind evil so as to "eliminate the initial cause" and relieve the airway spasms that result from the wind evil. The above medicinals all function mainly to dispel wind and diffuse the Lung, therefore *bái sháo* (Radix Paeoniae Alba), *wǔ wèi zǐ* (Fructus Schisandrae Chinensis), and *bái guǒ* (Semen Ginkgo) are also added in order to astringe and descend Lung qi. The intention is to coordinate the actions of diffusing plus descending, and opening plus closing. The use of all of the medicinals together can expel wind, relieve spasms, open the orifices, descend qi, clear phlegm, and calm panting. Thus, the wind can be dispelled, the phlegm eliminated, and the spasms relieved. Then the asthma will be naturally stopped. In clinic, the prescription may be modified according to pattern differentiation. For example, *shēng shí gāo* (Gypsum Fibrosum), *huáng qín* (Radix Scutellariae), and *sāng bái pí* (Cortex Mori) may be added for heat asthma. *Guì zhī* (Ramulus Cinnamomi) and *xì xīn* (Radix et Rhizoma Asari) may be added for cases with predominant cold manifestations. The prescription can be taken without modifications for cases with no prominent cold or heat manifestations.

(2) Regulating and Tonifying the Lung and Kidney during the Remission Stage of Asthma

Plain questions: Comment on Heat Diseases (素问·评热病论, *Sù Wèn · Píng Rè Bìng Lùn*) says "As one is invaded by evils his right qi must be deficient (邪之所凑，其气必虚)." Therefore the key for wind evil to invade the airway and repeatedly induce asthma is a deficiency of the right qi. Only under the condition of a relative deficiency of the body's right qi, can wind evil overwhelm the deficiency and enter the body, as it lacks the strength to resist the evils. This leads to spasms of the airway and disturbance of the Lung "tube", hence there is an acute asthmatic episode. During the remission stage of asthma, the airways of most patients are still in a hyper-responsive state, so there is usually a danger of relapse. Therefore the Lung and Kidney should be regulated and tonified while in the remission stage, so as to prevent a sudden asthma attack.

With asthma, a deficiency of the right qi is ascribed mainly to the Lung and Kidney. Therefore it is necessary to support the right qi during the remission stage of asthma. To prevent acute asthmatic episodes, one should also start with regulating and tonifying the Lung and Kidney. The Lung governs qi and controls respiration, and the Kidney is in charge of receiving qi. The function of the Lung in respiration relies upon the assistance of the Kidney's function in receiving qi. Therefore there are sayings: "The pathogenic wind must take the advantage of the body's weakness so that it can invade the body." and "The Lung is the governor of qi, and the Kidney is the root of qi". Regardless of whether the asthma is new or old, if there are signs of depletion of the Lung and Kidney, regulating and tonifying the Lung and Kidney should be emphasized during the remission stage of asthma. For new asthma, even with no Lung and Kidney deficiencies or impairment, one must regulate and tonify the Lung and Kidney. On the one hand, this aims to support the right qi and prevent flare-ups; on the other hand, this may also delay the later stages of the disease when one presents with the symptoms of Lung and Kidney deficiencies.

Bǔ Fèi Shèn Fāng (补肺肾方) may be used. The ingredients are:

冬虫夏草	dōng chóng xià cǎo	3g	Cordyceps Sinensis
西洋参	xī yáng shēn	3g	Radix Panacis Quinquefolii
女贞子	nǚ zhēn zǐ	10g	Fructus Ligustri Lucidi
枸杞子	gǒu qǐ zǐ	10g	Fructus Lycii
五味子	wǔ wèi zǐ	10g	Fructus Schisandrae Chinensis
山萸肉	shān yú ròu	10g	Fructus Corni Officinalis
淫羊藿	yín yáng huò	10g	Herba Epimedii

白果	bái guǒ	10g	Semen Ginkgo
丹参	dān shēn	12g	Radix et Rhizoma Salviae Miltiorrhizae
茯苓	fú líng	12g	Poria

This whole prescription is warm but not dry, and drains while tonifying. This is "seeking yin from yang" and "seeking yang from yin". For the convenience of patients taking long term medication, the formula can be ground into a fine powder and prepared with honey as pills.

[Han Chun-sheng, Zhang Hong-chun. Professor Chao En-xiang's Experience of Treating Asthma. *Beijing Journal of Traditional Chinese Medicine* 北京中医. 1996, (3): 18-20]

10. Professor Liu Wei-sheng: Three Steps in the Treatment of Asthma

Asthma attacks are based upon latent phlegm in the Lung, and induced by factors such as exogenous contraction, diet, emotion, and overstrain. This leads to the obstruction of the airway by the phlegm. It is a distinct disease, characterized clinically by repeated episodes of dyspnea and dry wheezing in the throat. The disease is stubborn and difficult to cure. Both the physician and patient should have confidence and patience, for over a long period of treating both the root and the branch, an effect can be achieved. A comprehensive therapy may be divided into the following three steps:

(1) Dispelling Wind, Transforming Phlegm and Calming Panting-Treating the Branch

For asthma in the acute attack stage, the treatment should be to dispel wind, transform phlegm and calm panting. In treating the branch during the acute stage, the treatment should be given in accordance with whether the pattern is cold or heat. Cold asthma should be treated with *Shè Gān Má Huáng Tāng* (射干麻黄汤) or *Xiǎo Qīng Lóng Tāng* (小青龙汤); while heat asthma should be treated with *Dìng Chuǎn Tāng* (定喘汤).

However, it should be remembered that "a warming method is indispensable in the treatment of asthma". In treating acute attack stage asthma, cold and cool remedies should not used too much. The commonly used medicinals are:

炙麻黄	zhì má huáng	12g	Herba Ephedrae Praeparata
北杏	běi xìng	12g	Armeniacae Semen Amarum
甘草	gān cǎo	9g	Radix et Rhizoma Glycyrrhizae
桑白皮	sāng bái pí	15g	Cortex Mori
黄芩	huáng qín	15g	Radix Scutellariae
苏子	sū zǐ	15g	Fructus Perillae
细辛	xì xīn	6g	Radix et Rhizoma Asari
干姜	gān jiāng	6g	Rhizoma ZingiberisTostum
紫菀	zǐ wǎn	15g	Radix et Rhizoma Asteris
地龙	dì lóng	16g	Lumbricus
白芷	bái zhǐ	15g	Radix Angelicae

For cold asthma, subtract *sāng bái pí* (Cortex Mori) and *huáng qín* (Radix Scutellariae); for heat asthma, subtract *gān jiāng* (Rhizoma ZingiberisTostum) and *xì xīn* (Radix et Rhizoma Asari).

(2) Tonifying the Lung and Kidney to Consolidate the Root

For asthma in the remission stage, the treatment should be mainly to consolidate the root (primary aspect) in order to prevent its relapse. At all times one should tonify the Lung and Kidney; at this stage it is even more necessary at the time to treat the "latent origin" of abiding phlegm. The commonly used medicinals are:

党参	dǎng shēn	15g	Radix Codonopsis
白术	bái zhú	15g	Rhizoma Atractylodis Macrocephalae
茯苓	fú líng	15g	Poria
炙甘草	zhì gān cǎo	9g	Radix et Rhizoma Glycyrrhizae Praeparata
川贝末	chuān bèi mò	3g	Bulbus Fritillariae Powder
法半夏	fǎ bàn xià	15g	Rhizoma Pinelliae Praeparatum

胆星	dǎn xīng	10g	Arisaema cum Bile
补骨脂	bǔ gǔ zhī	16g	Fructus Psoraleae
菟丝子	tù sī zǐ	10g	Semen Cuscutae
山萸肉	shān yú ròu	10g	Fructus Corni Officinalis

This formula should be taken for a long period of time to treat the root so as to prevent relapse.

(3) Dealing with the Aftermath of Asthma

After coughing and panting are relieved, dietary therapy should be given so as to improve health and reject disease. Recipe (#1) should be given first, and recipe (#2) should be given second. (#1) Take one chicken with the internal organs and skin removed, and put *bái guǒ* (Semen Ginkgo) 15 pieces, *xìng rén* (Armeniacae Semen Amarum) 10g, and *chén pí* (Pericarpium Citri Reticulatae) 3g into the chicken, then sew it shut with thread, and stew it in water. When it is ready, eat with without salt. (#2) Take *yú biāo jiāo* (Pseudosciaena crocea) 15g, *dōng chóng xià cǎo* (Cordyceps Sinensis) 10g, and lean pork meat 100g, and decoct them in water until they are well done. Eat both the meat and decoction with a little bit of salt. The dietary therapy should be taken twice a week. It is effective to apply this therapy over a long period of time.

(Guangdong Provincial Hospital of Traditional Chinese Medicine)

11. Professor Feng Wei-bin: Treating Asthma by Paying Attention to the Phase and Variability

Professor Feng Wei-bin believes that for the asthma in the attack stage, Chinese medical remedies should mainly eliminate the pathogenic evils and calm panting. For cold asthma due to exteriorly constraint of cold evil, the treatment should be to warm the Lung and dispel cold, expel phlegm and calm panting. The commonly chosen medicinals have an acrid flavor with diffusing and opening actions. These include *má huáng* (Herba Ephedrae), *guì zhī* (Ramulus Cinnamomi), *xì xīn* (Radix et Rhizoma Asari), *bǔ gǔ zhī* (Fructus Psoraleae), *shēng jiāng* (Rhizoma Zingiberis Recens) and *fáng fēng* (Radix Saposhnikoviae). For heat asthma due to heat evil attacking the Lung, the treatment should be to clear heat and expel phlegm, diffuse the Lung and calm panting. The commonly chosen medicinals have a bitter flavor and a cold nature, with actions of lowering and draining. These include *yú xīng cǎo* (Herba Houttuyniae), *dì lóng* (Lumbricus), *sāng bái pí* (Cortex Mori), *wěi jīng* (Coulis Phragmitis), *pú gōng yīng* (Herba Taraxaci), *shí gāo* (Gypsum Fibrosum), and *qīng tiān kuí* (Nervilia Fordii). Among them *yú xīng cǎo* (Herba Houttuyniae) plus *sāng bái pí* (Cortex Mori) have a good effect to clear heat, expel phlegm, diffuse the Lung, and calm panting. *Shí gāo* (Gypsum Fibrosum) plus *qīng tiān kuí* (Nervilia Fordii) have a good effect on lowering heat. For asthma in the remission stage, the treatment with Chinese medicine should mainly be to tonify the Lung, Spleen, and Kidney. Tonifying the Lung can consolidate the exterior so as to prevent invasion of the pathogenic evils and reduce relapse. *Yù Píng Fēng Sǎn* (玉屏风散) is the most famous formula this function. The Spleen is the origin of the acquired (post-heaven) constitution. More attention to methods of strengthening the Spleen and supplementing the middle should be given for young patients so that the acquirement [post-heaven qi] can be reinforced. Thus the source of generation of phlegm (or "latent origin") can be removed. In this way, after growing up, the illness will not recur. The representative formula is *Chén Xià Liù Jūn Zǐ Tāng* (陈夏六君子汤). The Kidney is the origin of congenital (pre-heaven) constitution, therefore supporting the Spleen and warming the Kidney is also very important.

Attack stage asthma can be divided into four categories-cold asthma (corresponding to allergic asthma), heat asthma (corresponding to infectious asthma), phlegm and stasis obstruction, and sudden desertion of yang qi. In addition, there is also a pattern of external cold and internal heat that corresponds to mixed asthma in terms of biomedicine. In the treatment, in addition to dispelling and scattering wind-cold, clearing phlegm and calming panting, medicinals that clear internal heat should also be used, thus the effects will be good. During the remission stage, although the Lung, Spleen, and Kidney can appear singly deficiency, it is more common in clinic for there to be a composite deficiency, like Lung and Kidney dual deficiency, Spleen and Kidney dual deficiency, or Lung, Spleen and Kidney all deficiencies. Therefore distinguish treatment appropriately. Even for the same asthmatic patient, there may be different symptoms with different episodes because of invasion by different six pathogenic agents. It may be cold asthma, heat asthma, or cold-and-heat mixed asthma due to internal transformation of cold into heat. Exterior resolving medicinals are required, but they cannot be used too much. With regards to the use of heat-clearing medicinals, substances that are too bitter and cold should be avoided. These cautions should be more seriously noted particularly for those patients who are emaciated and weak, or suffer from vacuity obesity from long-term corticosteroids. Adding *wǔ wèi zǐ* (Fructus Schisandrae Chinensis) or *bái sháo* (Radix Paeoniae Alba) in the formulas to treat asthma can prevent too much acridity and dispersion. This is because they are medicinals with sour and astringent natures, and can protect the yang qi.

(Zhong Shi-jie. Introduction of Academic Thinking of Professor Feng Wei-bin. In Treatment of Bronchial Asthma. *Chinese Journal of Clinical Practical Medicine* 中华临床实用医药杂志 . 2003, 4: 114)

12. Professor Ren Ji-xue: The Treatment of Asthma is Based upon the Recognition that Wheezing and Panting are Similar

Ancient physicians usually hold that wheezing (哮 , *xiào*) and panting (喘 , *chuǎn*) are different patterns. Professor Ren, through his 40 years of clinical observations, believes that wheezing and panting have no strict difference, and that they are not easily differentiated. There is a differentiation in the *Orthodox Medical Record* (*Yī Xué Zhèng Zhuàn*, 医学正传) that "panting is named according to its breathing condition; while wheezing is defined based on its sound". But Wang Ken-tang of the Ming dynasty did not agree with this idea. He put forth that "wheezing and panting are similar". This opinion is consistent with the clinical condition. Therefore together they can be called *xiào chuǎn bìng* (哮喘病, asthma).

This disease is mostly caused by exogenous contraction of six pathogenic evils or pestilent evils. Then the evils are not expelled and stay deep in the Lung because of wrong or delayed treatment. This disease may also be caused by residual measles toxin accumulating in the Lung. There are also cases in which the Lung membrane and collaterals are damaged because of prolonged cough. When the trachea and the Lung are involved, and the collaterals are damaged, the blood circulation will be hindered, so there are acute pathological changes such as spasms. Then the fluid cannot be distributed normally, the nutritive qi and defensive qi fail to harmonize, thus the exterior *wei* becomes unconsolidated and the Lung qi fails to diffuse. Therefore, over a long time the disease mechanism becomes chest qi congested and blocked, phlegm in the diaphragm sticky and bound, and abnormal contraction of exterior evils, hence the illness appears. Thus, the treatment should mainly be to diffuse the Lung, expel phlegm, regulate qi, and relieve spasms. The medicinals used are: *tiān zhú zǐ* (Fructus Nandinae Domesticae), *quán xiē* (Scorpio), *bái jiè zǐ* (Semen Sinapis Albae), *tán xiāng* (Lignum Santali Albi), *qīng pí* (Pericarpium Citri Reticulatae Viride), *chuān xiōng* (Rhizoma Chuanxiong), *jiāo mù* (Semen Zanthoxyli Bungeani), *wū méi* (Fructus Mume), *hē zǐ ròu* (Fructus Terminaliae Chebulae), *bái guǒ rén* (Semen Ginkgo), *xìng rén* (Armeniacae Semen Amarum), and *hǎi fú shí* (Os Costaziae).

天烛子	tián zhú zǐ	Fructus Nandinae Domesticae
全蝎	quán xiē	Scorpio
白芥子	bái jiè zǐ	Semen Sinapis Albae
檀香	tán xiāng	Lignum Santali Albi
青皮	qīng pí	Pericarpium Citri Reticulatae Viride
川芎	chuān xiōng	Rhizoma Chuanxiong
椒目	jiāo mù	Semen Zanthoxyli Bungeani
乌梅	wū méi	Fructus Mume
诃子肉	hē zǐ ròu	Fructus Terminaliae Chebulae
白果仁	bái guǒ rén	Semen Ginkgo
杏仁	xìng rén	Armeniacae Semen Amarum
海浮石	hǎi fú shí	Os Costaziae

Decoct the medicinals with water, and take orally. For cases of cold phlegm, add *xiān máo* (Rhizoma Curculiginis), *ròu guì* (Cortex Cinnamomi), and *yín yáng huò* (Herba Epimedii). For cases of heat phlegm, add *shēng shí gāo* (Gypsum Fibrosum) and *huáng qín* (Radix Scutellariae). After the panting has been calmed, use *tāi pán* (Placenta Hominis), *dōng chóng xià cǎo* (Cordyceps Sinensis), *hē zǐ ròu* (Fructus Terminaliae Chebulae), *bái guǒ rén* (Semen Ginkgo), *hǎi mǎ* (Hippocampus), *gé jiè* (Concha Meretricis seu Cyclinae), *chén xiāng* (Lignum Aquilariae Resinatum), and *shān yú ròu* (Fructus Corni Officinalis) to support the right qi.

胎盘	tāi pán	Placenta Hominis
冬虫夏草	dōng chóng xià cǎo	Cordyceps Sinensis
诃子肉	hē zǐ ròu	Fructus Terminaliae Chebulae
白果	bái guǒ	Semen Ginkgo
海马	hǎi mǎ	Hippocampus
蛤蚧	gé jiè	Concha Meretricis seu Cyclinae
沉香	chén xiāng	Lignum Aquilariae Resinatum
山茱萸	shān yú ròu	Fructus Corni Officinalis

One can also put *bái fán* (Alumen), and *shēng fǎ bàn xià* (Rhizoma

Pinelliae Praeparatum) into a pig's foot, and calcine it in an earthenware pot, then add a little *shè xiāng* (Secretio Moschi) and grind them into a fine powder. Take 5-10g orally with boiled water twice a day. Thus a cure can be affected.

(Ren Ji-xue. *Experience Collection of China Famous Veteran Physicians of Traditional Chinese Medicine* 中国名老中医经验集萃 . Beijing Science and Technology Publishing House, 1993. 190)

PERSPECTIVES OF INTEGRATIVE MEDICINE

Challenges and Solutions

Bronchial asthma is a disease that is difficult to cure. It was recognized very early, and many therapeutic experiences in treating it have been accumulated, but because an asthma attack is sudden in onset, rapid in development, and very quick to evolve into dyspnea, it can bring on enormous pain to the patient, and in some cases even become life-threatening. Therefore relevant issues such as prevention, how to reduce its relapse, and how to carry out treatment by integrative medicine can be challenging to us. Therefore these are a series of problems on treatment difficulties, and how to carry out integrated Chinese medical and biomedical treatments.

CHALLENGE #1: HOW TO PREVENT THE OCCURRENCE OF ASTHMA

Because the etiology of the asthma is complex and the patients' constitutional factors are different, asthma can be divided into exogenous asthma, endogenous asthma and mixed asthma. Therefore, in prevention, attention should be paid to the elimination of pathogens and the control of infection.

(1) Eliminating the Pathogens

Exogenous asthma (allergic asthma) is associated with exposure to allergens. Those who are sensitive to fish, meat, crabs, egg, and milk should stop eating such foods. Those whose asthmatic episodes are induced by bacteria, pollen, indoor dust, industrial dust, animal dander, or feathers should try to pay attention to environmental hygiene, and improving or changing the living environment in order to avoid contact with the allergens. For those whose asthmatic episodes are induced by mites, cockroaches, fungal spores, a corresponding vaccine should be applied to reduce the allergy.

(2) Controlling the Infection

Endogenous (infectious) asthma is related to infection, Endogenous asthma is not caused by infection, but it is very easily complicated by pulmonary infection. In addition, many cases of mixed asthma also involve pulmonary infection. Therefore it is really necessary to control infection.

In general, infections are usually either bacterial or viral. Chinese medicine has a better effect in controlling viral infections. Such exterior-relieving medicinals with acrid and warm natures as *má huáng* (Herba Ephedrae), *guì zhī* (Ramulus Cinnamomi), *fáng fēng* (Radix Saposhnikoviae), *jīng jiè* (Herba Schizonepetae), *zǐ sū* (Folium Perillae), *shēng má* (Rhizoma Cimicifugae); and such exterior-relieving medicinals with acrid and cool natures as *jīn yín huā* (Flos Lonicerae), *lián qiào* (Fructus Forsythiae), *sāng yè* (Folium Mori), *xiāng rú* (Herba Elsholtziae Seu Moslae), and *bò hé* (Herba Menthae) all have a definite effect on viral infections of the airway. For viral infections presenting with wind-cold tightening the Lung, select the exterior-relieving medicinals with acrid and warm natures; for viral infections presenting with wind-heat attacking the Lung, select the exterior-relieving medicinals with acrid and cold natures.

Viral infection is usually followed by bacterial infection. *Huáng qín*

(Radix Scutellariae), *pú gōng yīng* (Herba Taraxaci), *yú xīng cǎo* (Herba Houttuyniae), *bài jiàng cǎo* (Herba Patriniae) all have a better effect on Gram-positive bacteria; while *shè gān* (Rhizoma Belamcandae), *qín pí* (Cortex Fraxini), *mù xiāng* (Raadix Aucklandiae), *hòu pò* (Cortex Magnoliae Officinalis), *bǎi bù* (Radix Stemonae), *bái zhǐ* (Radix Angelicae), *dīng xiāng* (Flos Caryophylli), and *wū méi* (Fructus Mume) have a definitive effect on Gram-negative bacteria. For patients with chronic infections and weak physique, tonifying and antibacterial medicinals like *huáng qí* (Radix Astragali), *dāng guī* (Radix Angelicae Sinensis), *chuān xiōng* (Rhizoma Chuanxiong), *bái sháo* (Radix Paeoniae Alba), *tiān mén dōng* (Radix Asparagi), *mài mén dōng* (Radix Ophiopogonis), and *huáng jīng* (Rhizoma Polygonati) can be used. If the above medicinals are appropriately applied based on treatment according to pattern differentiation, the infection can be controlled promptly and effectively, and the morbidity rate of exogenous asthma and mixed asthma will be effectively reduced.

CHALLENGE #2: HOW TO REDUCE THE RELAPSE OF ASTHMA

Repeated episodes of asthma are a common issue of concern for patients, their relatives and medical personnel. These episodes are also a point of difficultly in treating asthma.

Most asthmatics, because of low immune function, are predisposed to attack by exogenous and endogenous pathogenic factors. The medicinals in Chinese medicine with actions of boosting qi, fortifying the Spleen, and tonifying the Kidney have the effect to raise immune function. These include *huáng qí* (Radix Astragali), *dǎng shēn* (Radix Codonopsis), *bái zhú* (Rhizoma Atractylodis Macrocephalae), *dāng guī* (Radix Angelicae Sinensis), *nǚ zhēn zǐ* (Fructus Ligustri Lucidi), *tù sī zǐ* (Semen Cuscutae), *shú fù zǐ* (Radix Aconiti Praeparata), *zǐ hé chē* (Placenta Hominis), *bǔ gǔ zhī* (Fructus Psoraleae), and *yín yáng huò* (Herba Epimedii). Their long-term use during the remission stage will have a very good effect to reduce episodes of asthma. This is consistent with theories in Chinese medicine of strengthening the right qi and eliminating evils, and preventing disease. *Yù Píng Fēng Sǎn* (玉屏风散) is a representative formula, being held in high esteem by all doctors and patients.

Since the 1980's, in the wake of increasingly in-depth research into the pathogenesis of asthma, asthma has been recognized not as an illness characterized by bronchial spasms, but as an inflammation of the respiratory tract causing a hyper-reactivity of the airway. Therefore, in regards to treatment, there was a change from simply resolving smooth muscle spasms, to preventing and treating the airway inflammation. Corticosteroids are considered to be the best medicine in eliminating chronic inflammation of the respiratory tract and reducing the hyper-reactivity of the airway. The following Chinese medicinals have steroid-like functions: *rén shēn* (Radix Ginseng), *dǎng shēn* (Radix Codonopsis), *lù róng* (Cornu Cervi Pantotrichum), *zǐ hé chē* (Placenta Hominis), *dōng chóng xià cǎo* (Cordyceps Sinensis), *ròu guì* (Cortex Cinnamomi), *dù zhòng* (Cortex Eucommiae), *xiān máo* (Rhizoma Curculiginis), *yín yáng huò* (Herba Epimedii), *qín jiāo* (Radix Gentianae Macrophyllae), and *qín pí* (Cortex Fraxini). Although their effect is not as powerful as corticosteroids, their side effects are also not as strong as corticosteroids. In addition, many of them have the function of tonifying the Lung, Spleen and Kidney, and thus can be used for a long time.

From a variety of large-scale researches, it has been reported that acupoint application therapy during the remission stage can enhance the immune function of the body, and prevent and reduce relapse of asthma (with an effectiveness rate between 70% and 90%).

Bǔ gǔ zhī (Fructus Psoraleae) acupoint injection therapy has a remarkable long-term effect on infectious asthmatics, and can reduce the episodes of asthma. *Bǔ gǔ zhī* (Fructus Psoraleae) can adjust the function of the hypothalamus-pituitary-adrenal cortex axis. It also has several other actions, including increasing the number of white blood cells, and inhibiting the growth of staphylococci staphylococcus aureus and fungi. This relates to the fact that *Bǔ gǔ zhī* (Fructus Psoraleae) warms the Kidney and invigorates yang so as to enhance the resistance of the body and reduce the opportunity for infection.

Acupoint injection therapy of Nucleotide and Casein Injection at RN 17 (*dàn zhōng*) and acupoint embedding therapy in rabbit pituitary glands has a better curative effect to prevent and treat asthma, and can achieve the goal of reducing asthma relapses.

Challenge #3: The Treatment of Critical Asthma

According to clinical manifestations, critical asthma is called "sudden desertion of yang qi". In previous Chinese medical literature there is very little discussion of critical asthma. In the discourse on asthma only two kinds (cold and heat) are mentioned, and the critical type is seldom dealt with. Perhaps because of insufficient experience, the necessity of Chinese medicine in the treatment of critical asthma is neglected. Some authors only present *Shēn Fù Tāng* (参附汤) or *Huí Yáng Jiù Jí Tāng* (回阳救急汤), but do not further expound upon them, thus leaving the reader, specially the beginner, feeling quite puzzled.

We believe that the majority of mild or moderate asthma may be relieved through Chinese medical treatment. But patients with more severe conditions should be treated with integrative medicine. For example, the use of antibiotics to treat infection, or antispasmodics to relieve asthma, is helpful in patient recovery.

Generally speaking, for a critical asthma we advocate integrative treatment. For serious dyspnea complicated by excessive sweating, cyanotic lips, cold limbs, or serious anoxia and respiratory failure due to a disturbance of ventilation function, (which belongs to sudden desertion of yang qi in Chinese medicine), oxygen therapy, fluid infusions, correction of electrolyte imbalances, and the use of antispasmodics, antibiotics, and corticosteroids should be considered in accordance with the condition. There should be concurrent use of Chinese medical therapies to restore yang so as to save the patient from collapse, like boosting qi and calming panting. In these moments, the Chinese medicine *Huí Yáng Dìng Chuǎn Tāng* (回阳定喘汤) can be used, and the effect is usually good.

【Prescription】

熟附子	shú fù zǐ	Radix Aconiti Lateralis Praeparata
干姜	gān jiāng	Rhizoma Zingiberis Officinalis
炙麻黄	zhì má huáng	Herba Ephedrae Praeparata
杏仁	xìng rén	Armeniacae Semen Amarum
肉桂	ròu guì	CortexCinnamomi

If the community hospital has insufficient resources, the patient should be transferred immediately to a hospital that is well equipped for medical care.

It is our experience that an asthma attack of a moderate degree, with symptoms like dyspnea with wheezing, and heavy perspiration that wets the clothes, or gasping with the shoulders raised, a thin weak voice and unclear speech, is critical asthma. This needs immediate treatment with integrative medicine, lest the opportunity for treatment be missed.

CHALLENGE #4: THE TREATMENT OF HORMONE-DEPENDENT ASTHMA

In recent years, in the wake of the establishment of respiratory tract inflammation theory, glucocorticoids with anti-inflammation functions have become the first choice in the treatment of asthma. However, in addition to general negative reactions that occur after long-term administration (like Cushing's disease, peptic ulcers, and osteoporosis), a dependency on the hormones can develop. The treatment of patients with hormone-dependent asthma is a big problem for clinicians. Currently, immunosuppressants are used to replace steroid therapy. However these medications have greater toxic side effects and the treatment effect is not reliable, therefore in clinic patients do not readily accept this treatment.

We believe that bronchial asthma is related to the Lung, Spleen and Kidney. Clinically, the majority of patients with hormone dependent asthma present with depletion of Kidney yin and yang (especially Kidney yang). The manifestations are vacuity obesity, a pale complexion, soreness and weakness in the lower back and knees, nocturia, a pink tongue with a white coating, and a deep, thready and forceless pulse. In clinic, the patients are given *Jīn Guì Shèn Qì Wán* (金匮肾气丸) plus *bǔ gǔ zhī* (Fructus Psoraleae), *yín yáng huò* (Herba Epimedii), and *bā jǐ tiān* (Radix Morindae Officinalis) to take orally. In addition, to strengthen the curative effect, *rén shēn* (Radix Ginseng), *gé jiè* (Gecko), and *Tāi Pán Wán* (Placenta Pill) are given orally in the early morning and in the evening. As early as 1984 we discovered that *bǔ gǔ zhī* (Fructus Psoraleae) injection has a good effect to treat deficiency of Kidney yang. It can enhance the function of the hypothalamus-pituitary-adrenal cortex axis (HPA). In clinic, we have already been successful in withdrawing over 10 patients from corticosteroids, reducing the dosage and the side effects of corticosteroids. We have also discovered that some patients have simultaneous manifestations of yin and yang deficiency, Liver qi depression and binding constraint, and Spleen and Stomach qi deficiency. Therefore the treatment should be based on invigorating the Kidney yang, with the addition of *Liù Wèi Dì Huáng Wán* (六味地黄丸) to tonify yin in order to assist yang. *Rén shēn* (Radix Ginseng) can be added to boost qi and consolidate the exterior. *Yù jīn* (Radix Curcumae), and *fó shǒu* (Fructus Citri Sarcodactylis) can be added to course the Liver and resolve depression. *Rén shēn* (Radix Ginseng), *fú líng* (Poria), and *bái zhú* (Rhizoma Atractylodis Macrocephalae), can be added to boost qi and fortify the Spleen.

Insight from Empirical Wisdom

1. Asthma Outbreaks Occur in Stages

Asthma can be divided into two stages—the attack stage and the remission stage. During the attack stage, if the symptoms are not serious, it may treated by either Chinese medicine (based on the pattern differentiation) or Biomedical pharmacotherapy. During the attack stage the treatment with Chinese medicine should focus on dispelling evils and calming panting. For cold asthma due to invasion of the exterior by cold evil, the therapy is to warm the Lung and dispel cold, expel phlegm and calm panting. The medicinals used most are acrid natured ones with actions of dispelling, opening and diffusing. These include *má huáng* (Herba Ephedrae), *guì zhī* (Ramulus Cinnamomi), *xì xīn* (Radix et Rhizoma Asari), *bǔ gǔ zhī* (Fructus Psoraleae), *shēng jiāng* (Rhizoma Zingiberis Recens), *fáng fēng* (Radix Saposhnikoviae), and *jīng jiè* (Herba Schizonepetae). For heat asthma due to attack of the Lung by heat evil, the therapy is to clear heat and eliminate phlegm, diffuse the Lung and clam panting. The medicinals used most are bitter-cold natured ones with actions of descending and purging. These include *yú xīng cǎo* (Herba Houttuyniae), *tíng lì zǐ* (Semen Lepidii seu Descurainiae), *sāng bái pí* (Cortex Mori), *wěi jīng* (Coulis Phragmitis), *huáng qín* (Radix Scutellariae), *pú gōng yīng* (Herba Taraxaci), *shí gāo* (Gypsum Fibrosum), and *qīng tiān kuí* (Nervilia Fordii). *Yú xīng cǎo* (Herba Houttuyniae) combined with *sāng bái pí* (Cortex Mori) can clear Lung-heat, remove phlegm and calm panting. *Shí gāo* (Gypsum Fibrosum) plus *qīng tiān kuí* (Nervilia Fordii) are good at lowering fever. As for patients with serious asthma attacks manifesting as shortness of breath, wheezing, hyperinflation of the chest, gasping with the shoulders raised, and orthopnea [the inability to breathe easily unless one is sitting up straight or standing erect], and especially for those with a longer history of repeated episodes, integrative medical treatments should be considered. In terms of Biomedicine, intravenous glucocorticoids and aminophylline are usually employed for eliminating the airway inflammation, and relieving bronchial spasms. In terms of Chinese medicine, methods to strengthen the right qi may be employed so as to reinforce the Lung and tonify the Kidney. *Sū Zǐ Jiàng Qì Tāng* (苏子降气汤) can be give as the base, with the additions of *dǎng shēn* (Radix Codonopsis), *dāng guī* (Radix Angelicae Sinensis), *shú dì huáng* (Radix Rehmanniae Praeparata), or *ròu guì* (Cortex Cinnamomi) according to the pattern differentiation. In brief, the application of integrative medical treatments is beneficial to rapidly alleviating the condition and controlling asthmatic episodes. Critical asthma is an acute internal medical illness and requires active emergency treatment. For details of treatments, see **Challenge #3: Treatment of critical asthma**.

On remission stage, asthma can be treated primarily with Chinese medicine, namely by regulating and tonifying the Lung, Spleen and Kidney. Tonifying the Lung can consolidate the exterior so as to prevent attack by the six climatic evils, and reduce the number of asthma episodes. *Yù Píng Fēng Sǎn* (玉屏风散) is a representative formula. The Spleen-earth is the origin of acquired constitution; especially for younger patients, attention should be paid to fortifying the Spleen in order to reinforce the middle jiao. Thus the acquired constitution (post-heaven) can be nourished, and the growth and development will be strong and healthy, so that the source of phlegm will be stopped and "latent root" will be removed. Therefore appropriate regulation can put an end to recurrence of asthma after the patient has grown up. *Chén Xià Liù Jūn Zǐ Tāng* (陈夏六君子汤) and *Xiāng Shā Liù Jūn Zǐ Tāng* (香砂六君子汤) are the representative formulas. The Kidney is the origin of congenital constitution, and the Kidney yin and yang are both opposite and complementary. Therefore there is a saying: "He who is good at nourishing yang must seek yang from yin ... He who is good at nourishing yin must seek yin from yang (善补阳者必从阴中求阳 … 善补阴者必从阳中求阴)." Ye Tian-shi in his book *Case Records as a Guide to Clinical Practice* (临证指南医案, *Lín Zhèng Zhǐ Nán Yī Àn*) says that the treatment of asthma "should mainly be to warm and open the Lung, and benefit the Kidney essence. For a long illness with deficiency of the middle jiao, fortifying and boosting the middle qi should also be considered (以温通肺脏，下护及肾真为主，久发中虚岁又必补益中气)." This also emphasizes the key of tonifying the Lung, Spleen and Kidney during the remission stage.

In clinical practice, the persistent treatment of asthma in the remission stage can help greatly to reduce relapse. Especially for juveniles it may achieve the goal of removing the root of asthma by strengthening both the congenital and acquired constitution. If treatment is delayed until after the child is grown, "removal of the root" will be difficult.

2. The Complexity of Pattern Types

Asthma in the attack stage can be divided into four types: cold asthma (corresponding to allergic asthma), heat asthma (corresponding to infectious asthma), obstruction of mixed phlegm and stasis, and sudden collapse of yang qi. In addition, there are some cases of external cold and internal heat that are induced by catching colds in the winter or in a cold environment. This presents with aversion to cold, thin nasal discharge, sneezing, cough with yellow and thick sputum that is difficult to cough up, and thirst. In biomedicine this corresponds to mixed asthma. In the treatment, besides dispelling wind and cold, expelling phlegm, and calming panting, medicinals that clear internal heat should also be used, thus a good effect will be achieved.

In the remission stage there are cases of simple deficiency of the Lung, or Spleen, or Kidney; but most cases are a compound expression, such as deficiency of both the Lung and Kidney, deficiency of both the Spleen and Kidney, or deficiency of both the Lung and Spleen. Therefore treatment should come from careful pattern differentiation.

3. The Variability of Pattern Types

For one asthmatic patient, there may be different symptoms amongst different episodes of asthma because of invasion by the different six pathogenic agents. It may manifest as a cold asthma, heat asthma, or cold-and-heat mixed asthma due to transformation of heat internally.

In the course of treatment, pay attention to protecting yang qi. Asthmatics often have repeated episodes and usually take exterior-resolving or heat-clearing medicinals, which are apt to damage yang qi of the body. Furthermore, patients often sweat profusely during the attack, and yang qi will emerge following perspiration, thus easily leading to a sudden desertion of yang qi. These are the most dangerous changes in asthma symptoms. The method of pattern differentiation is to: ① Check whether there is improvement or change in the patient's state of consciousness and anoxia; ② Observe whether there is improvement in the patient's dyspnea; ③ Examine via auscultation whether the wheezing sounds over the patient's lungs has increased or disappeared. If the patient is in a confused state with no improvement of dyspnea, and the wheezing sounds over the lungs conversely becomes lower or disappears, this is a critical sign of yang-collapse that needs our constant vigilance. Therefore in the treatment, one should pay attention to application of the exterior-resolving medicinals, as the overuse of acrid-natured agents with dispersing actions should be avoided. In the application of heat-clearing medicinals, those that are too bitter and cold natured should be avoided. Especially for those patients who are emaciated and weak, or have vacuity obesity, from long term corticosteroids medication, all of these cautions should be followed more seriously. In Zhong-jing's formulae for treating asthma there is often *wǔ wèi zǐ* (Fructus Schisandrae Chinensis) or *bái sháo* (Radix Paeoniae Alba). This is to prevent too much acridity and over-dispersion, for these medicinals have sour-astringent natures and can protect yang qi.

4. Experience of Using Medicinals in the Treatment of Asthma

Asthma attack is due mainly to airway inflammation associated with mast cells and eosinophils, which cause swelling of the mucous membranes, spasms of the bronchial smooth muscles and increased secretions such that the airway becomes narrow. Therefore there are a series of symptoms including dyspnea. There are three important segments to treat asthma: eliminating airway inflammation, relieving bronchial smooth muscle spasms, and clearing away secretions such as turbid phlegm and liquids.

Referring to medical books, reports, and periodicals, in combination with our clinical experience, we believe that the following Chinese medicinals have a certain therapeutic effects with regard to the above three treatment points. In clinic they can be chosen according to the identification of different patterns.

(1) Acrid-Warm Exterior-Resolving Medicinals

These include *má huáng* (Herba Ephedrae), *xì xīn* (Radix et Rhizoma Asari), *zǐ sū* (Folium Perillae), *jīng jiè* (Herba Schizonepetae), *shēng jiāng* (Rhizoma Zingiberis Recens), *xīn yí* (Flos Magnoliae), *ài yè* (Folium Artemisiae), *huò xiāng* (Herba Agastachis), *bái zhǐ* (Radix Angelicae), and *gǎo běn* (Rhizoma et Radix Ligustici). They can function to eliminate airway inflammation and smooth the airway through resolving the exterior, removing evils, diffusing the Lung, and benefiting qi.

(2) Phlegm-Expelling and Cough-Stopping Medicinals

These include *xìng rén* (Armeniacae Semen Amarum), *bǎi bù* (Radix

Stemonae), *bǎi hé* (Bulbus Lilii), *bái guǒ* (Semen Ginkgo), *kuǎn dōng huā* (Flos Farfarae), *xuán fù huā* (Flos Inulae), *bái jiè zǐ* (Semen Sinapis Albae), *qián hú* (Radix Peucedani), *shān dòu gēn* (Radix et Rhizoma Sophorae Tonkinensis), *mǎ dōu líng* (Fructus Aristolochiae), *pí pa yè* (Folium Eriobotryae), *ǎi dì chá* (Herba Ardisiae Japonicae), *zǐ jīn niú* (Ardisia Japonica), *zǐ huā dù juān* (Rhododendron Hance), and *tíng lì zǐ* (Semen Lepidii seu Descurainiae). They can function to remove secretions and turbidity that have blocked the airway, and thus, through their inherent nature and flavor, smooth the airway by resolving turbid phlegm.

(3) Qi-Regulating and Stomach-Warming Medicinals

These include *hú jiāo* (Fructus Piperis Nigri), *jiāo mù* (Semen Zanthoxyli Bungeani), *chén pí* (Pericarpium Citri Reticulatae), *fó shǒu* (Fructus Citri Sarcodactylis), *dīng xiāng* (Flos Caryophylli), *bái dòu kòu* (Fructus Amomi), *gān sōng* (Radix et Rhizoma Nardostachyos), *mù xiāng* (Radix Aucklandiae Lappae), *gāo liáng jiāng* (Rhizoma Alpiniae Officinarum), and *wú zhū yú* (Fructrus Evodiae). They can function to warm the Lung and Stomach, fortify the Spleen in transporting dampness, strengthen the right qi, expel evils, eliminate inflammation, and reduce production of airway secretions like phlegm.

(4) Heat-Clearing and Detoxifying Medicinals

These include *kǔ shēn* (Radix Sophorae Flavescentis), *qín pí* (Cortex Fraxini), *bái máo gēn* (Rhizoma Imperatae), *huáng qín* (Radix Scutellariae), *bàn biān lián* (Herba Lobeliae Chinensis), *bàn zhī lián* (Herba Scutellariae Barbatae), and *cè bǎi yè* (Cacumen Platycladi). They can clear heat and toxins, and eliminate turbidity and stop panting. Therefore they are the most suitable to treat heat asthma.

(5) Antispasmodic and Anti-asthmatic Medicinals

For example *dì lóng* (Lumbricus), *gōu téng* (Ramulus Uncariae cum

Uncis), *shí chāng pú* (Rhizoma Acori Tatarinowii), *lú huì* (Herba Aloes), *cǎo jué míng* (Semen Cassiae), *chán sū* (Venenum Bufonis), and *xiè bái* (Bulbus Allii Macrostemi) all have definite effects.

According to studies, *má huáng* (Herba Ephedrae), *fù zǐ* (Radix Aconiti Lateralis Praeparata), *xì xīn* (Radix et Rhizoma Asari), *wú zhū yú* (Fructrus Evodiae), *jiāo mù* (Semen Zanthoxyli Bungeani), *gāo liáng jiāng* (Rhizoma Alpiniae Officinarum), and *dīng xiāng* (Flos Caryophylli) contain racemic noraconitine and have β_2 receptor excitability functions. *Shí chāng pú* (Rhizoma Acori Tatarinowii) also has the ability to excite to β_2 receptors, and thus can relieve spasms and asthma. *Bǔ gǔ zhī* (Fructus Psoraleae), *kǔ shēn* (Radix Sophorae Flavescentis), *dì lóng* (Lumbricus), *gōu téng* (Ramulus Uncaria), *máo gēn* (Rhizoma Imperatae), *lú huì* (Herba Aloes), *mài mén dōng* (Radix Ophiopogonis), and *bǎi hé* (Bulbus Lilii) have the function of resisting bronchial spasms induced by histamines. *Yín yáng huò* (Herba Epimedii), *dāng guī* (Radix Angelicae Sinensis), *xì xīn* (Radix et Rhizoma Asari), *lú huì* (Herba Aloes), and *shān dòu gēn* (Radix et Rhizoma Sophorae Tonkinensis) can relieve bronchial spasms induced by bradykinins. *Lián qiào* (Fructus Forsythiae), *bái máo xià kū cǎo* (Herba Ajugae), *cǎo jué míng* (Semen Cassiae), and *chuān xiōng* (Rhizoma Chuanxiong) can reduce degeneration of cAMP through inhibiting di-phosphate ester enzyme. Thus they have a function similar to aminophylline in dilating the bronchi to stop asthma. *Bàn biān lián* (Herba Lobeliae Chinensis), *yáng jīn huā* (Flos Daturae), and *shí chāng pú* (Rhizoma Acori Tatarinowii) have anti-cholinergic functions. *Dāng guī* (Radix Angelicae Sinensis), *chuān xiōng* (Rhizoma Chuanxiong), *bái zhǐ* (Radix Angelicae) *gǎo běn* (Rhizoma et Radix Ligustici), *qián hú* (Radix Peucedani), and *chì sháo* (Radix Paeoniae Rubra) act as calcium antagonists, and thus can relax the bronchial smooth muscle.

We believe that in the treatment of asthma, the above medicinals can be chosen and used in a prescription based on different pattern differentiations. For example, for patients suffering from cold asthma due to invasion of wind-cold complicated with cold due to Stomach qi deficiency manifesting as symptoms of chest oppression, nausea, and vomiting phlegm, we can give *Xiǎo Qīng Lóng Tāng* (小青龙汤) based on a pattern of differentiation of cold asthma. On this basis, other medicinals can be added, such as the qi rectifying and Stomach-warming herbs mentioned above that have certain antispasmodic functions. These include *chén pí* (Pericarpium Citri Reticulatae), *gāo liáng jiāng* (Rhizoma Alpiniae Officinarum), and *wú zhū yú* (Fructrus Evodiae). As another example, the following herbs can be added to *Dìng Chuǎn Tāng* (定喘汤) for patients with heat asthma: *bái máo gēn* (Rhizoma Imperatae), *bàn biān lián* (Herba Lobeliae Chinensis) and *dì lóng* (Lumbricus). By doing this, we can select medicinals that not only have the advantage of treating according to pattern differentiation, but also treating in combination with the results of modern pharmacological studies. Thus the treatment is more targeting and the curative effects are increased.

5. Knowledge from Experience Regarding the Use of *Má Huáng* (Herba Ephedrae)

During the attack stage of asthma, *má huáng* (Herba Ephedrae) can be used for many types of patients. Generally, *shēng má huáng* (Herba Ephedrae Recens) may be chosen for cases with an exterior pattern; its effect is to resolve the exterior disperse evil. For cases without an exterior pattern, *zhì má huáng* (Herba Ephedrae Praeparata) can be used so as to reduce its dry and harsh nature. However, for cases of yin deficiency with hyperactivity of yang, *má huáng* (Herba Ephedrae) should be used with caution. For critical asthma, we advocate using *Huí Yáng Dìng Chuǎn Tāng* (回阳定喘汤), in which *zhì má huáng* (Herba Ephedrae Praeparata) is used to descend qi and calm panting. However, some people worry about that using *má huáng* (Herba Ephedrae) in cases with sweating is disobeying ancient precepts, and that *má huáng* (Herba Ephedrae) with its harsh and dry nature could result in sweating and thus damage the yang. Also, some people believe that using *má huáng* (Herba Ephedrae) may induce heart failure by making the heart beat faster. But we believe that the above clinical manifestations of critical asthma are due mainly to a disturbance of ventilation caused by airway inflammation and spasms of the small bronchi. *Huí Yáng Dìng Chuǎn Tāng* (回阳定喘汤) has in it large dosages of *shú fù zǐ* (Radix Aconiti Lateralis Praeparata), *ròu guì* (Cortex Cinnamomi), *gān jiāng* (Rhizoma Zingiberis Officinalis), and *dǎng shēn* (Radix Codonopsis), to warm and tonify the Lung, Spleen and Kidney, on which the use of honey-fried *zhì má huáng* (Herba Ephedrae Praeparata) is based. This can reduce its side effects and decrease its harsh and dry nature. Therefore *zhì má huáng* (Herba Ephedrae Praeparata) will not increase perspiration and increase the heart rate, on the contrary, it can improve the ventilation function through relieving spasms and calming panting, leading to improvement of clinical symptoms, decreasing the heart rate, and alleviating sweating following the improvement of dsypnea.

6. IF ANY OF THE BELOW CONDITIONS ARE ENCOUNTERED, TREAT WITH BIOMEDICINE OR INTEGRATIVE MEDICINE AS SOON AS POSSIBLE

(1) Critical Asthma.

(2) Serious Asthma in the Acute Attack Stage.

(3) Non-acute Stage of Asthma, but the Patient Needs the Inhalation of β_2-Receptor Agonists or Long-acting Bronchodilators Everyday, or Long-term Medication by Glucocorticoids (by Inhalation or Orally).

(4) Asthma in the Mild or Moderate Acute Attack Stage which cannot be Remitted by Various Active Chinese Medical Treatments

(5) Asthma in a Non-acute Attack Stage which cannot be Controlled by Various Active Chinese Medical Treatments.

Summary

In recent years, there has been significant progress in the research into the pathogenesis of asthma. The understanding of asthma has changed from being a simple allergy to being a chronic airway inflammation associated with several kinds of cells and characterized clinically by airway hyper-reactivity. Treatment by simple application of bronchodilators is not enough, and dependence on bronchodilators (for example, β_2-agonists) is harmful. This is because they do not have anti-inflammation functions, and this symptomatic treatment can conceal the development of inflammation, leading to exacerbation of airway hyper-reactivity. Therefore the use of anti-inflammation drugs is required. At present, glucocorticoids are the most effective anti- inflammation drugs for treating asthma. However, the inappropriate and long-term use of high-dosage glucocorticoids also can bring on many problems. These include, dual infection due to concurrent treatment with broad spectrum antibiotics, obesity, increase in blood sugar, increase in blood pressure, water and sodium retention, edema, decrease in blood potassium, gastric and duodenal ulcers, and osteoporosis. Thus the clinical use of glucocorticoids is limited, and the clinician needs to pay attention to these details.

The anti-asthmatic effects of Chinese medicinals are not as rapid and effective as those of biomedical treatments, but the curative results for mild and moderate asthma are pretty good. However, a serious episode or status asthmaticus usually needs the treatment of integrated medicine. How to rapidly and effectively relieve asthma is an important topic facing medical staff. We should go a step further and seek and unearth (sift through) a number of Chinese medicinals and formulas that show promise, and change the form, dose and administrative route of these medicines so that the drugs can more quickly have a marked effect.

Chinese medicinal therapy, compared with biomedicine therapy, has obvious superiority in treating the remission stage of asthma. Chinese medicine can be efficacious if treatment is based on the patient's different clinical manifestations. For example, in young patients treatment emphasizes regulating and tonifying the Spleen and Kidney, which are the origin of the acquired and the congenital (pre- and post-heaven). Therefore this treatment can promote the patient's healthy growth in order to achieve the goal of "removing the root". For middle and older aged patients, treatment emphasizes regulating and tonifying the Lung and Kidney so as to consolidate the defensive power of the body, strengthen the right qi and enhance the resistance against invasion by the six climate evils. Thus it reduces asthmatic episodes. For some patients that are dependent upon long-term glucocorticoids, or patients with side effects like Cushing's disease, the method of invigorating the Kidney (according to the principle of treatment based on pattern differentiation), may be adopted to achieve the treatment goals.

In the past ten years, there have been numerous and varied domestic studies on asthma. In terms of clinical treatments, the reports are mostly on acupuncture and moxibustion, acupoint injection, and acupoint application. These studies report very good results. In particular, acupoint medicinal treatment and acupuncture treatments have roughly the same results, suggesting that the therapeutic effect is stable, and the repeatability is strong. However, in some research the inclusion and exclusion criteria for subjects are not strictly followed, Also, the strict objective indexes for effective evaluation, especially for pulmonary function tests, immunity, and biochemistry are left wanting. In some institutions with good research conditions, the newest achievements in modern medicine should be fully utilized to do the assays of essential inflammatory media, and to determine airway hyper-reactivity (because the airway hyper-reactivity is closely associated with the airway inflammation). Thus the therapeutic effects can be more objectively and accurately evaluated, and the results will be reliable, which can further guide clinical treatment. In experimental studies, the research work on chronic airway inflammation (including the release of inflammation media and repair of airway epithelium) and airway hyper-reactivity should be further enhanced. The screening of single medicinals or compound formulas for treating asthma needs to be developed so as to find Chinese medicinals that are effective for reducing inflammation. In addition, the research and development of aerosol preparations should be carried out further, thus establishing a series of anti-asthmatics and therapies with the characteristics of Chinese medicine.

In summary, we believe that the majority of cases of mild or moderate asthma can be alleviated through treatment with Chinese medicine, but we advocate integrated therapies of Chinese medicine and biomedicine for serious or critical cases of asthma. Particularly in cases of serious dyspnea accompanied by profuse sweating, cyanotic lips, cold limbs, and a disturbance of ventilation leading to serious hypoxia or respiratory failure, (which in Chinese medicine is a sudden collapse of yang qi), oxygen therapy, fluid infusion, anti-spasmodics antibiotics, corticosteroids, or artificial ventilation should be administered promptly. Chinese medicinal therapies of restoring yang to save the patient from collapse, boosting qi, and calming panting should be taken in combination with the biomedical treatments. Taken at the time, the Chinese medicinal remedy *Huí Yáng Dìng Chuǎn Tāng* (回阳定喘汤) can have a good curative effect. The ingredients are *shú fù zǐ* (Radix Aconiti Lateralis Praeparata), *gān jiāng* (Rhizoma Zingiberis), *zhì má huáng* (Herba Ephedrae Praeparata), *xìng rén* (Armeniacae Semen Amarum), and *ròu guì* (Cortex Cinnamomi).

【Prescription】

熟附子	shú fù zǐ	Radix Aconiti Lateralis Praeparata
干姜	gān jiāng	Rhizoma Zingiberis
炙麻黄	zhì má huáng	Herba Ephedrae Praeparata
杏仁	xìng rén	Armeniacae Semen Amarum
肉桂	ròu guì	Cortex Cinnamomi

Our experience shows that for patients with a moderate attack of asthma (manifesting as sudden dyspnea, wheezing, profuse perspiration, gasping with the shoulders raised, a weak and low voice, or intermittent and blurred speech) or a critical attack of asthma, prompt treatment with integrative medicine should be given without delay, lest the opportunity for a cure be missed.

SELECTED QUOTES FROM CLASSICAL TEXTS

Compilation and Supplement to Diagnosis and Treatment - Volume 5 - Wheezing (证治汇补·卷5·哮病, *Zhèng Zhì Huì Bǔ · Juàn 5 · Xiào Bìng*):

"内有壅塞之气，外有非时之感，膈有胶固之痰……，闭拒气道，搏击有声，发为哮病。"

"Internally there is congested and blocked qi, externally there is contraction at the wrong time, the diaphragm has stubborn phlegm …, the airway is blocked, and this contention of qi and phlegm produces sound, hence the *xiào bìng* (asthma)."

Orthodox Medical Record - Asthma (医学正传·哮喘, *Yī Xué Zhèng Zhuàn · Xiào Chuǎn*):

"哮以声响言，喘以气息言。"

"Wheezing is named based on sound, panting is named based on the breath."

Essentials from the Golden Cabinet - Volume 1 - Pulse, Symptoms and

Treatment of Phlegm-fluid Retention and Cough - No 12 (金匮要略·卷上·痰饮咳嗽病脉证并治第十二, *Jīn Guì Yào Luè · Juàn Shàng · Tán Yǐn Ké Sòu Bìng Mài Zhèng Bìng Zhì Dì Shí Èr*):

"膈上病痰,满喘咳吐,发则寒热,背痛腰疼,目泣而出,其人振振身瞤剧,必有伏饮。"

"Phlegm disease on the diaphragm, fullness, panting, coughing, vomiting, then a contraction of cold or heat, the back is sore and the lumbar aches, the eyes tear, the patient's body shakes severely – there must be latent fluids."

Key to Diagnosis and Treatment Secretly Handed Down - Volume 6 - Asthma (秘传证治要诀·卷6·哮喘, *Mì Chuán Zhèng Zhì Yào Jué · Juàn 6 · Xiāo Chuǎn*):

"喘气之病,哮吼如水鸡之声,牵引胸背,气不得息,坐卧不安,此谓嗽而气喘,或宿有此根……遇寒暄则发……"

"The disease has panting, bellowing like the sound of a frog, involving the chest and back, the breathing is ceaseless, and there is restlessness. This is called coughing and panting, or there is an latent root cause…when cold or heat is encountered there will be an attack."

Plain questions - Volume 2 - Additional Discussion on Yin-Yang - No 7 (素问·卷第二·阴阳别论篇第七, *Sù Wèn · Juàn Dì Èr · Yīn Yáng Bié Lùn Piān Dì Qī*):

"阴争于内,阳扰于外,魄汗未藏,四逆而起,起则熏肺,使人喘鸣。"

"The yin contends internally, the yang disturbs externally, the sweats of the *po* (corporeal soul), that is, the sweats of the Lung channel does not store, but counterflow from the four limbs, upwards attacking and steaming the Lung, which causes people to have a panting or stridor sound."

Magical Effects of Seasonal Prescriptions - Asthma (时方妙用·哮证, *Shí Fāng Miào Yòng · Xiào Zhèng*):

"哮喘之病，寒邪伏于肺俞，痰窠结于肺膜，内外相应，一遇风寒暑湿燥火六气之伤即发，伤酒、伤食亦发; 动怒、动气亦发; 劳役、房劳亦发。"

"In the disease of asthma, cold evil is hidden in the BL 13 (*fèi shù*), and phlegm is burrowed and bound in the Lung membrane. Internal and external correspond, and when one encounters the six qi of cold, summer heat, dampness, dryness, or fire there is damage and then an induction [disease flare up]. Damage from drinking and damage from eating can also induce; the loss of temper and the movement of qi can induce; damage from labor and damage from sex can also induce."

Discussion of the Origins of the Symptoms of Disease - Symptoms of Dyspnea, Wheezing and Panting in Manifestations of Qi Disorders (诸病源候论·气病诸候·上气鸣息候, *Zhū Bìng Yuán Hòu Lùn · Qì Bìng Zhū Hòu · Shàng Qì Míng Xī Hòu*):

"肺主于气，邪乘于上肺，则肺痕，痕则肺管不利，不利则气道涩，故气上喘逆，喘息不通。"

"The Lung governs qi, evil overwhelms the Lung, then the Lung is distended. Distention then leads to an inhibition of the Lung tubes, and in turn, to obstruction of the airway, therefore the qi ascends in panting counterflow, and there is panting and obstruction."

Collected Treatises of Jing-yue - Symptoms and Treatment of Excess Panting in Panting and Dyspnea (景岳全书·喘促·实喘证治, *Jǐng Yuè Quán Shū · Chuǎn Cù · Shí Chuǎn Zhèng Zhì*):

"喘有夙根，遇寒即发者，亦名哮喘。未发时以扶正为主，既发时以攻邪为主，扶正者，须辨阴阳，阴虚者补其阴，阳虚者补其阳。攻邪气者，须分微甚，或散其风，或温其寒，或清其痰火。然发久者，气无不虚，故于消散中宜酌加温补，或于温补中宜量加消散，此等证候，当眷眷以元气为念。必致元气渐充，庶可望其渐愈，若攻之太过，未有不致日甚而危者。"

"Panting has a long standing root, its episode occurs when there is an encounter with cold, this is also called *xiào chuǎn* (asthma). Supporting the right qi should be the main treatment between episodes, while eliminating the evils should the main treatment during an episode. As for supporting the right qi, yin and yang must be differentiated. For yin deficiency, tonify yin. For yang deficiency, tonify yang. As for attacking the evil qi, divide the slight from the severe; or scatter the wind, or warm the cold, or clear the phlegm-fire accordingly. However in cases of long standing episodes, there must be qi deficiency, so warming and tonifying medicinals should be added into an eliminating and purging remedy; or eliminating and purging medicinals should be appropriately added into a warming and tonifying remedy. With these patterns, constantly bear in mind the original qi. Must gradually make the original qi full, and the illness can be cured. If the purging remedy is over used, the illness will deteriorate and even endanger life."

Teachings of Dan-xi - Volume 2 - Asthma (丹溪心法·卷二·哮喘, *Dān Xī Xīn Fǎ · Juàn Èr · Xiào Chuǎn*):

"哮喘必用薄滋味，专主于痰。"

"[In the treatment] of asthma, must use mild flavors, because asthma is particularly caused by phlegm."

Essentials from the Golden Cabinet - Volume 1 - The Pulse, Symptoms and Treatment of Lung Wilting, Lung Abscess, Cough and Dyspnea - No 7 (金匮要略·卷上·肺痿肺痈咳嗽上气脉症并治第七, *Jīn guì Yào Luè · Fèi Wěi Fèi Yōng Ké Sòu Shàng Qì Mài Zhèng Bìng Zhì Dì Qī*):

"咳而上气，喉中水鸡声，射干麻黄汤主之。"

"For cough with rising qi, and stridor in the throat like the sound of frog, *Shè Gān Má Huáng Tāng* (射干麻黄汤) governs."

MODERN RESEARCH

Clinical Research

1. Pattern Differentiation and Corresponding Treatment

(1) Cold and Heat Pattern Differentiation, with Emphasis on Phlegm and Stasis

Wang Zhi-ying and his coworkers[1] think that the basic pathomechanism of asthma is the blockage of phlegm-qi, and failure of the Lung to descend and diffuse. Phlegm, qi, and stasis are the main pathological results. Wang Zhi-ying and his coworkers propose transforming phlegm, dispelling stasis, descending qi, and calming panting as the fundamental methods to treat asthma. For cold asthma, they used *Hán Xiào Píng Kǒu Fú Yè* (寒哮平口服液). This is composed of *zhì má huáng* (Herba Ephedrae Praeparata), *tíng lì zǐ* (Semen Lepidii seu Descurainiae), *xìng rén* (Armeniacae Semen Amarum), *sū zǐ* (Fructus Perillae), *fǎ bàn xià* (Rhizoma Pinelliae Praeparatum), *gān jiāng* (Rhizoma Zingiberis), *xì xīn* (Radix et Rhizoma Asari), *táo rén* (Semen Persicae), *bái jiāng cán* (Bombyx Batryticatus), and *yáng jīn huā* (Flos Daturae), 10ml in each, containing crude medicinals 24.1g. Taken orally, three times a day.

炙麻黄	zhì má huáng	Herba Ephedrae Praeparata
葶苈子	tíng lì zǐ	Semen Lepidii seu Descurainiae
杏仁	xìng rén	Armeniacae Semen Amarum
苏子	sū zǐ	Fructus Perillae
法半夏	fǎ bàn xià	Rhizoma Pinelliae Praeparatum
干姜	gān jiāng	Rhizoma Zingiberis
细辛	xì xīn	Radix et Rhizoma Asari
桃仁	táo rén	Semen Persicae
白僵蚕	bái jiāng cán	Bombyx Batryticatus
洋金花	yáng jīn huā	Flos Daturae

For heat asthma, they used *Rè Xiào Píng Kǒu Fú Yè* (热哮平口服液). It consists of *zhì má huáng* (Herba Ephedrae Praeparata), *huáng qín* (Radix Scutellariae), *sāng bái pí* (Cortex Mori), *shè gān* (Rhizoma Belamcandae), *qián hú* (Radix Peucedani), *zhú lì* (Succus Bambusae), *bàn xià* (Rhizoma Pinelliae), *táo rén* (Semen Persicae), *píng dì mù* (Herba Ardisiae Japonicae), *dì lóng* (Lumbricus), 10ml in each, containing crude medicinals 28.7g, taken orally, three times a day.

炙麻黄	zhì má huáng	Herba Ephedrae Praeparata
黄芩	huáng qín	Radix Scutellariae
桑白皮	sāng bái pí	Cortex Mori
射干	shè gān	Rhizoma Belamcandae
前胡	qián hú	Radix Peucedani
竹沥	zhú lì	Succus Bambusae
半夏	bàn xià	Rhizoma Pinelliae
桃仁	táo rén	Semen Persicae
平地木	píng dì mù	Herba Ardisiae Japonicae
地龙	dì long	Lumbricus

For the control group they used *Guì Lóng Ké Chuān Níng Jiāo Náng* (桂龙咳喘宁胶囊), 0.3 g in each capsule, 5 capsules taken orally, three times a day. In each group 10 days made up a course of treatment. Results: the treatment group clinical control had a significant effective rate of 72.38% and a total effective rate of 89.52%. For the control group the rates are 40.39% and 73.08% respectively.

(2) Treatment Based on Pattern Differentiation of Different Stages of Asthma

Li Chuan and his coworkers[2] classified acute attack stage asthma into cold asthma and heat asthma. For cold asthma, the treatment principles were to diffuse the Lung and scatter cold, and the formula was *Shè Gān Má Huáng Tāng* (射干麻黄汤) with modifications. For cases of exterior cold and interior fluid retention with more serious cold sings,

Xiǎo Qīng Lóng Tāng (小青龙汤), with modifications, was selected. For heat asthma, the treatment principles were to clear heat and diffuse the Lung, transform phlegm and calm panting. The formula was *Dìng Chuǎn Tāng* (定喘汤) with modifications. The course of treatment was 3 weeks for all patients. Pattern differentiation in the remission stage was divided into qi deficiency of both the Lung and Spleen, or deficiency of both the Lung and Kidney. For qi deficiency of both the Lung and Spleen, treatment principles were to fortify the Spleen, transform phlegm, and tonify Earth to engender Metal. They used a prescription of *huáng qí* (Radix Astragali), *fáng fēng* (Radix Saposhnikoviae), *bái zhú* (Rhizoma Atractylodis Macrocephalae), *guì zhī* (Ramulus Cinnamomi), *bái sháo* (Radix Paeoniae Alba), *shēng jiāng* (Rhizoma Zingiberis Recens), *dǎng shēn* (Radix Codonopsitis), *fú líng* (Poria), *xìng rén* (Armeniacae Semen Amarum), *chén pí* (Pericarpium Citri Reticulatae), *bàn xià* (Rhizoma Pinelliae), and *zhì gān cǎo* (Radix et Rhizoma Glycyrrhizae Praeparata).

黄芪	huáng qí	Radix Astragali
防风	fáng fēng	Radix Saposhnikoviae
白术	bái zhú	Rhizoma Atractylodis Macrocephalae
桂枝	guì zhī	Ramulus Cinnamomi
白芍	bái sháo	Radix Paeoniae Alba
生姜	shēng jiāng	Rhizoma Zingiberis Recens
党参	dǎng shēn	Radix Codonopsitis
茯苓	fú líng	Poria
杏仁	xìng rén	Armeniacae Semen Amarum
陈皮	chén pí	Pericarpium Citri Reticulatae
半夏	bàn xià	Rhizoma Pinelliae
炙甘草	zhì gān cǎo	Radix et Rhizoma Glycyrrhizae Praeparata

For deficiency of both the Lung and Kidney, the treatment principles were to tonify the Lung and Kidney to receive qi. They used a formula of *dǎng shēn* (Radix Codonopsis), *bái zhú* (Rhizoma Atractylodis

Macrocephalae), *fú líng* (Poria), *shēng shú dì huáng* (Radix Rehmanniae Glutinosae and Radix Rehmanniae Praeparata), *shān yào* (Rhizoma Dioscoreae), *shān zhū yú* (Fructus Corni Officinalis), *zé xiè* (Rhizoma Alismatis), *dān pí* (Cortex Moutan), *zhì gān cǎo* (Radix et Rhizoma Glycyrrhizae Praeparata).

党参	dǎng shēn	Radix Codonopsitis
白术	bái zhú	Rhizoma Atractylodis Macrocephalae
茯苓	fú líng	Poria
生地黄	shēng dì huáng	Radix Rehmanniae Glutinosae
熟地黄	shú dì huáng	Radix Rehmanniae Praeparata
山药	shān yào	Rhizoma Dioscoreae
山茱萸	shān zhū yú	Fructus Corni Officinalis
泽泻	zé xiè	Rhizoma Alismatis
丹皮	dān pí	Cortex Moutan
炙甘草	zhì gān cǎo	Radix et Rhizoma Glycyrrhizae Praeparata

The course of treatment was 5 weeks for all patients. In total, 48 patients were treated. After the treatment, clinically controlled cases are 26, accounting for 54.2%; improved cases 18, accounting for 37.5%: and non-effective cases 4, accounting for 8.3%. The total effective rate was 91.7%.

(3) Additional Pattern Differentiation

In recent years, there has been an appearance of many new viewpoints of clinical pattern differentiation. In the medical field there has also been a deepening of understanding of the etiology and pathology of bronchial asthma. Zeng De-you[3] divided asthma into different types. These were: cold evil lying deep in the Lung, obstruction of the Lung by heat-phlegm, qi depression and phlegm obstruction, phlegm stasis and qi obstruction, and deficiency of both the Lung and Kidney. For the type of cold evil lying deep in the Lung, *Xiǎo Qīng Lóng Tāng* (小青龙汤) was the formula used, plus *shè gān* (Rhizoma Belamcandae), *bǎn lán gēn* (Radix Isatidis), *dì lóng* (Lumbricus), and *chán tuì* (Periostracum Cicadae). For the type of obstruction of the Lung by heat-phlegm, the formula used was *Dìng Chuǎn Tāng* (定喘汤) plus *dì lóng* (Lumbricus) and *chán tuì* (Periostracum Cicadae). For the type of qi depression and phlegm obstruction, the formula used was *Sì Nì Sǎn* (四逆散) plus *Xiǎo Qīng Lóng Tāng* with additions of *dì lóng* (Lumbricus) and *bái jiāng cán* (Bombyx Batryticatus). For the type of the phlegm stasis and qi obstruction, the formula used was *Dí Tán Tāng* (涤痰汤) plus *Táo Hóng Sì Wù Tāng* (桃红四物汤) with additions of *dān shēn* (Radix et Rhizoma Salviae Miltiorrhizae), and *dì lóng* (Lumbricus). For the type of deficiency of both the Lung and Kidney, the formula used was *Jīn Shuǐ Liù Jūn Jiān* (金水六君煎) plus *Sān Niù Tāng* (三拗汤) with additions of *dì lóng* (Lumbricus) and *dōng chóng xià cǎo* (Cordyceps). For the control group 3,200,000 units of penicillin were given intravenously, twice a day. Aminophylline 0.1 g was taken orally, 3 times a day, and chlorpheniramine 4mg was taken orally, 3 times a day. For both of the groups, one week made up a course of treatment. The results: In the trial group there were 78 cases, 34 of which were cured, 33 of which improved, and 11 of which had no response. The total effective rate was 85.9%. In the control group of 42 cases, 9 cases were cured, 16 cases improved, and 17 cases did respond to treatment. The total effective rate was 59.52%. The result for trial group was obviously better than that for the control group (P<0.05).

2. Specific Formulas

(1) *Huó Xuè Huà Yū Tāng* (活血化瘀汤)

Jiang Shu-guang[4] believes that the pathological key of asthma is the cementation of the blood stasis. Tang Rong-chuan first initiated the simultaneous treatment of phlegm and stasis, believing that "phlegm-water will disappear following removal of the stasis". He composed the following formula *Huó Xuè Huà Yū Tāng* (活血化瘀汤). The ingredients are *dāng guī* (Radix Angelicae Sinensis) 16g, *dān shēn* (Radix et Rhizoma Salviae Miltiorrhizae) 15g, *táo rén* (Semen Persicae) 10g, *hóng huā* (Flos Carthami) 5g, *chì sháo* (Radix Paeoniae Rubra) 10g, *gān dì lóng* (Lumbricus) 10g, *dì biē chóng* (Eupolyphaga seu steleophaga) 10g, and *huáng qí* (Radix Astragali) 20g.

当归	dāng guī	16g	Radix Angelicae Sinensis
丹参	dān shēn	15g	Radix et Rhizoma Salviae Miltiorrhizae
桃仁	táo rén	10g	Semen Persicae
红花	hóng huā	5g	Flos Carthami
赤芍药	chì sháo yào	10g	Radix Paeoniae Rubra
干地龙	gān dì lóng	10g	Lumbricus
地鳖虫	dì biē chóng	10g	Eupolyphaga seu steleophaga
黄芪	huáng qí	20g	Radix Astragali

For cold asthma, he adds *má huáng* (Herba Ephedrae) 10g and *dàn gān jiāng* (Rhizoma Zingiberis) 10g. For heat asthma, he adds *shēng shí gāo* (Gypsum Fibrosum) 30g, and *sāng bái pí* (Cortex Mori) 12g. The total effective rate was 96.8%.

(2) *Sì Chóng Qū Fēng Gù Běn Tāng* (四虫祛风固本汤)

Wu Xing-he[5] treated 64 cases of asthma with his self-composed *Sì Chóng Qū Fēng Gù Běn Tāng* (四虫祛风固本汤). The basic formula was *quán xiē* (Scorpio), *dì lóng* (Lumbricus), *bái jiāng cán* (Bombyx Batryticatus), *chán tuì* (Periostracum Cicadae) 12g each, *dì fū zǐ* (Fructus Kochiae), *shé chuáng zǐ* (Fructus Cnidii), *zhì sū zǐ* (Fructus Perillae Praeparata), *kǔ shēn* (Radix Sophorae Flavescentis), *xuán fù huā* (Flos Inulae) (wrapped with gauze) 12g each, *yú xīng cǎo* (Herba Houttuyniae), *sān yè qīng* (Tetrastlgma hemsleyanum) 30g each, *zhì kuǎn dōng huā* (Flos Farfarae Praeparata), *chǎo dǎng shēn* (Radix Codonopsis Tostum) 15g each; *chǎo bái zhú* (Rhizoma Atractylodis Macrocephalae Tostum) 15g, and *zhì gān cǎo* (Radix et Rhizoma Glycyrrhizae Praeparata) 6g.

全蝎	quán xiē	12g	Scorpio
地龙	dì lóng	12g	Lumbricus
白僵蚕	bái jiāng cán	12g	Bombyx Batryticatus
蝉蜕	chán tuì	12g	Periostracum Cicadae
地肤子	dì fū zǐ	12g	Fructus Kochiae
蛇床子	shé chuáng zǐ	12g	Fructus Cnidii
炙苏子	zhì sū zǐ	12g	Fructus Perillae Praeparata
苦参	kǔ shēn	12 g	Radix Sophorae Flavescentis
旋复花	xuán fù huā	12 g	Flos Inulae (wrapped with gauze)
鱼腥草	yú xīng cǎo	30 g	Herba Houttuyniae
三叶青	sān yè qīng	30 g	Tetrastlgma hemsleyanum
炙款冬花	zhì kuǎn dōng huā	15g	Flos Farfarae Praeparata
炒党参	chǎo dǎng shēn	15g	Radix Codonopsitis Tostum
炒白术	chǎo bái zhú	15g	Rhizoma Atractylodis Macrocephalae Tostum
炙甘草	zhì gān cǎo	6g	Radix et Rhizoma Glycyrrhizae Praeparata

For the control group of 60 patients, the first 4 medicinals in the basic formula were removed, and the quantities of the remaining medicinals were the same as those in the basic formula. According to Chinese medical pattern differentiation, if the patients in either of the two groups had an exterior pattern of wind-cold, 12g each of *sū yè* (Folium Perillae), *jīng jiè* (Herba Schizonepetae), and *fáng fēng* (Radix Saposhnikoviae) were added. If the pattern belonged to wind-heat, 12g each of *jīn yín huā* (Flos Lonicerae Japonicae), *lián qiào* (Fructus Forsythiae), and *huáng qín* (Radix Scutellariae) were added. If the pattern was yin deficiency of the Lung and Kidney, 30g each of *yù zhú* (Rhioma Polygonati Odorati), and *huáng jīng* (Rhizoma Polygonati) were added. One dose was given every day, and one week made up a course of treatment. After 3 courses of treatment, the results are statistically analyzed. The results were: 33 cases of complete remission for the trial group, and 16 cases for the control group. 23 cases in the trial group and 24 cases in the control group showed a remarkable effect. 3 cases in the trial group and 11 cases in the control group improved. 5 cases in the trial group and 9 cases in the control group did not respond to treatment. The results in the trial group were obviously better than that in the control group.

(3) *Píng Chuǎn Tāng* (平喘汤)

Liu liu[6] treated 100 cases of bronchial asthma with his self-composed *Píng Chuǎn Tāng* (平喘汤). The ingredients were *dì lóng* (Lumbricus), *bái jiāng cán* (Bombyx Batryticatus), *quán xiē* (Scorpio), *chán tuì* (Periostracum Cicadae), and *fú líng* (Poria) 10g each, *xú cháng qīng* (Radix et Rhizoma Cynanchi Paniculati) 30g, *sū zǐ* (Fructus Perillae), *bái jiè zǐ* (Semen Sinapis Albae), *lái fú zǐ* (Semen Raphani), and *xuán fù huā* (Flos Inulae) 12g each, and *yě qiáo mài gēn* (Radix et Rhizoma Fagopyri Cyrosi) 15g.

地龙	dì lóng	10g	Lumbricus
白僵蚕	bái jiāng cán	10g	Bombyx Batryticatus
全蝎	quán xiē	10g	Scorpio
蝉蜕	chán tuì	10g	Periostracum Cicadae
茯苓	fú líng	10g	Poria
徐长卿	xú cháng qīng	30g	Radix et Rhizoma Cynanchi Paniculati
苏子	sū zǐ	12g	Fructus Perillae
白芥子	bái jiè zǐ	12 g	Semen Sinapis Albae
莱菔子	lái fú zǐ	12 g	Semen Raphani
旋复花	xuán fù huā	12 g	Flos Inulae
野荞麦根	yě qiáo mài gēn	15 g	Radix et Rhizoma Fagopyri Cyrosi

For a pattern of exterior cold, he added *jīng jiè* (Herba Schizonepetae), *fáng fēng* (Radix Saposhnikoviae), and *xì xīn* (Radix et Rhizoma Asari). For an exterior pattern due to wind-heat, he added *jīn yín huā* (Flos Lonicerae Japonicae), *jú huā* (Flos Chrysanthemi), and *sāng yè* (Folium Mori). For cases of yin deficiency, he added *yù zhú* (Rhioma Polygonati Odorati), *mài mén dōng* (Radix Ophiopogonis), and *huáng jīng* (Rhizoma Polygonati). The formula was given one dose per day, divided into 3 portions, and taken orally when the decoction was warm. One course of treatment consisted of 10 days. The curative result was good .

(4) Modified *Xìng Rén Tāng* (加味杏仁汤)

Wang Yu-yu[7] treated 56 cases of bronchial asthma with his self composed modified *Xìng Rén Tāng* (杏仁汤). The ingredients were *xìng rén* (Armeniacae Semen Amarum) 15g, *sū zǐ* (Fructus Perillae) 15g, *chuān bèi mǔ* (Bulbus Fritillariae Cirrhosae) 15g, *huáng qín* (Radix Scutellariae) 15g, *zhì kuǎn dōng huā* (Flos Farfarae Praeparata) 15 g, *hòu pò* (Cortex Magnoliae Officinalis) 15, *zhǐ qiào* (Fructus Aurantii) 15g, *huáng qí* (Radix Astragali) 15g, *bái zhú* (Rhizoma Atractylodis Macrocephalae) 15g, *fáng fēng* (Radix Saposhnikoviae) 15g, *suān zǎo rén* (Semen Ziziphi Spinosae) 20g, and *gān cǎo* (Radix et Rhizoma Glycyrrhizae) 10g.

杏仁	xìng rén	15g	Armeniacae Semen Amarum
苏子	sū zǐ	15g	Fructus Perillae
川贝母	chuān bèi mǔ	15g	Bulbus Fritillariae Cirrhosae
黄芩	huáng qín	15g	Radix Scutellariae
炙款冬花	zhì kuǎn dōng huā	15g	Flos Farfarae Praeparata
厚朴	hòu pò	15g	Cortex Magnoliae Officinalis
枳壳	zhǐ qiào	15g	Fructus Aurantii
黄芪	huáng qí	15 g	Radix Astragali
白术	bái zhú	15 g	Rhizoma Atractylodis Macrocephalae
防风	fáng fēng	15 g	Radix Saposhnikoviae
酸枣仁	suān zǎo rén	20g	Semen Ziziphi Spinosae
甘草	gān cǎo	10g	Radix et Rhizoma Glycyrrhizae

For cases with remarkable signs of cold, he added *má huáng* (Herba Ephedrae) and *guì zhī* (Ramulus Cinnamomi). For cases with remarkable signs of heat, he added *shí gāo* (Gypsum Fibrosum), and *sāng bái pí* (Cortex Mori). For cases with remarkable signs of phlegm-dampness, he added *fǎ bàn xià* (Rhizoma Pinelliae Praeparatum), *tíng lì zǐ* (Semen Lepidii seu Descurainiae), and *fú líng* (Poria). For cases with remarkable signs of blood stasis, he added *dāng guī* (Radix Angelicae Sinensis), and *dān shēn* (Radix et Rhizoma Salviae Miltiorrhizae). For cases with remarkable signs of internal heat, he added *dà huáng* (Radix et Rhizoma Rhei), and *máng xiāo* (Natrii Sulfas). One dose was given per day, divided into 3 portions, and taken orally when the decoction was warm. *Liù Wèi Dì Huáng Wán* (六味地黄丸) was also given in combination; one pill, 3 times a day. A course of treatment was 2 weeks. The results: 37 cases were controlled, 8 cases showed a remarkable effect, 10 cases were improved, and 1 case did not respond. The controlled rate was 66%, and the effective rate was 98%.

(5) *Ké Chuǎn Líng* (咳喘灵)

Xuan Jiang-da[8] treated 150 cases of asthma with *Ké Chuǎn Líng* (咳喘灵). The ingredients were *zhì má huáng* (Herba Ephedrae Praeparata) 6g, *cè bǎi yè* (Cacumen Platycladi) 10g, *sāng bái pí* (Cortex Mori) 10g, *zǐ wǎn* (Radix et Rhizoma Asteris) 12g, *zhì bǎi bù* (Radix Stemonae Praeparata) 15g, *shè gān* (Rhizoma Belamcandae) 10g, *kuǎn dōng huā* (Flos Farfarae) 10g, *yě qiáo mài gēn* (Radix et Rhizoma Fagopyri Cyrosi) 30g, and *bái jiāng cán* (Bombyx Batryticatus) 10g.

炙麻黄	zhì má huáng	6g	Herba Ephedrae Praeparata
侧柏叶	cè bǎi yè	10g	Cacumen Platycladi
桑白皮	sāng bái pí	10g	Cortex Mori
紫菀	zǐ wǎn	12g	Radix et Rhizoma Asteris
炙百部	zhì bǎi bù	15g	Radix Stemonae Praeparata
射干	shè gān	10g	Rhizoma Belamcandae
款冬花	kuǎn dōng huā	10g	Flos Farfarae
野荞麦根	yě qiáo mài gēn	30 g	Radix et Rhizoma Fagopyri Cyrosi
白僵蚕	bái jiāng cán	30g	Bombyx Batryticatus

For cases with profuse sputum, he added *jiāng bàn xià* (Rhizoma Pinelliae Preparata), *zhè bèi mǔ* (Bulbus Fritillariae) 12g each. For cases with excess heat, he added *huáng qín* (Radix Scutellariae) and *yú xīng cǎo* (Herba Houttuyniae) 30g each. For cases of yin deficiency, he added *běi shā shēn* (Radix Glehniae), and *mài mén dōng* (Radix Ophiopogonis) 12g each. The medicinals were decocted in water, divided into 2 portions for one pack a day. It was taken orally for 6 successive doses, which made up a course of treatment. The results: 118 cases were clinically controlled, 12 cases showed a remarkable effect, 7 cases improved, and 3 cases did not respond. The total effective rate was 96.3%.

(6) *Wēn Dǎn Tāng* (温胆汤)

Li Hui[9] treated 56 cases of asthma with *Wēn Dǎn Tāng* (温胆汤). The ingredients were *zhì bàn xià* (Rhizoma Pinelliae Preparata) 9g, *zhú rú* (Caulis Bambusae in Taeniis) 15 g, *zhǐ shí* (Fructus Aurantii Immaturus) 12g, *chén pí* (Pericarpium Citri Reticulatae) 6g, *fú líng* (Poria) 18g, *gān cǎo* (Radix et Rhizoma Glycyrrhizae) 5g, *zhì má huáng* (Herba Ephedrae Praeparata) 10g, *sū zǐ* (Fructus Perillae) 12g, and *dì lóng* (Lumbricus) 10g.

制半夏	zhì bàn xià	9g	Rhizoma Pinelliae Preparata
竹茹	zhú rú	15g	Caulis Bambusae in Taeniis
枳实	zhǐ shí	12g	Fructus Aurantii Immaturus
陈皮	chén pí	6g	Pericarpium Citri Reticulatae
茯苓	fú líng	18g	Poria
甘草	gān cǎo	5g	Radix et Rhizoma Glycyrrhizae
炙麻黄	zhì má huáng	10g	Herba Ephedrae Praeparata
苏子	sū zǐ	12g	Fructus Perillae
地龙	dì lóng	10g	Lumbricus

For cases with predominant signs of heat, he added *sāng bái pí* (Cortex Mori) 15g, and *huáng qín* (Radix Scutellariae) 10g. For cases with predominant signs of cold, he added *xì xīn* (Radix et Rhizoma Asari) 3g, and *gān jiāng* (Rhizoma Zingiberis) 8g. One dose was given each day, divided into 2 portions, and taken orally for 2 successive weeks. The results: 17 cases were clinically controlled, 24 cases showed remarkable effects, 10 cases improved, and 5 cases showed no response. The total effective rate was 91.1%.

(7) *Lái Fú Zǐ Sǎn* (莱菔子散)

Zheng Guo-hua[10] used his self-composed *Lái Fú Zǐ Sǎn* (莱菔子散). The ingredients were *lái fú zǐ* (SemenRaphani Sativi) 500g (well steamed and dried), and *zhū yá zào jiǎo* (Spina Gleditsiae Abnormalis) 15g (with the peel and back spine removed).

| 莱菔子 | lái fú zǐ | 500g | SemenRaphani Sativi (well steamed and dried) |
| 猪牙皂角 | zhū yá zào jiǎo | 15g | Spina Gleditsiae Abnormalis (with the peel and back spine removed) |

The two medicinals were ground together into a fine powder, and put into an air-tight bottle. 3g was taken orally, with a good curative effect.

(8) *Ké Chuǎn Gù Běn Tāng* (咳喘固本汤)

Zhang Zheng-yuan [11] treated 112 cases of asthma with his self-composed *Ké Chuǎn Gù Běn Tāng* (咳喘固本汤). The ingredients were *dǎng shēn* (Radix Codonopsitis), *huáng qí* (Radix Astragali), *fáng fēng* (Radix Saposhnikoviae), *shú dì huáng* (Radix Rehmanniae Praeparata), *shān zhū yú* (Fructus Corni Officinalis), *bǔ gǔ zhī* (Fructus Psoraleae), *táo rén* (Semen Persicae), *fù zǐ* (Radix Aconiti Lateralis Praeparata), *má huáng* (Herba Ephedrae), *guì zhī* (Ramulus Cinnamomi), *sū zǐ* (Fructus Perillae), *fǎ bàn xià* (Rhizoma Pinelliae Praeparatum), *mài mén dōng* (Radix Ophiopogonis), *tiān mén dōng* (Radix Asparagi), *fú líng* (Poria), *bīng láng* (Semen Arecae), *tíng lì zǐ* (Semen Lepidii seu Descurainiae), and *dān shēn* (Radix et Rhizoma Salviae Miltiorrhizae).

党参	dǎng shēn	Radix Codonopsis
黄芪	huáng qí	Radix Astragali
防风	fáng fēng	Radix Saposhnikoviae
熟地黄	shú dì huáng	Radix Rehmanniae Praeparata
山茱萸	shān zhū yú	Fructus Corni Officinalis
补骨脂	bǔ gǔ zhī	Fructus Psoraleae
桃仁	táo rén	Semen Persicae

附子	fù zǐ	Radix Aconiti Lateralis Praeparata
麻黄	má huáng	Herba Ephedrae
桂枝	guì zhī	Ramulus Cinnamomi
苏子	sū zǐ	Fructus Perillae
法半夏	fǎ bàn xià	Rhizoma Pinelliae Praeparatum
麦门冬	mài mén dōng	Radix Ophiopogonis
天门冬	tiān mén dōng	Radix Asparagi
茯苓	fú líng	Poria
槟榔	bīng láng	Semen Arecae
葶苈子	tíng lì zǐ	Semen Lepidii seu Descurainiae
丹参	dān shēn	Radix et Rhizoma Salviae Miltiorrhizae

The medicinals were ground and prepared with honey into soybean-sized pills. 10g was taken orally, three times per day. The 75 cases in the control group were given 1mg of Ketotifen, orally, 2 times per day. The observation period was 15 months. The results were: in the trial group, 60 cases were cured, 39 cases showed a remarkable effect, and 12 cases showed no effect. The total effective rate was 88.4%. In the control group, 31 cases were cured, 24 cases showed a remarkable effect, and 29 cases showed no effect. The total effective rate was 65.5%.

(9) Guì Zhī Jiā Hòu Pò Xìng Zǐ Tāng (桂枝加厚朴杏子汤)

Yu Xia and his coworkers [12] treated 68 cases of cough-variant asthma. Among them 37 cases were treated with Guì Zhī Jiā Hòu Pò Xìng Zǐ Tāng (桂枝加厚朴杏子汤). The ingredients were guì zhī (Ramulus Cinnamomi) 9g, sháo yào (Radix Paeoniae) 6g, hòu pò (Cortex Magnoliae) 6g, xìng rén (Armeniacae Semen Amarum) 9g, zhì gān cǎo (Radix et Rhizoma Glycyrrhizae Praeparata) 6g, shēng jiāng (Rhizoma Zingiberis) 9g, and dà zǎo (Fructus Jujubae) 12 pieces.

桂枝	guì zhī	9g	Ramulus Cinnamomi
芍药	sháo yào	6g	Radix Paeoniae

厚朴	hòu pò	6g	Cortex Magnoliae
杏仁	xìng rén	9g	Armeniacae Semen Amarum
炙甘草	zhì gān cǎo	6g	Radix et Rhizoma Glycyrrhizae Praeparata
生姜	shēng jiāng	9g	Rhizoma Zingiberis
大枣	dà zǎo	12 pieces	Fructus Jujubae

The medicinals were decocted in water, and one dose was taken orally each day for 2 months. The remaining 31 cases in the control group were treated with Loperamide. The course of treatment was two months. The results: in the trial group the rate of remarkable effect was 89.1%, but in the control group it was only 51.6%. The effect of the trial group was obviously better than that of control group ($P<0.05$).

(10) *Gù Běn Shí Wèi Sǎn* (固本十味散)

Sun Shi-tian and his coworkers[13] used the self-composed *Gù Běn Shí Wèi Sǎn* (固本十味散) to treat bronchial asthma during the remission stage. The ingredients were *huáng qí* (Radix Astragali) 300g, *dǎng shēn* (Radix Codonopsitis) 300g, *rén shēn* (Radix Ginseng) 100g, *bái zhú* (Rhizoma Atractylodis Macrocephalae) 100g, *fáng fēng* (Radix Saposhnikoviae) 80g, *gé jiè* (Gecko) 5 pairs, *dì lóng* (Lumbricus) 80g, *bái guǒ* (Semen Ginkgo Bilobae) 100g, *sū zǐ* (Fructus Perillae) 100g, and *zǐ hé chē* (Placenta Hominis) 1 piece.

黄芪	huáng qí	300g	Radix Astragali
党参	dǎng shēn	300g	Radix Codonopsis
人参	rén shēn	100g	Radix Ginseng
白术	bái zhú	100g	Rhizoma Atractylodis Macrocephalae
防风	fáng fēng	80g	Radix Saposhnikoviae
蛤蚧	gé jiè	5 pairs	Gecko
地龙	dì lóng	80g	Lumbricus
白果	bái guǒ	100g	Semen Ginkgo Bilobae
苏子	sū zǐ	100g	Fructus Perillae
紫河车	zǐ hé chē	1 piece	Placenta Hominis

This dosage was per person. The medicinals were ground together into a fine powder. Each dose was 6g, taken twice a day, in the early morning and evening. Modifications: he added *cāng ěr zǐ* (Fructus Xanthii), *bái zhǐ* (Radix Angelicae), *xīn yí* (Flos Magnoliae) for cases of allergic rhinitis. He added *shēng dì huáng* (Radix Rehmanniae Glutinosae), *mài mén dōng* (Radix Ophiopogonis), and *huáng qín* (Radix Scutellariae) for cases of yin deficiency of the Lung and Kidney with obvious Lung-heat. He added *bā jǐ tiān* (Radix Morindae Officinalis), *bái jiè zǐ* (Semen Sinapis Albae), *hú táo ròu* (Semen Juglandis Regiae), *fǎ bàn xià* (Rhizoma Pinelliae Praeparatum) for cases of yang deficiency of the Kidney with obvious Lung-cold. In total, 176 cases were treated, and among them 45 cases were completely cured, 77 cases showed remarkable effect, 36 cases showed some effect, and 18 cases were non-responsive. The total effective rate was 89.77%.

(11) *Píng Gān Xiào Chuǎn Tāng* (平肝哮喘汤)

Su Cai-feng and his co-workers[14] used *Píng Gān Xiào Chuǎn Tāng* (平肝哮喘汤) to treat 60 cases of bronchial asthma. The ingredients are *má huáng* (Herba Ephedrae), *jiāng cán* (Bombyx Batryticatus), *chán tuì* (Periostracum Cicadae), *quán xiē* (Scorpio), *bàn xià* (Rhizoma Pinelliae), *sū zǐ* (Fructus Perillae), and *chén xiāng* (Lignum Aquilariae Resinatum).

麻黄	má huáng	Herba Ephedrae
僵蚕	jiāng cán	Bombyx Batryticatus
蝉蜕	chán tuì	Periostracum Cicadae
全蝎	quán xiē	Scorpio
半夏	bàn xià	Rhizoma Pinelliae
苏子	sū zǐ	Fructus Perillae
沉香	chén xiāng	Lignum Aquilariae Resinatum

The total effective rate was 91.7%. This result suggests that the method has the effect of calming the Liver, rectifying qi, transforming phlegm and calming panting.

3. Additional Treatment Modalities

(1) Anti-asthma Gauze Mask

Wang Xiu-qin [15] and his co-workers made up an anti-asthma gauze mask. The medicinal composition was *zhì má huáng* (Herba Ephedrae Praeparata), *zǐ wǎn* (Radix et Rhizoma Asteris), *kuǎn dōng huā* (Flos Farfarae), *mǎ dōu líng* (Fructus Aristolochiae), *yáng jīn huā* (Flos Daturae), *chǎo dì lóng* (Lumbricus Tostum), and dexamethasone.

炙麻黄	zhì má huáng	Herba Ephedrae Praeparata
紫菀	zǐ wǎn	Radix et Rhizoma Asteris
款冬花	kuǎn dōng huā	Flos Farfarae
马兜铃	mǎ dōu líng	Fructus Aristolochiae
洋金花	yáng jīn huā	Flos Daturae
炒地龙	chǎo dì lóng	Lumbricus Tostum

There was an appropriate dose for each medicinal. For serious patients during the attack stage, in addition to treatments with conventional hormones and anti-inflammatories, wearing the mask continuously was required. For patients in the control group, *Gé Jiè Dìng Chuǎn Wán* (蛤蚧定喘丸) was given orally, and for serious patients conventional hormonal anti-inflammatory therapies were added as an auxiliary treatment. The results: The clinical effective rates were 87.5% and 60% respectively. The effect of the trial group was obviously better that that of the control group ($P<0.01$).

(2) *Tíng Lì Píng Chuǎn Shuān* (葶苈平喘栓)

Li Zhen-qian[16] made his own *Tíng Lì Píng Chuǎn Shuān* (葶苈平喘栓). The ingredients were *tíng lì zǐ* (Semen Lepidii seu Descurainiae) 24g, *zào jiá* (Fructus Gleditsiae Sinensis) 10g, *má huáng* (Herba Ephedrae) 12g, *xìng rén* (Armeniacae Semen Amarum) 6g, *dà huáng* (Radix et Rhizoma Rhei) 12g, *máng xiāo* (Natrii Sulfas) 3g, and *dà zǎo* (Fructus Jujubae) 3g.

葶苈子	tíng lì zǐ	24g	Semen Lepidii seu Descurainiae
皂荚	zào jiá	10g	Fructus Gleditsiae Sinensis
麻黄	má huáng	12g	Herba Ephedrae
杏仁	xìng rén	6g	Armeniacae Semen Amarum
大黄	dà huáng	12g	Radix et Rhizoma Rhei
芒硝	máng xiāo	3g	Natrii Sulfas
大枣	dà zǎo	3g	Fructus Jujubae

They were prepared as suppository, each containing 10g of original crude medicinals. 3 pieces were used a day. 7 days made up a course of treatment. For patients in the control group: *Guì Lóng Níng Jiāo Náng* (桂龙宁胶囊) (0.3g for each capsule), was given. 5 capsules were taken orally, 3 times a day. 7 days made up a course of treatment. The trial group had 151 cases, and the control group had 51 cases. The rates of remarkable control were 57.93% and 40.48% respectively. The total effective rate was 89.68% and 76.19% respectively.

(3) Intravenous Medication

Shen Jia[17] treated 65 cases of asthma with *Huáng Qí Zhù Shè Yè* (黄芪注射液) 20—50ml in a glucose injection or 0.9% sodium chloride injection in 250 ml of fluid, and *Yú Xīng Cǎo Zhù Shè Yè* (鱼腥草注射液) 50—100 ml in a 5% glucose injection or 0.9% sodium chloride injection in 250 ml of fluid. The medication was given intravenously. At the same time, conventional medicines were used, like β_2 agonists, aminophylline, or steroids, and appropriate antibiotics in cases complicated by infection. For patients in the control group neither *Huáng Qí Zhù Shè Yè* (黄芪注射液) nor *Yú Xīng Cǎo Zhù Shè Yè* (鱼腥草注射液) were used, and the western medicine pharmacotherapies were the same as that for the trial group. The results shows that the curative effect of the trial group was obviously better that that of the control group ($P<0.01$).

4. Acupuncture and Moxibustion

In recent years, acupuncture and moxibustion have been commonly applied to treat asthma. The treatments are easily popular because they are various in technique, unique in manipulation, simple, and safe.

(1) Acupuncture

Cheng Jiang-sheng[18] used LU 10 (*yú jì*) bilaterally, with a 1 *cun* perpendicular insertion. After strong stimulation leading to arrival of qi, the needles were retained for 30 minutes, with rotating every 10 minutes. The therapy was performed once a day. In total 60 cases of acute attack of asthma were treated. The results show that within 30 minutes, there were 36 cases which showed remarkable effects, 23 cases which showed some effect, and 1 case which had response. The total effective rate was 98.3%.

Jiang Xiang-dong[19] needled SJ 17 (*yì fēng*) to treat 60 cases of acute asthma attack. He used an even supplement and drainage technique by using the lifting and thrusting method. The needle manipulation was performed for 3 minutes. Strong stimulation was applied when the needles were removed, and there was no needle retention. After one minute of needling, 58 cases showed an effect, and 2 cases showed no effect. The effective rate was 97%.

Fu Wen-bin and his coworkers[20] treated 30 cases of acute asthma attack with eye acupuncture. They selected points in *fèi qū* (Lung region), and *shàng jiāo qū* (upper jiao region). The acupuncture was performed for 15 minutes. The results showed that 20 cases were clinically controlled, 5 cases had a remarkable effect, 3 cases had some effect, and 2 cases got no effect. The effective rate was 90%.

Huang He-sheng[21] used many kinds of therapies. He selected the bilateral *xiōng qiāng qū* (chest region) in scalp acupuncture; *bǎi láo*, RN 22 (*tiān tū*), RN 17 (*dàn zhōng*) and LU 14 (*hé gǔ*) in body acupuncture; the middle triangular fossa (TF3) and *shén mén* (TF4) in ear acupuncture; and the Lung channel, Lung acupoint and coughing-gasping point in hand acupuncture. He used all of these different points to treat 154 cases of asthma, with an effective rate of 79.2%.

(2) Moxibustion

Wu Jian-ming and his coworkers[22] used *Jié Chuǎn Gāo* (截喘膏) plasters at DU 14 (*dà zhuī*), BL 13 (*fèi shù*), BL 17 (*gé shù*), BL 23 (*shèn shù*), RN 22 (*tiān tū*), RN 17 (*dàn zhōng*) and KI 1 (*yǒng quán*). The ingredients in the plaster were *yán hú suǒ* (Rhizoma Corydalis), *xì xīn* (Radix et Rhizoma Asari), *gān suí* (Radix Kansui), *fáng fēng* (Radix Saposhnikoviae), and *bái zǎo xiū* (Rhizhoma Paridis).

延胡索	yán hú suǒ	Rhizoma Corydalis
细辛	xì xīn	Radix et Rhizoma Asari
甘遂	gān suí	Radix Kansui
防风	fáng fēng	Radix Saposhnikoviae
白蚤休	bái zǎo xiū	Rhizhoma Paridis

These were ground into a powder, and prepared with ginger juice. 260 cases of allergic asthma were treated. Each treatment was for 4—6 hours. The first application was done on the first day of the initial period of the greatest heat days in summer and once more 10 days later. Three times made up one course of treatment. The effective rate was 85.4%.

Liu Ming-qi and his coworkers[23] selected points in groups: (1) RN 22 (*tiān tū*), DU 14 (*dà zhuī*), *dìng chuǎn*, BL 12 (*fēng mén*), and BL 13 (*fèi shù*); (2) BL 43 (*gāo huāng*), DU 9 (*zhì yáng*), BL 13 (*fèi shù*), and BL 23 (*shèn shù*); (3) RN 17 (*dàn zhōng*), LU 7 (*liè quē*), RN 4 (*guān yuán*), and ST 40 (*fēng lóng*). Every 10 days one of the groups of points were selected, alternating among the 3 groups. 30 days made up a course of treatment. Pustulating moxibustion was applied at these points. In 33 cases of bronchial asthma, 15 cases were cured, 16 cases showed remarkably effect, and 2 cases showed some effect. The effective rate was 100%.

Xu Lü-ping and his coworkers [24] made an extract from the following medicinals: *bái jiè zǐ* (Semen Sinapis Albae) and *gān suí* (Radix Kansui) each accounting for 30%, *xì xīn* (Radix et Rhizoma Asari) and *yán hú suǒ* (Rhizoma Corydalis) each accounting for 15%, and *shēng má huáng* (Herba Ephedrae) accounting for 10%. This extract was used for medicinal moxibustion. The medicinal extract was applied at BL 13 (*fèi shù*), *dìng chuǎn*, and RN 22 (*tiān tū*) on the first day of the first of the three ten-day periods of the hot season; at BL 12 (*fēng mén*), BL 14 (*jué yīn shù*), and RN 17 (*dàn zhōng*) on the first day of the second of the three ten-day periods of the hot season; and at BL 11 (*dà zhù*), BL 15 (*xīn shù*), and RN 20 (*huá gài*) on the first day of the third of the three ten-day periods of the hot season. They used this to treat 218 case of asthma. The total effective rate was 96.8%.

(3) Other Acupoint Therapies

1) Acupoint application

Yang Zhen-han[25] and his coworkers treated 55 cases of asthma. The patients in the trial group were given the self-composed *Má Xìng Zhǐ Xiào Sǎn* (麻杏止哮散). The ingredients were *mǎ qián zǐ* (Semen Strychni) 20g, *dì biē chóng* (Eupolyphaga seu steleophaga) 15g, and *běi xìng rén* (Armeniacae Semen Amarum) 15g, smashed and ground into a fine powder.

马钱子	mǎ qián zǐ	20g	Semen Strychni
地鳖虫	dì biē chóng	15g	Eupolyphaga seu steleophaga
北杏仁	běi xìng rén	15g	Armeniacae Semen Amarum

Then they added water to prepare the medicicnals into a paste. The paste was applied externally on KI 1 (*yǒng quán*), bilaterally, for 24 hours while the patient lay in bed. Each week the therapy was performed once, with discontinuance of other medication. The patients were advised to stop smoking. During the acute attack stage of asthma, the inhaled medication Becotide was be added and taken via aerosolization, 200μg each time, twice a day. The patients in the control group were only given 200μg of inhaled Becotide via aersolization, twice a day. The treatments for the two groups were conducted continuously for one month, and the observations were conducted for 3—6 months. The results showed that the 1 second forced expiratory volume (FEV_1) in the trial group increased markedly more than that of the control group.

Tao Hong[26] treated 70 cases of asthma with his self-made medicinal cakes. The ingredients were *bái jiè zǐ* (Semen Sinapis Albae), *xì xīn* (Radix et Rhizoma Asari), *gān suí* (Radix Kansui), *é zhú* (Rhizoma Curcumae), *yán hú suǒ* (Rhizoma Corydalis), and *liú huáng* (Sulphur) in the proportions of 6:5:4:3:2:1.

自芥子	bái jiè zǐ	6	Semen Sinapis Albae
细辛	xì xīn	5	Radix et Rhizoma Asari
甘遂	gān suí	4	Radix Kansui
莪术	é zhú	3	Rhizoma Curcumae
延胡索	yán hú suǒ	2	Rhizoma Corydalis
硫黄	liú huáng	1	Sulphur

First the medicinals were ground into a powder, next *shè xiāng* (Secretio Moschi) 0.9g was added into each 100g of medicinal powder, and they it was mixed evenly with fresh ginger juice before application. An appropriate quantity of *bīng piàn* (Borneolum Syntheticum) was dissolved into a 75% ethanol saturated solution, then the ginger juice compound was mixed with the *bīng piàn*-ethanol solution in a proportion of 5:1 This was made into medicinal cakes in the size and thickness of 5 *fen* coin. They were applied on DU 14 (*dà zhuī*), *dìng chuǎn* (bilaterally), BL 13 (*fèi shù*) (bilaterally), BL 43 (*gāo huāng*) (bilaterally), and BL 15 (*xīn shù*) (bilaterally). The duration of application was 4—6 hours each time; 2 hours for young children. It was best when the local skin appeared to have ecchymoses or blisters. The time that this was done was on the first days of the 1st, 2nd and 3rd periods of the greatest heat days in summer respectively. It was applied once. A total of 3 times made up one course of treatment. This was carried out, continuously for 3 years. The results: The total effective rate was 91.4%.

2) Medicated thread [suture] embedding at acupoints

Lu Ai-ping[27] embedded sheep medicated threads soaked in *Dìng Chuǎn Fāng* (定喘方) (*zhì fù zǐ* [Radix Aconiti Lateralis Praeparata], and *bái zhú* [Rhizoma Atractylodis Macrocephalae]) into the following points: *dìng chuǎn* and BL 13 (*fèi shù*). The stimulation was intense and long-lasting. In total 68 cases of asthma were treated. The total effective rate was 93%. The results for treating deficienct asthma was better than that for treating excess asthma (P<0.05).

3) Small needle knife therapy

Qin Chong-ning and his coworkers[28] used a small needle knife therapy to treat 40 cases of bronchial asthma. They were also given *Píng Chuǎn Jiàng Qì Tāng* (平喘降气汤) orally, in combination with the knife therapy. The total effective rate was 90%; and the effect was better than that of the pure biomedical treatments in the control group. In addition, the method was simple, and had no side effects.

4) Medicated thread (suture)-embedding therapy

Li Yue and his coworkers[29] took sutures and *xī xiān cǎo* (Herba Siegesbeckiae) and boiled them together for 30min. They then cut the sutures into sections 0.5cm long and implanted them into RN 17 (*dàn zhōng*) to treat 306 cases of asthma. The embedding was conducted once a month, for 3 continuous months. 3 times made up a course of treatment. The results: 256 cases were clinically controlled, 42 cases showed effective results, and 8 cases showed no effective results. The effective rate was 97.4%. Yang Pei-zhi[30] implanted the sutures into BL 13 (*fèi shù*), BL 12 (*fēng mén*), ST 40 (*fēng lóng*), *dìng chuǎn*, BL 20 (*pí shù*), and BL 23 (*shèn shù*) to treat asthma.

5) Acupoint-tapping therapy

Leng Yu-ling and his coworkers[31] used BL 13 (*fèi shù*), and *dìng chuǎn* as the chief acupoints. For cases of wind-cold, they added LU 7 (*liè quē*), and BL 12 (*fēng mén*). For cases of excessive phlegm, they added RN 17 (*dàn zhōng*), and ST 40 (*fēng lóng*). For cases of deficiency, they added LU 9 (*tài yuān*), KI 3 (*tài xī*), RN 6 (*qì hǎi*) and BL 23 (*shèn shù*). Tapping was conducted with a magnetic round-point needle. A bird-pecking technique was used on the points, and each point was tapped for 3min, once a day. 10 days made up a course of treatment. In 64 cases of asthma, 38 cases were cured, 24 cases showed remarkably effective results, and 2 cases were non-responsive. The effective rate was 96.9%.

6) Intradermal needle therapy

Tian Cong-huo and his coworkers[32] selected BL 13 (*fèi shù*), *dìng chuǎn*, and back tender points for excess patterns; and BL 17 (*gé shù*), BL 23 (*shèn shù*), and back tender points for deficiency patterns. On these point they did intadermal needle-embedding. The needles were kept in for 3–5 days, 1 or 2 times per week, altogether for 4 weeks. The results showed that there were 25 cases controlled by first retention, 28 cases that showed remarkable effects, and 17 cases with no response. The effective rate was 75.72%. The ventilation function of the lung was also remarkably improved, with a better effect in treating excess patterns.

7) Plum-blossom needling therapy

Du Shan-xia and his coworkers[33] used plum blossom needles to lightly tap on the bladder channels along both sides of the thoracic vertebrae. They did this up and down 3 times. They then tapped on the Ren Vessel from RN 22 (*tiān tū*) to RN 17 (*dàn zhōng*), until the skin beamed flushed. In addition, moxibustion was carried out at DU 14 (*dà zhuī*), BL 12 (*fēng mén*), BL 13 (*fèi shù*), RN 22 (*tiān tū*), and RN 17 (*dàn zhōng*) for 15min, every 3 days. 3 times made up one course of treatment.

In total, 120 cases of asthma were treated, and follow-up was conducted 1 year later. The results were that 14 cases were cured, 86 cases had improvement, and 20 cases showed no effect. The effective rate was 91.7%.

8) Lipid cutting therapy

Zhang Su-ya[34] applied lipid cutting therapy to treat 200 cases of asthma. The point selected was RN 17 (*dàn zhōng*). After local anesthesia, the incision was done deeply to the fat level. The local fat was cut out, then the site was debrided and sutured. The stitches were removed one week later. Three times made up a course of treatment. Half year later he did a reexamination. The results were that 100 cases were cured, 95 cases were improved in the short-term, and 5 cases showed no effect. The total effective rate was 97.50%.

9) Acupoint injection

Du xue-song and his coworkers[35] injected dexamethasone and vitamin K into BL 13 (*fèi shù*), and *dìng chuǎn*, and Gentamicin into LI 11 (*qū chí*) to treat 60 cases of bronchial asthma. Among them 29 cases showed a remarkable effect, 16 cases showed some effect, 10 cases showed improvement, and 5 cases were not responsive. The effective rate was 91.67%. Liu Nai-ji[36] selected BL 13 (*fèi shù*) and LI 20 (*yíng xiāng*), and injected Triamcinolone Acetonide, 654-2, placental tissue extract, and Lidocaine respectively, into the points to treat 53 cases of asthma. For the first time, he selected BL 13 (*fèi shù*) or nearby tender points, and for the second time (15 days later) he used LI 20 (*yíng xiāng*). The two times made up a course of treatment. After 1 or 2 courses of treatment, 22 cases recovered (and had no relapses within 3 years), 23 cases had remarkable effects, 6 cases improved, and 3 cases showed no response. The total effective rate was 94.3%.

Experimental Studies

1. Research on the Efficacy of Single Chinese Medicinals

(1) Study on the Anti-asthmatic Action of Polyglucosides from *Niú Xī* (Radix Achyranthis Bidentatae Polysccharide)

A study by Hu Xiao-guang and his coworkers[37] showed that Achyranthis Bidentatae polysaccharide (ABPS) could treat airway inflammation by adjusting the imbalance of TH1/TH2 in animal asthma models. The effect of Achyranthan, with regards to IL-4 and IFN-r, is almost the same as that of dexamethasone. So at the least it may be used as a substitute for dexamethasone in partly treating asthma, thus avoiding a series of side effects from dexamethasone.

(2) Study on the Anti-asthmatic Mechanism of Polyglucosides from *Léi Gōng Téng* (Radix Tripterygii Wilfordi)

Son Hong-tao and his coworkers[38] found an obvious decrease in the number of eosinophils in bronchoalveolar lavage fluid (BALF) ($P<0.01$) in asthmatic rat models that were treated with polyglucosides from *léi gōng téng* (Radix Tripterygii Wilfordi). Thus they believe that the polyglucosides of *léi gōng téng* (Radix Tripterygii Wilfordi) might suppress eosinophils so as to have a therapeutic effect.

(3) Study on the Anti-asthmatic Action of *Pī Shí* (Arsenicum)

Yao Wei-min and his coworkers[39] found that remarkably elevated levels (compared to those in a control group) of leukotrines-B4 (LTB4) in bronchoalveolar lavage fluid (BALF) in experimental asthmatic mice. They also found an increase in the expression level of 5-lipoxidase (5-Lo) gene of the lung tissue. The researchers found that *pī shí* (Arsenicum), in 4 kinds of dosages, was able to suppress the LTB4 level in BALF in asthmatic mice. *Pī shí* (Arsenicum), through suppressing of the 5-Lo mRNA expression in the lung, can inhibit the production of LTB4 on the transcription level. This might be one of the reasons that *pī shí* (Arsenicum) reduced the level of BALF LFB4 in asthmatic mice.

2. Research on the Efficacy of Herbal Prescription

(1) Anti-inflammatories

Jian Xiao-yun and his coworkers[40] found that, on the basis of conventional therapy of biomedicine for asthmatic patients during the acute attack stage, the administration of *Dìng Chuǎn Tāng* (定喘汤) could more quickly alleviate the condition than conventional biomedicine (control group) (P<0.05). The ingredients were *má huáng* (Herba Ephedrae), *xìng rén* (Armeniacae Semen Amarum), *bàn xià* (Rhizoma Pinelliae), *sū zǐ* (Fructus Perillae), *kuǎn dōng huā* (Flos Farfarae), *huáng qín* (Radix Scutellariae), *bái guǒ* (Semen Ginkgo), *sāng bái pí* (Cortex Mori), and *gān cǎo* (Radix et Rhizoma Glycyrrhizae).

麻黄	má huáng	Herba Ephedrae
杏仁	xìng rén	Armeniacae Semen Amarum
半夏	bàn xià	Rhizoma Pinelliae
苏子	sū zǐ	Fructus Perillae
款冬花	kuǎn dōng huā	Flos Farfarae
黄芩	huáng qín	Radix Scutellariae
白果	bái guǒ	Semen Ginkgo
桑白皮	sāng bái pí	Cortex Mori
甘草	gān cǎo	Radix et Rhizoma Glycyrrhizae

They also found that the levels of TNF-α and IL-6 in the trial group were obviously lower than those in the control group (P<0.05). The effective mechanism might be related to the decrease of TNF-α and IL-6, and the alleviation of airway inflammation.

Hu Zuo-wei and his coworkers[41] observed that *Zhǐ Xiào Píng Chuǎn Tāng* (止哮平喘汤) could reduce the number inflammatory cells in the peripheral blood and local airways of experimental guinea pigs, with an anti-inflammatory effect on the airway. The ingredients were *bàn xià* (Rhizoma Pinelliae), *guā lóu* (Fructus Trichosanthis), *xiè bái* (Bulbus Allii Macrostemonis), *bái sháo* (Radix Paeoniae Alba), *chái hú* (Radix Bupleuri), *huáng qín* (Radix Scutellariae), *má huáng* (Herba Ephedrae), *zhǐ qiào* (Fructus Aurantii), *gān cǎo* (Radix et Rhizoma Glycyrrhizae), and *shè gān* (Rhizoma Belamcandae)

半夏	bàn xià	Rhizoma Pinelliae
瓜蒌	guā lóu	Fructus Trichosanthis
薤白	xiè bái	Bulbus Allii Macrostemonis
白芍	bái sháo	Radix Paeoniae Alba
柴胡	chái hú	Radix Bupleuri
黄芩	huáng qín	Radix Scutellariae
麻黄	má huáng	Herba Ephedrae
枳壳	zhǐ qiào	Fructus Aurantii
甘草	gān cǎo	Radix et Rhizoma Glycyrrhizae
射干	shè gān	Rhizoma Belamcandae

This confirms that the airway anti-inflammation effect of *Zhǐ Xiào Píng Chuǎn Tāng* (止哮平喘汤) is via the adjustment of T lymphocyte immune function (during asthma) by promoting or inducing apoptosis of T lymphocytes.

The studies by Gao Bao-an and his coworkers[42] show that, *Qín Yí Hé Jì* (芩夷合剂) could promote eosinophil apoptosis in the airway and reduce the recruitment of eosinophils, thus relieving airway inflammation. The ingredients were *huáng qín* (Radix Scutellariae), *xīn yí* (Flos Magnoliae), *xiè bái* (Bulbus Allii Macrostemonis), *má huáng* (Herba Ephedrae), *jīn yín huā* (Flos Lonicerae Japonicae), *xìng rén* (Armeniacae Semen Amarum), *chuān xiōng* (Rhizoma Chuanxiong), and *dì lóng* (Lumbricus).

黄芩	huáng qín	Radix Scutellariae
辛夷	xīn yí	Flos Magnoliae

薤白	xiè bái	Bulbus Allii Macrostemonis
麻黄	má huáng	Herba Ephedrae
金银花	jīn yín huā	Flos Lonicerae Japonicae
杏仁	xìng rén	Armeniacae Semen Amarum
川芎	chuān xiōng	Rhizoma Chuanxiong
地龙	dì lóng	Lumbricus

(2) Influence on Hormone Levels

A study by Xu Jian-hua and his coworkers[43] indicated that *Bǔ Shèn Dìng Chuǎn Tāng* (补肾定喘汤) could cause a drop in the high glucocorticoid levels of lung tissue (P<0.05), and cause an increase in the levels of serum ACTH and corticosterone (P<0.01). This shows an excitatory effect in the pituitary gland-adrenal gland cortex system. The ingredients were *Liù Wèi Dì Huáng Tāng* (六味地黄汤) plus *lù jiǎo piàn* (Cornu Cervi Slice), *ròu cōng róng* (Herba Cistanches), *bā jǐ tiān* (Radix Morindae Officinalis), *é guǎn shí* (Balanophyllia), *shú fù zǐ* (Radix Aconiti Lateralis Praeparata), and *ròu guì* (Cortex Cinnamomi).

鹿角片	lù jiǎo piàn	Cornu Cervi Slice
肉苁蓉	ròu cōng róng	Herba Cistanches
巴戟天	bā jǐ tiān	Radix Morindae Officinalis
鹅管石	é guǎn shí	Balanophyllia
熟附子	shú fù zǐ	Radix Aconiti Lateralis Praeparata
肉桂	ròu guì	Cortex Cinnamomi

Mao Changchun and his coworkers[44] did research and thus believe that the inhibition of the HPA axis in experimental asthmatic rats may be related to deficiency of Kidney yang. *Bǔ Shèn Dìng Chuǎn Tāng* (补肾定喘汤) and *Bǔ Shèn Yáng Fāng* (补肾阳方) (subtract from the above formula *Liù Wèi Dì Huáng Tāng* [六味地黄汤]) can effectively improve the inhibitory state of the HPA axis in asthmatic rats at the hypothalamus level. The therapeutic method of tonifying the Kidney yang can improve the interaction between the immune system and the nerve endocrine system in asthma patients. Consequently, it is possible to achieve a long term curative effect in treating asthma, thus preventing seasonal episodes.

(3) Influence on Immune Function

Studies by Yang Jun-ping[45] indicate that, after the application of *Jiàng Qì Dìng Chuǎn Tāng* (降气定喘汤) the IL-12 level was obviously higher than before the treatment ($P<0.05$), and the IL-4 and IgE levels were obviously lower than those before the treatment ($P<0.05$ or $P<0.01$). The ingredients were *má huáng* (Herba Ephedrae), *xìng rén* (Armeniacae Semen Amarum), *chán tuì* (Periostracum Cicadae), *dì lóng* (Lumbricus), *shè gān* (Rhizoma Belamcandae), *bàn xià* (Rhizoma Pinelliae), *jú hóng* (Exocarpium Citri Rubrum), *wǔ wèi zǐ* (Fructus Schisandrae Chinensis), *fú líng* (Poria), *yín yáng huò* (Herba Epimedii), *dān shēn* (Radix et Rhizoma Salviae Miltiorrhizae), *lái fú zǐ* (Semen Raphani), *gān cǎo* (Radix et Rhizoma Glycyrrhizae), and *xì xīn* (Radix et Rhizoma Asari).

麻黄	má huáng	Herba Ephedrae
杏仁	xìng rén	Armeniacae Semen Amarum
蝉蜕	chán tuì	Periostracum Cicadae
地龙	dì lóng	Lumbricus
射干	shè gān	Rhizoma Belamcandae
半夏	bàn xià	Rhizoma Pinelliae
橘红	jú hóng	Exocarpium Citri Rubrum
五味子	wǔ wèi zǐ	Fructus Schisandrae Chinensis
茯苓	fú líng	Poria
淫羊藿	yín yáng huò	Herba Epimedii
丹参	dān shēn	Radix et Rhizoma Salviae Miltiorrhizae
莱菔子	lái fú zǐ	Semen Raphani
甘草	gān cǎo	Radix et Rhizoma Glycyrrhizae
细辛	xì xīn	Radix et Rhizoma Asari

Thus they deduced that *Jiàng Qì Dìng Chuǎn Tāng* (降气定喘汤) could elevate the IL-12 level and lower the IL-4 and IgE levels so as to regulate the immune function of the body. The results of the study from Yao Yuyou and his coworkers[46] showed that *Ké Chuǎn Níng Fěn Jì* (咳喘宁粉剂) (*bái sháo* [Radix Paeoniae Alba] and *mò yú gú fěn* [Puilvis Os Sepiella seu Sepiae]) not only could improve lung function of the asthmatic child, but also decrease high levels of IgE, and result is a better clinical control rate. It could also remarkably delay the asthma-inducing period in guinea pigs and reduce the NO and the EF-1 levels of bronchoalveolar lavage fluid.

(4) Regulating AMP/GMP

Observations on asthmatic guinea pigs by Li Chu and his coworkers[47] showed that the application of *Yú Mián Píng Chuǎn Fāng* (鱼棉平喘方) could remarkably delay the asthma-inducing period, elevate the plasma AMP level, and reduce the plasma GMP level. The ingredients were *yú xīng cǎo* (Herba Houttuyniae), *mián gēn pí* (Cortex Radix Gossypii), *má huáng* (Herba Ephedrae), *mǎ dōu líng* (Fructus Aristolochiae), *dì lóng* (Lumbricus), *yín xìng yè* (Folium Ginkgo), *shí wěi* (Folium Pyrrosiae), *tíng lì zǐ* (Semen Lepidii seu Descurainiae), and *gān cǎo* (Radix et Rhizoma Glycyrrhizae).

鱼腥草	yú xīng cǎo	Herba Houttuyniae
棉根皮	mián gēn pí	Cortex Radix Gossypii
麻黄	má huáng	Herba Ephedrae
马兜铃	mǎ dōu líng	Fructus Aristolochiae
地龙	dì lóng	Lumbricus
银杏叶	yín xìng yè	Folium Ginkgo
石韦	shí wěi	Folium Pyrrosiae
葶苈子	tíng lì zǐ	Semen Lepidii seu Descurainiae
甘草	gān cǎo	Radix et Rhizoma Glycyrrhizae

Thus, through adjusting the AMP/GMP ratio, it suppressed the degranulation of eosinophils and mastocytes, checked the release of allergic media, and relaxed the bronchial smooth muscle. Therefore it participated in many important functions like anti-inflammation and immune regulation. In elevating the AMP/GMP ratio, the effect in the large dose group was remarkably higher than that in the small dose group (P<0.05), which suggests there may exist a dose-dependency correlation.

3. Studies on Forms of Chinese Medicinals

(1) Capsules

Wang Zhen and his coworkers[48] found that *Gé Jiè Dìng Chuǎn Jiāo Náng* (蛤蚧定喘胶囊) could remarkably reduce the blood serum total IgE contents and platelet activating factors in experimental asthmatic guinea pigs (P<0.01).

(2) Mixtures

Peng Hong-xing and coworkers[49] evaluated the plasma cAMP levels of asthmatic guinea pigs after treatment with *Hǎi Shí Hé Jì* (海石合剂) (*má huáng* [Herba Ephedrae], *xìng rén* [Semen Pruni Armeniacae]), etc.). The result was that the plasma cAMP level of the asthmatic guinea pigs increased. Thus the goal of relieving asthma was achieved, and the effect was similar to that of aminophylline.

Fang Xiang-ming and his coworkers[50] found that after asthmatic guinea pigs were treated with *Píng Chuǎn Hé Jì* (平喘合剂) (*má huáng* [Herba Ephedrae], *xì xīn* [Radix et Rhizoma Asari], etc.), the T cell apoptosis rate in the bronchoalveolar lavage fluid was remarkably increased (P<0.05).

REFERENCES

[1] Wang Zhi-ying, Zhou Zhong-ying, Jin Miao-wen, et al. Clinical Study on Bronchial Asthma Treated with Method of Resolving phlegm and Removing Stasis, Lowering the Adverse Flow of Qi and Calming Panting (化痰祛瘀·降气平喘治疗支气管哮喘的临床研究). *Journal of Emergency in Traditional Chinese Medicine* (中国中医急症). 2000, 9 (4): 137, 138.

[2] Li Chuan, Chang Wei-zhi. Treatment of 48 Cases of Bronchial Asthma with

Chinese Medicine (中医药治疗支气管哮喘48例). *Acta Chinese Medicine and Pharmacology* (中医药学报). 2005, 33 (4): 52-53.

[3] Zeng De-you. Treatment of 48 Cases of Acute Bronchial Asthma According to Pattern Differentiation (分型论治急性支气管哮喘78例). *Hunan Guiding Journal of Traditional Chinese Medicine and Pharmacology* (湖南中医药导报). 2000, 6 (7): 29-30.

[4] Jiang Shu-guang. Effective Observation on 35 Cases of Bronchial Asthma Treated with Method of Invigorating Blood and Removing Stasis (活血化瘀法治疗支气管哮喘35例疗效观察). *Hunan Journal of Traditional Chinese Medicine* (湖南中医杂志). 2001, 17 (5): 15-16.

[5] Wu Xing-he. Clinical Observation on 64 Cases of Bronchial Asthma in the Acute Attack Stage Treated with *Sì Chóng Qū Fēng Gù Běn Tāng* (四虫祛风固本汤治疗支气管哮喘急性发作期64例临床观察). *Journal of Traditional Chinese Medicine* (中医杂志). 2001, 42 (8): 476-477.

[6] Liu Liu. Treatment of 100 Cases of Bronchial Asthma with *Píng Chuǎn Tāng* (平喘汤治疗支气管哮喘100例). *Shanxi Journal of Traditional Chinese Medicine* (陕西中医). 2002, 23 (4): 342.

[7] Wang Yu-yu, Ni Zhi-jian. Experiences of 56 Cases of Bronchial Asthma Treated with *Jiā Wèi Xìng Rén Tāng* (加味杏仁汤治疗支气管哮喘56例体会). *Yunnan Journal of Traditional Chinese Medicine and Materia Medica* (云南中医中药杂志). 2002, 23 (4): 20.

[8] Xuan Jiang-da, Huang Zhao-wang. Treatment of 150 Cases of Bronchial Asthma with *Ké Chuǎn Líng* (咳喘灵治疗哮喘150例). *Journal of Zhejiang College of Traditional Chinese Medicine* (浙江中医学院学报). 2003, 27 (4): 55.

[9] Li Hui, Gao Min. Treatment of 56 Cases of Bronchial Asthma with *Wēn Dǎn Tāng* (温胆汤加减治疗支气管哮喘56例) with Modifications. *Hebei Journal of Traditional Chinese Medicine* (河北中医). 2004, 24 (5): 365.

[10] Zheng Guo-hua, Wang Yi-zhen. Treatment of Bronchial Asthma with *Lái Fú Zǐ Sǎn* (莱菔子散治疗支气管哮喘). *Shanxi Journal of Traditional Chinese Medicine* (陕西中医). 2002, 23 (3): 270.

[11] Zhang Zheng-yuan. Treatment of 112 Cases of Bronchial Asthma with *Ké Chuǎn Gù Běn Wán* (咳喘固本丸治疗支气管哮喘112例). *Hunan Guiding Journal of Traditional Chinese Medicine and Pharmacology* (湖南中医药导报). 2002, 8 (2): 61.

[12] Yu Xia, Wu Yu-chang, Bai Jie. Treatment of 37 Cases of Cough-Variant Asthma with *Guì Zhī Jiā Hòu Pò Xìng Zǐ Tāng* (桂枝加厚朴杏子汤治疗咳嗽变异型哮喘37例), *Chinese Journal of the Practical Chinese with Modern Medicine* (中华实用中西医杂志). 2005, 18 (20): 1319.

[13] Sun Shi-tian, Zhang Fu-qin, Song Li-xiang, et al. Clinical Observations on Treatment of 76 Cases of Bronchial Asthma in the Remission Stage with *Gù Běn Shí Wèi*

Sǎn (固本十味散治疗支气管哮喘缓解期176例临床观察). *Hebei Journal of Traditional Chinese Medicine* (河北中医). 2005, 27 (9): 667.

[14] Su Cai-feng, Cui Xiao-ping. Treatment of 60 Cases of Bronchial Asthma with *Píng Gān Xiào Chuǎn Tāng* (平肝哮喘汤治疗支气管哮喘60例). *Shanxi Journal of Traditional Chinese Medicine* (陕西中医). 2005.12.05; 26 (12): 1271.

[15] Wang Xiu-qin, Peng Xiu-fen, Li Ying-quan, et al. Treatment of 80 Cases of Bronchial Asthma with Antiasthmatic Gauze Mask (止喘口罩治疗支气管哮喘80例). *Shandong Journal of Traditional Chinese Medicine* (山东中医杂志). 2001, 20 (7): 398-399.

[16] Li Zhen-qian, Wei Su-li, Chen Xuan-jing, et al. Treatment of 151 Cases of Bronchial Asthma with *Tíng Lì Píng Chuǎn Shuān* (葶苈平喘栓治疗支气管哮喘151例). *Shanxi Journal of Traditional Chinese Medicine* (陕西中医). 2003, 24 (10): 881-882.

[17] Shen Jia. Analysis of 65 Cases of Bronchial Asthma Treated with *Huáng Qí Zhù Shè Yè* Plus *Yú Xīng Cǎo Zhù Shè Yè* (黄芪鱼腥草注射液为主治疗支气管哮喘65例分析). *Journal of Practical Traditional Chinese Internal Medicine* (实用中医内科杂志). 2002, 16 (2): 98-99.

[18] Cheng Jian-sheng. Treatment of Acute Attack of Asthma by Needling LU 10 (yú jì) (针刺鱼际穴治疗急性哮喘发作). *Chinese Acupuncture & Moxibustion* (中国针灸). 2001, 21 (9): 547.

[19] Jiang Xiang-dong. Treatment of 60 Cases of Acute Attack of Asthma by Needling SJ 17 (yì fēng) (针刺翳风治疗哮喘急性发作60例). *Chinese Acupuncture & Moxibustion* (中国针灸). 2002, 22 (9): 611.

[20] Fu Wen-bin, Chen Xiu-hua. Clinical Observation on Control of Acute Attack of Asthma with Eye Acupuncture (眼针控制哮喘急性发作的临床观察). *Shanghai Journal of Acupuncture and Moxibustion* (上海针灸杂志). 2002, 21 (5): 20-22.

[21] Huang He-sheng. Effective Analysis on Treatment of 154 Cases of Asthma Attack Treated with Several Kinds of Acupuncture (多种针法治疗哮喘发作154例疗效分析). *Yunnan Journal of Traditional Chinese Medicine and Materia Medica* (云南中医中药杂志). 2000, 21(2): 109.

[22] Wu Jian-ming, Wang Xian-xi. Study on Factors of Effects of Moxibustion with Acupoint Applications in 260 Cases of Allergic Asthma (穴位贴灸过敏性哮喘260例疗效因素研究). *Chinese Acupuncture & Moxibustion* (中国针灸). 2000, 20 (2): 75-76.

[23] Liu Ming-qing, Huang Qi-song, You Bin. Observation on Clinical Effects of Pustulating Moxibustion on Bronchial Asthma (化脓灸治疗支气管哮喘的临床疗效观察). *Chinese Acupuncture & Moxibustion* (中国针灸). 2002, 22 (8): 537-539.

[24] Xu Lǜ-ping, Zhou Jin-fang. Treatment of 218 Cases of Bronchial Asthma with

Acupoint Application (穴位贴敷治疗哮喘218例). *Shanghai Journal of Acupuncture and Moxibustion* (上海针灸杂志). 2002, 21 (1): 24.

[25] Yang Zhen-han, Xie Zhi-zhong, Song Ai-qun. Treatment of 55 Cases of Bronchial Asthma with *Má Xìng Zhǐ Xiào Sǎn* Application. (麻杏止哮散外敷治疗支气管哮喘55例) *Chinese New Medicine* (中华新医学). 2003, 4 (16): 1478-1479.

[26] Tao Hong, Xu Zi-hang, Hong Jun. Clinical Observation on 70 Cases of Bronchial Asthma Treated with Self-Made Medicinal Cake Application (自制中药饼穴位贴敷治疗支气管哮喘70例临床观察). *Anhui Clinical Journal of Traditional Chinese Medicine* (安徽中医临床杂志). 2000, 12 (2): 94-95.

[27] Lu Ai-ping. Treatment of 68 Cases of Bronchial Asthma with Acupoint Medicated Catgut Embedding Therapy (穴埋药线治疗支气管哮喘68例). *Heilongjiang Journal of Traditional Chinese Medicine* (黑龙江中医药). 2001, 4: 52.

[28] Qin Chong-ning, He Jian. Treatment of 68 Cases of Bronchial Asthma with Chinese Medicinals plus Small Needle Knife Therapy (中药加小针刀疗法治疗支哮68例). *Journal of Zhejiang College of Traditional Chinese Medicine* (广西中医学院学报). 2002, 5 (4): 35-36.

[29] Li Yue, Li Xing, Wang Li-ping, et al. Clinical Observation on 360 Cases of Simple Bronchial Asthma Treated with Medicated Catgut Embedding Therapy (穴位药线植入治疗单纯性支气管哮喘360例临床观察). *Chinese Acupuncture & Moxibustion* (中国针灸). 2001, 21(1): 11-12.

[30] Yang Pei-zhi. Clinical Effect Observation of Chronic Bronchial Asthma Treated with Acupoint Catgut Implantation (穴位植入疗法治疗慢性支气管哮喘的临床疗效观察). *Clinical Journal of Acupuncture and Moxibustion* (针灸临床杂志). 2003, 19 (9): 44-45.

[31] Leng Yu-ling, Pan Qing-rong. Clinical Observation on 64 Cases of Bronchial Asthma Treated with Magnet Round-Point Needle-Tapping Therapy (磁圆针叩击法治疗哮喘64例临床观察). *Clinical Journal of Acupuncture and Moxibustion* (针灸临床杂志). 2002, 18 (12): 32-33.

[32] Tian Cong-huo, Li Yi-song, Yang Hong. Preliminary Observation on Treatment of Bronchial Asthma with Intradermal Needle Therapy (皮下埋针治疗哮喘的初步观察). *Chinese Acupuncture & Moxibustion* (中国针灸). 2002, 22 (3): 153-154.

[33] Du Shan-xia, Guan Yan-xun, Cui Lian-min. Treatment of 120 Cases of Bronchial Asthma with Plum Blossom Needling Therapy with Moxibustion (梅花针加艾灸治疗哮喘120例). *Chinese Acupuncture & Moxibustion* (中国针灸). 2002, 22 (4): 221.

[34] Zhang Su-niu. Treatment of 200 Cases of Bronchial Asthma with Lipid Cutting Therapy (割脂治疗哮喘200例). *Shanghai Journal of Acupuncture and Moxibustion* (上海针灸杂志). 2002, 21 (1): 26.

[35] Du Xue-song, Wang Peng. Treatment of 60 Cases of Bronchial Asthma with Acupoint Injection (穴位注射治疗支气管哮喘60例). *Liaoning Journal of Traditional Chinese Medicine* (辽宁中医杂志). 2002. 29 (7): 431.

[36] Liu Nai-ji. Treatment of 53 Cases of Bronchial Asthma with BL 13 (fèi shù) and LI 20 (yíng xiāng) Acupoint Injection (肺俞迎香穴位注射治疗哮喘53例). *Chinese Acupuncture & Moxibustion* (中国针灸). 2002, 22 (1): 11.

[37] Hu Xiao-guang, Li Chang-chong, Wang Su-e, et al. Effect of Achyranthan and Dexamethasone on TH1/TH2 Imbalance in Asthma (哮喘TH1／TH2失衡及牛膝多糖和地塞米松的作用). *Zhejiang Journal of Integrated Traditional Chinese and Western Medicine* (浙江中西医结合杂志). 2004, 14 (2): 77.

[38] Sun Hong-tao, Lin Jiang-tao, He Wen-wen. Effect of Tripterygium and Glucocorticoid on the Eosinophils of Bronchoalveolar Lavage Fluid in Asthmatic Rat (雷公藤和糖皮质激素对哮喘大鼠支气管肺泡灌洗液中嗜酸性粒细胞的影响). *Modern Journal of Integrated Traditional Chinese and Western Medicine* (现代中西医结合杂志). 2003, 12 (14): 347.

[39] Yao Wei-min, Liang Biao, Liu Yu-yu. Effects of *Pī Shí* (Arsenicum) on Gene Expression of Leukotrines-B4 and 5-Lipoxidase (砒石对哮喘小鼠白三烯B4及5-脂氧合酶基因表达的影响). *Chinese Journal of Clinical Pharmacology and Therapeutics* (中国临床药理学与治疗学). 2004, 9 (2): 193.

[40] Jian Xiao-yun, Huang Zhao-qi, Lai Xin, et al. Effects of *Dìng Chuǎn Tāng* on TNF-α and IL-6 of Patients with Asthmatic Attack (定喘汤对哮喘发作患者TNF-α、IL-6的影响). *Modern Journal of Integrated Traditional Chinese and Western Medicine* (现代中西医结合杂志). 2002, 11 (14): 1307.

[41] Hu Zuo-wei, Zhou Yan-ping, Wang Peng. Effect of *Zhǐ Xiào Píng Chuǎn Fāng* on Apoptosis of T lymphocytes of Asthmatic Guinea Pigs (止哮平喘方对哮喘豚鼠T淋巴细胞凋亡的作用). *China Journal of Basic Traditional Chinese Medicine* (中国中医基础医学杂志). 2004, 10 (1): 31.

[42] Gao Bao-an, Liu Long-di, Jiang Bi-wu, et al. Influence of *Qín Yí Hé Jì* on Eosinophil Apoptosis in the Airway of Asthmatic Guinea Pig (芩夷合剂吸入对哮喘豚鼠气道嗜酸粒细胞凋亡的影响). *China Journal of Basic Traditional Chinese Medicine* (中国中医基础医学杂志). 2003, 9 (5): 39.

[43] Xu Jian-hua, Fan Zhong-ze, Wu Dun-xu, et al. Effect of *Bǔ Shèn Dìng Chuǎn Tāng* on Serum Glucocorticoid Receptor and Corticosterone and ACTH of Lung Tissue in Asthmatic Rats (补肾定喘汤对哮喘大鼠肺组织糖皮质激素受体及血浆皮质酮ACTH的影响). *China Journal of Basic Traditional Chinese Medicine* (中国中医基础医学杂志). 2003, 9 (1): 27.

[44] Mao Chang-chun, Xu Jian-hua, Guan Dong-yuan, et al. Influence of Different Invigorating-Kidney Method to the HPA Axis in Asthmatic Rat Models (不同补肾法对哮喘模型大鼠HPA轴的影响). *Shanghai Journal of Chinese Medicine and Medicinals* (上海中医药杂志). 2003, 37 (4): 3.

[45] Yang Jun-ping, Qiu Li-ying, Xuan Jiang-lei, et al. Research on *Jiàng Qì Dìng Chuǎn Tāng* in the Adjustment of Blood Serum IL-2 and IL-4 and the IgE levels of Childhood Asthma (降气定喘汤调节哮喘患儿血清IL-2、IL-4与IgE水平的研究). *Jiangxi Journal of Traditional Chinese Medicine* (江西中医药). 2003, 3-4 (12): 9.

[46] Yao Yu-you, Wu Qing-si, Yao Hai-yun. Clinical and Experimental Study on Treatment of Bronchial Asthma with *Ké Chuǎn Níng Fěn Jì* (咳喘宁粉剂治疗支气管哮喘的临床与实验研究). *Chinese Journal of Clinical Pharmacology and Therapeutics* (中国临床药理学与治疗学). 2003, 8 (4): 438.

[47] Li Chu, Long Zi-jiang, Hu Bao-cheng. Antiasthmatic Effect of *Yú Mián Píng Chuǎn Fāng* and Its Influence on Plasma cAMP and cGMP levels in Asthmatic Guinea Pigs (鱼棉平喘方对哮喘豚鼠的平喘作用及血浆cAMP、cGMP水平的影响). *Journal of Nanjing University of Traditional Chinese Medicine* (南京中医药大学学报). 2001, 17 (6): 36.

[48] Wang Zhen, Li Chu. Experimental Study on Antiasthmatic Effect of *Gé Jiè Dìng Chuǎn Jiāo Náng* and Its Mechanism (蛤蚧定喘胶囊的平喘作用及其作用机制的实验研究). *Journal of Clinical Healthcare* (临床中老年保健). 2001, 4 (4): 250-251.

[49] Peng Hong-xing, Chen Tao-hou. Influence of *Hǎi Shí Hé Jì* on Cyclic Nucleotide in Allergic Asthmatic Guinea Pigs (海石合剂对过敏性哮喘豚鼠环核苷酸的影响). *Modern Diagnosis & Treatment* (现代诊断与治疗). 2003, 14 (1): 4-5.

[50] Fang Xiang-ming, Cao Shi-hong. Effect of *Píng Chuǎn Hé Jì* on Apoptosis of T lymphocytes in Asthmatic Guinea Pigs (平喘合剂对哮喘豚鼠T淋巴细胞凋亡的影响). *China Journal of Basic Traditional Chinese Medicine* (中国中医基础医学杂志). 2003, 9 (3): 24-26.

Index by Disease Names and Symptoms

A

abdominal distention 117, 169, 170, 174, 175, 259, 269
accumulation of cold-phlegm in the Lung 055
Accumulation of Cold Phlegm 049
accumulation of Lung heat 123
accumulation of phlegm-fire 276
Accumulation of Phlegm-Heat 069
Accumulation of Phlegm-Heat 019, 271
Accumulation of Phlegm-Heat Mixed with Stasis 089
Accumulation of phlegm-heat mixed with stasis 090
Accumulation of Phlegm-Stasis 021
Accumulation of Turbid-Phlegm 277
acid regurgitation 251
acral coldness 169
acute bronchitis 156
Acute respiratory failure 168
adverse rising of Lung qi 219
agitation 019, 147, 171, 178, 184
Alimentary tract hemorrhage 168
allergic asthma 312, 325
Allergic Bronchial Asthma 265
allergic rhinitis 353
anasarca 016
anorexia 138
anoxemic PAH 200
anoxia 144, 187, 195, 320
Anoxic Pulmonary Hypertension 208
anxiety 047
apathy 147
ascites 016
asthmatic bronchitis 060, 100, 254, 297, 298
asthmatic prostration 220
aversion to cold 017, 051, 120, 144, 221, 325
aversion to wind 029, 086

B

belching 117, 251
bitter taste 082, 223
blockage of cold phlegm 032
blockage of damp-phlegm 034
blockage of phlegm-qi 339
blood deficiency 060
breathlessness 028, 097
bronchial asthma 050, 322
bronchial spasms 329
bronchiectasis 065
bronchitis 064, 154, 176

C

cardiac arrhythmia 012
cardiac dullness 009
cardiac insufficiency 093
cementation of the blood stasis 343
chest fullness 096
chest hyperinflation 296
chest oppression 009, 051
chest pain 269

chest stuffiness 096
Chest vexation 082
childhood asthma 288
chills 130, 223, 256
chronic bronchitis 048, 104, 195
chronic cough 125, 158
chronic larygopharyngitis 058
Chronic Obstructive Pulmonary Disease 127, 204
chronic respiratory failure 158
chuǎn 313
chuǎn tuō 168, 171, 220
chuǎn zhèng 012
coagulation and stagnation of phlegm and stasis 054
coarse breathing 096, 098
cold 028, 064
cold-and-heat mixed asthma 313, 326
Cold-excess 097
Cold-Phlegm Obstructing the Lung 268
cold-phlegm trasforming into heat 056
Cold Asthma 221, 255, 256
cold enveloping fire 284
cold evil lying deep in the Lung 342
cold extremities 063
cold fluid retention 071, 125
Cold Fluids Transforming to Heat 125
Cold in the Exterior and Fluid Retention in the Interior 017
Cold in the Lung and Heat in the Diaphragm 265
cold limbs 032, 067, 074, 091, 122, 168, 258, 320, 334
cold panting 045, 066
cold sweats 024
coma 016, 147
Concurrent deficiency and excess 263
congested throat 259
constipation 021, 056, 082, 083, 099, 107, 174, 198, 223, 281
Contraction of Wind-Heat 086
COPD 009, 014, 016
cor pulmonale 010
Cough-Variant Asthma 370
cough-variant asthma 351
counterflow of qi 223, 259
critical asthma 320, 321, 324, 330, 331
Cushing's disease 321, 333
cyanosis 013, 017, 021, 024, 147, 165, 170
cyanotic lips 138, 320, 334
panting 266

D

debilitation 138
debility 152, 153
deficienct asthma 360
deficiency asthma 126, 233, 282, 286
deficiency cold 133, 134
deficiency fullness 177
deficiency of both Kidney yin and Kidney yang 294
Deficiency of Both Qi and Yin 058
deficiency of both the Lung and Kidney 057, 144, 199, 326, 341, 342, 343
Deficiency of both the Lung and Spleen 048
deficiency of both the Lung and Spleen 038, 107, 326
deficiency of both the Spleen and Kidney 326
deficiency of both the Spleen and Stomach 107
Deficiency of Both Yin and Yang 171
deficiency of Kidney qi 044
Deficiency of Kidney yang 263
Deficiency of Kidney yin 263

Deficiency of Lung Qi 028, 226
Deficiency of Spleen Qi 228
deficiency of the Lung 188, 271
deficiency of the Lung, Spleen and Kidney 185
Deficiency of the Lung and excess of the Stomach 263
deficiency of the Spleen and Lung 085
Deficiency of the Spleen and Stomach 013
deficiency panting 034, 036, 168, 177
delirious speech 147, 180
delirium 023
depletion of Kidney essence 296
depletion of Kidney yang 032
depletion of Kidney yin and yang 322
diarrhea 066, 075, 128, 133, 184, 272
DIC 174
difficult breath 223
difficulty in laying flat 257, 265
dizziness 074, 076, 081, 083, 094, 197, 297
drowsiness 131
dry cough 064, 154, 183
Dry heat in the Lung 262

dry mouth 017, 020, 027, 077, 082, 088, 105, 122, 146, 147, 150, 170, 223, 249, 251
dryness of the Lung and Stomach 130
dry stools 069, 075, 080
dry throat 197, 262
dry tongue 262
Dual deficiency of both the Lung and Spleen 084
dual deficiency of Lung and Kidney 194
Dual Deficiency of Qi and Yin 074
Dual Deficiency of the Lung and Kidney 031, 057, 145
Dual Deficiency of the Lung and Spleen 029, 084, 146
dual deficiency of the Spleen and Kidney 094, 095, 164
dull pain in the epigastrium 251
dyspnea 009, 101, 254, 309

E

edema 009, 014, 073, 091, 101, 220, 332
emaciation 044, 147, 168, 169, 228, 263, 281
emphysema 048, 049, 050, 070, 109, 133, 144, 149, 247

endogenous asthma 316
enuresis 128
excess-heat 134
excess asthma 360
Excess Heat with Symptoms of Cold 126
excess in the Lung and deficiency in the Kidney 063
exhaustion of both qi and yin 028
exogenous asthma 316
exogenous cold and internal fluid retention 120
expiratory dyspnea 217
exterior cold and interior fluid retention 340
exterior cold and interior heat 034, 299
exterior cold with interior fluids 284
exterior constrainr of wind-cold 280
exterior deficiency 227, 230
exterior heat 098
exteriorly constraint of cold evil 311
external cold and internal heat 312, 325
extrinsic asthma 217

F

facial edema 128
failure of the clear yang to rise 076

failure of the defensive exterior to consolidate 109
failure of the Kidney to receive qi 109, 281, 294, 304
failure of the Lung qi to diffuse 258
Failure of the Lung to Clear and Depurate 080
failure of the Lung to clear and depurate 080
fatigue 170
fèi zhàng 012, 039, 220
fēng wēn 112
feverish sensation in the chest 263
flaring nose 179
fluid retention 017, 119, 123, 124, 293, 300
flushed cheeks 027
food retention 123, 124
forehead sweats 026
frequent urination 077
fullness 336

G

Gallbladder cough 128
gasping 265, 296, 321, 323, 335
gastric and duodenal ulcer 332
gastric distention 263
gastrointestinal congestion 174
gastrointestinal excess 261
general arthralgia 223
general debility 227
general edema 119
general pain 017, 145
general weakness 038

H

hacking cough 262
halitosis 019, 099
headache 073, 081,221, 255, 271
Heart cough 128
heart failure 009, 012, 157, 174, 331
Heat-excess 098
heat asthma 234, 295, 302, 307, 340
heat damaging the Lung yin 088
heat evil attacking the Lung 312
heat in the Large Intestine causing fluid exhaustion 082
heat panting 260, 264
heat phlegm 315
heavy sweating on the head 303
hemoptysis 198
hemorrhoids 082
hepatomegaly 009
hiccup 145
hoarse breathing 296
hormone-dependent asthma 321

hyperactivity of Liver-yang 081, 083
hypercapnia 010, 157
hyperhidrosis 266
hyperinflation of the chest 323
hypochondriac pain 117, 259
hypoxemia 009, 010, 157
hypoxia 165, 174, 204, 334

I

infectious asthma 312, 325
Insecurity of the lower origin 281
insomnia 036, 077, 093, 147, 171
insufficiency of both the Lung and Kidney 269
interior obstruction of turbid phlegm 258
Interior retention of cold fluids 262
Internal accumulation of phlegm-heat 261
internal fluid retention 287
internal heat with yin deficiency 067
Internal Obstruction of Turbid Phlegm 144
internal obstruction of turbid phlegm 144
internal retention of latent phlegm 219
intolerance of cold 032,

063, 138, 168, 169, 231, 263, 271, 273
intolerance of wind 153, 226
intrinsic asthma 217
Invasion of Wind-Cold 050
itching 059, 127, 136, 154, 252
itching and stridor in the throat 258
itching throat 053, 147

K

Kidney asthma 296
Kidney cough 128
Kidney deficiency and exterior excess 263
Kidney deficiency and fluid exhaustion 183
Kidney Deficiency Failing to Receive Qi 061
Kidney essence depletion 219
Kidney qi deficiency 122, 169, 299
Kidney yang deficiency 153, 189
Kidney yin deficiency 118, 153
knee weakness 297

L

laryngeal edema 114
lassitude 107, 151, 231
Latent cold fluids upwardly invading the Lung 070
lethargy 016
leukocytosis 274
lip cyanosis 052
listlessness 107
Liver-wind internally stirring 024
Liver cough 128
Liver qi depression and binding constraint 322
loose stools 029, 068, 084, 107, 115, 138, 146, 175, 228, 231, 272
low fever 060, 271
lumbago 094
lumbar pain 101
lumbar soreness 118, 168, 169, 231, 269, 297
Lung, Spleen and Kidney all deficiencies 313
Lung-cold 353
Lung-dryness 263
Lung-heat 263, 353
Lung Abscess 338
Lung affected by Liver fire 198
Lung and Kidney qi deficiency 188
Lung and Spleen qi deficiency 193, 263
Lung cough 128
Lung deficiency 100, 109, 118, 141, 153
Lung deficiency cold 178
Lung Deficiency and Phlegm-Damp 086

Lung distention 012, 039, 144, 177, 220
Lung excess with heat and panting 178
Lung exhaustion 180
Lung heat depression and blockage 121
Lung Qi Deficiency 144
Lung qi deficiency 045, 169, 173, 189, 197, 202
Lung qi obstruction and counterflow 296
Lung Wilting 338
Lung yang deficiency 125, 126
Lung yin deficiency 250

M

masses 050
measles 290, 314
melancholy 047
middle-cold failing to warm Lung qi 130
mixed asthma 313, 325
muscle soreness 271, 273

N

nasal discharge 128, 149, 259, 325
nasal obstruction 051, 149, 280
nausea 093, 131, 330
night sweats 231, 250
nocturia 168, 322
non-consolidation of the exterior 228

O

obstruction of mixed phlegm and stasis 325
obstruction of the Lung by heat-phlegm 342, 343
oliguria 077, 078
oppression in the chest 258, 276
Original Yang about to Expire 026
orthopnea 323
osteoporosis 321, 332

P

pain 263
pain and distention of the head 259
pain in the throat 252
palpitation 147, 148, 171, 262, 297
Panting 029, 057, 061, 069, 096, 179, 221, 309, 338, 369
panting 013, 016, 020, 070, 074, 092, 099, 144, 170
panting collapse 168, 171
paroxysmal choking cough 127
peptic ulcers 321
perspiration 227, 326, 331
pertusis 060
pharyngeal congestion 060
pharyngodynia 086
pharyngolaryngitis 141
Phlegm-Damp Cough 068
phlegm-damp internally flourishing 105
phlegm-damp internally smoldering 107
Phlegm-Damp Obstructing 084
phlegm-damp obstruction in the middle jiao 084
Phlegm-Drool Congestion 260
Phlegm-excess 099
Phlegm-Fire Assailing the Lung 274
Phlegm-fire assailing the Lung 275
Phlegm-Fluid Retention 013
phlegm-fluid retention 016, 066, 074, 080, 104, 119, 123, 144, 301
phlegm-fluid retetion 072
phlegm-heat 017, 034, 064, 066, 081, 083, 088, 099, 105, 106, 120, 161, 174, 197
phlegm-heat accumulated in the Lung 193
phlegm-heat blocking the Lung 150
phlegm-heat cough 117
Phlegm-Heat Internally Accumulating 080
Phlegm-heat internally accumulating 080
phlegm-heat obstructing the Lung 082, 083, 175
phlegm-heat obstruction in the Lung 204
Phlegm-Heat Retention 209
phlegm panting 295
Phlegm-Stasis Obstruction in the Lung 170
phlegm-stasis stagnating in the Lung 125, 126
phlegm-turbidity obstruction 296
phlegm and fluid retention 284
Phlegm and Fluids Lodged in the Lung 061
phlegm and stasis in the Lung 056
phlegm and stasis obstruction 312
phlegm asthma 295
Phlegm Clouding the Spirit-orifice 023
Phlegm Obstructing the Lung Collaterals 261
phlegm obstruction 118, 149, 172, 190, 196, 219
phlegm stasis and qi obstruction 342, 343
Phlegm Turbidity Assailing the Lung 151
phlegm wheezing 221, 223
physical fatigue 094
pneumonia 123
Pneumoniae gravis 168

polydipsia 020
poor appetite 009, 029, 060, 074, 076, 101, 105, 146, 151, 162, 168, 169, 170, 198, 251, 259
poor digestion 169
postcapillary pulmonary hypertension 166
potential collapse due to qi deficiency 026
pre-capillary pulmonary artery hypertension 165
preference for hot drinks 255, 257
primary pulmonary hypertension 166
productive cough 036
profuse perspiration 335
prolonged expiration 217
puffy limbs 122
Pulmonary Artery Hypertension 165, 209
pulmonary emphysema 074, 077, 089, 092
pulmonary heart disease 092, 138, 164
Pulmonary Hypertension 205, 206
pulmonary tuberculosis 138

Q

qi counterflow 099, 130, 149, 151, 178, 180, 183, 228
qi deficiency 066, 080, 091, 162, 173, 190, 260, 286, 338
qi deficiency and blood stasis 039
qi deficiency of both the Lung and Kidney 144
qi deficiency of both the Lung and Spleen 169, 341
qi deficiency of the Lung, Spleen and Kidney 168, 170
qi deficiency of the Lung and Kidney 038
qi deficiency of the Lung and Spleen 188, 263
Qi Depression 152
qi depression and phlegm obstruction 342
qi stagnation 123, 253

R

rapid breathing 269
reluctance to talk 251, 262
respiratory failure 011, 040, 157
Respiratory Muscle Fatigue 206
respiratory muscle fatigue 160, 193, 219
respiratory tract infection 274
restlessness 023, 102, 121, 183, 258, 276, 336
retention of damp-heat in the interior of the Lung 282
retention of phlegm and fluids in the Lung 280
Retention of Water due to Yang Deficiency 024
right-sided heart failure 040, 166
right cardiomegaly 010
right qi deficiency 145
runny nose 277, 280

S

Senile Asthma 295
shortness of breath 009, 014, 022, 029, 046, 061, 076, 086, 093, 094, 100, 101, 107, 121, 145, 153, 177, 194, 226, 228, 250, 258, 281, 297, 323
shuǐ gǔ 016
Sinking of the Gathering Qi 170
slurred speech 023
sneezing 277, 278, 280, 325
sore throat 300
spasm 268, 291, 314, 331
spasmodic cough 295
Spleen and Kidney dual deficiency 313
Spleen and Lung qi deficiency 195
Spleen and Stomach qi deficiency 322
Spleen cough 128
Spleen deficiency 101,

131, 132, 138
Spleen qi deficiency 162, 169
Spleen yang deficiency 189, 197
spontaneous cold sweats 026
spontaneous perspiration 226, 231, 250, 296
spontaneous sweating 028, 029, 060, 089, 091, 170, 197
stagnated cold transforming into heat 125
stagnated heat in the Lung 064
stagnation and obstruction of the Lung collaterals 271
Stagnation of Phlegm and Stasis 054
stagnation of wind-phlegm 154
Status asthmaticus 247
steaming bones 118
Stomach affecting the Lung 128
Stomach qi deficiency 251, 330
stridor 021, 077, 145, 151, 255, 280, 298, 336
stuffy nose 259
sudden collapse of yang qi 325, 334
sudden desertion of yang qi 312, 320, 326
sweating 017, 019, 022, 029, 102, 111, 120, 131, 142, 145, 153, 168, 171, 178, 181, 223, 228, 258, 266, 320, 330, 334
sweats 230
swelling 110, 258, 259

T

tachypnea 009, 056, 093, 112, 148
taiyang wind stroke 120
tán yǐn 016
taxation fatigue 219
thirst 069, 077, 098, 121, 221, 255, 275, 296, 325
thoracic fluid retention 071
thoracic hyperinflation 217
tidal fever 118, 171
tinnitus 094, 118, 197
tonsillitis 258, 259
trachitis 058
tuberculosis 084
turbid phlegm retention 146
turbid phlegm smoldering in the Lung 087

U

ulcer 174
unconsciousness 012, 016
unsmooth breathing 219
unsmooth defecation 263, 277
upper respiratory infection 156

V

vacuity obesity 322, 326
vertigo 146
vexation 019, 020, 027, 059, 077, 122, 131, 147, 171, 184, 275, 284
vexing heat 150
vexing oppression 296
vexing thirst 225
viscous sweats 027
vomiting 093, 131, 145, 183, 336
vomiting phlegm 330

W

Warm evil transforming into heat, contending with cold fluids 077
Water Flooding into the Flesh and Skin 147
water overflowing to form phlegm 131
weakness 170
weight loss 009
wheezing 009, 086, 099, 103, 114, 149, 181, 217, 274, 290, 295, 296, 335
whooping cough 295
wind-cold 017, 097, 106, 120, 142, 150, 154, 182, 220, 223, 225, 273, 278, 296, 299, 313, 330, 345, 361
wind-cold fettering the

exterior 150, 296
Wind-Cold Fettering the
   Lung 257
wind-cold settling in the
   Lung 258
wind-cold tightening the
   Lung 317
wind-cold to transform
   into heat 156
wind-heat 017, 086, 150,
   161, 273, 300, 345, 346
wind-heat attacking the
   Lung 317
wind-warm 112
wind evils invading the
   Lung 156
Wood and Fire Torturing
   Metal 147

X

xiào 313
xiào bìng 335
xiào chuǎn 276, 280, 290,
   297, 338
xiào chuǎn bìng 314
xiào zhèng 219
xuán yǐn 016, 119
xū chuǎn 168

Y

yang-collapse 326
yang deficiency 072, 126,
   162, 173, 288, 338
yang deficiency affecting
   yin 056
Yang Deficiency and
   Phlegm-Stasis Turning
   to Heat 126
yang deficiency and water
   counterflow 122
yang deficiency and water
   overflowing 138
yang deficiency of the
   Kidney 353
Yang deficiency of the
   Spleen and Kidney 173
Yang Deficiency with
   Water Flooding 092
Yang deficiency with
   water flooding 093

Yang qi deficiency 126
yin and yang deficiency
   322
yin cold internally
   blocking 187
yin deficiency 059, 122,
   175, 301, 338, 346
yin deficiency and
   insufficient blood 131
yin deficiency and
   phlegm-heat 289
yin deficiency of both the
   Lung and Kidney 039
yin deficiency of the Liver
   and Kidney 282
yin deficiency of the Lung
   252
yin deficiency of the Lung
   and Kidney 241, 250,
   345, 353
yin deficiency with heat
   260
yin deficiency with hyperactivity of yang 330
yì yǐn 016

Index by Chinese Medicinals and Formulas

A

ǎi dì chá 038, 328
ài yè 199, 327
Alumen 068, 103, 288, 292, 315
Ān Dá Píng Kǒu Fú Yè 033
Ardisia Japonica 328
Arisaema cum Bile 023, 060, 078, 103, 114, 136, 256, 288, 294, 311
Armeniacae Semen Amarum 032, 038, 039, 043, 053, 062, 069, 071, 073, 077, 083, 098, 120, 124, 130, 134, 137, 142, 149, 150, 159, 180, 188, 198, 222, 225, 239, 245, 252, 256, 257, 266, 274, 278, 288, 291, 293, 301, 310, 311, 314, 321, 327, 334, 339, 341, 347, 351, 358, 364
Armeniacae Semen Amarum Tostum 084
Armenicae Semen Amarum 019, 021, 030

Arsenicum 103, 363, 364
Asarum and Brassicae Albae Semen Plaster 236

B

bǎi bù 039, 049, 060, 134, 150, 159, 202, 318, 327
bǎi bù cǎo 053
bái dòu kòu 068, 328
Bái fán 068, 103, 288, 292, 315
bái guǒ 043, 121, 247, 249, 264, 292, 307, 311, 328, 352, 364
Bái Guǒ Dìng Chuǎn Tāng 284
bái guǒ rén 291, 314, 315
Bái Guǒ Tāng 296
bǎi hé 043, 116, 189, 249, 328
Bǎi Hé Gù Jīn Tāng 147
bái jí 118
bái jiāng cán 112, 258, 339
bài jiàng cǎo 318
bái jiāng chán 259
Bái jiè zǐ 055, 062, 256
Bǎi Líng Jiāo Náng 033, 190

bái máo xià kū cǎo 329
bái qián 053, 065, 136, 187, 278
bái sháo 024, 133, 264, 307, 313, 318, 327, 341, 365
bái shēn 109, 260
bái tóu wēng 163
bái zǎo xiū 357
bái zhǐ 310, 318, 327, 329, 353
Bái zhú 032, 227
bǎi zǐ rén 046, 175
bā jǐ tiān 231, 232, 260, 322, 353, 366
Balanophyllia 048, 302, 366
Bambusae Succus 023
bàn biān lián 328, 330
bǎn lán gēn 060, 136, 191, 342
Bàn xià 062, 065, 071
bàn xià 029, 114, 123, 149, 180, 193, 225, 340
bàn xià qū 085, 103
bàn zhī lián 328
Bǎo Fèi Dìng Chuǎn Chōng Jì 192, 206

Bǎo Fèi Tāng 133
Bǎo Hé Wán 124
Bá Wèi Dì Huáng Wán 133
Bā Wèi Wán 131
bèi mǔ 114, 186, 190
Běi Qí Zhù Shè Yè 162
běi shā shēn 084, 262, 348
běi xìng 310
biē jiǎ 060
bīng láng 098, 350
bīng piàn 237, 359
bì táo gān 049
bò hé 098, 120, 225, 317
Bombyx Batryticatus 060, 112, 258, 307, 339
Borneolum Syntheticum 237, 359
Bǔ Fèi Shèn Fāng 308
Bǔ Fèi Tāng 145, 202, 208
Bǔ Fèi Yì Shèn Gāo 046
Bǔ Fèi Yì Shèn Kē Lì 188, 205
bǔ gǔ zhī 108, 311
Bulbus Allii 120
Bulbus Allii Macrostemi 329
Bulbus Fritillariae 053, 114, 186, 190, 348
Bulbus Fritillariae Cirrhosae 032, 044, 078
Bulbus Fritillariae Powder 310
Bulbus Fritillariae Thunbergii 019, 051, 150

Bulbus Lilii 043, 116, 189, 190, 249, 328, 329
Bǔ Shèn Fáng Chuǎn Piàn 095
Bǔ Shèn Fáng Chuǎn Tāng 366, 373
Bǔ Shèn Yáng Fāng 366
bù zhā yè 049
Bǔ Zhōng Yì Qì Tāng 160, 162, 164, 170, 171
Bǔ Zhōng Yì Qì Wán 139

C

Cacumen Platycladi 328, 348
Cāng ěr zǐ 064
cāng ěr zǐ 259, 353
cāng zhú 022, 067, 105
cǎo hé chē 065
cǎo jué míng 329
Carapax Trionycis 060
Caulis Bambusae in Taeniis 081, 083, 104, 137, 349
Caulis Dendrobii 088
Caulis Perillae 263
cè bǎi yè 328, 348
Chái Chén Jiān 130
chái hú 117, 130, 365
Chāng Pú Yù Jīn Tāng 023
chán sū 329
Chán yī 307
chǎo bái jiè zǐ 121
chǎo bái zhú 091, 344
chǎo biǎn dòu 115
chǎo chén pí 090

chǎo dāng guī 091
chǎo dǎng shēn 344
chǎo dì lóng 354
chǎo èr yá 190
chǎo gān jiāng 131
chǎo lái fú zǐ 093, 121
chǎo niú bàng zǐ 259
chǎo pí pá yè 090, 091
chǎo sū zǐ 052, 093
chǎo tíng lì zǐ 142
chǎo xìng rén 084
chǎo yuǎn zhì 085
chǎo zhǐ qiào 082, 092
Chá yè 098
chén dǎn xīng 288
Chén Xià Liù Jūn Zǐ Tāng 312, 324
chén xiāng 056, 108
chē qián cǎo 090, 192
chē qián zǐ 025, 026, 039, 077, 078
chì sháo 025, 032, 039, 159, 167, 173, 184, 202, 329
Chì Sháo Zhù Shè Yè 167
Chì Shí 128
chì xiāo dòu 279
chuān bèi 032, 270, 288
chuān bèi mò 310
chuān bèi mǔ 044, 078, 084, 134, 186, 246
Chuān Hǔ Níng Zhù Shè Yè 196
chuān jiāo 103
chuān jiāo mù 192
chuān wū 103, 288

chuān xiōng 039, 167, 247
Chuān Xiōng Qín Zhù Shè Yè 167
Chú Yún Zhǐ Ké Tāng 052, 053
cì jí lì 081
Cinnabaris 036
cí shí 032, 102
Colla Corii Asini 077, 118, 133, 281
Colla Cornus Cervi 032, 054, 055, 187, 194
Concha Margaritifera 094
Concha Meretricis seu Cyclinae 020, 078, 087, 262, 302, 315
Concha Ostreae 081, 122, 171, 228, 268
Concha Ostreae Calcinatun 026, 267
Concretio Silicea Bambusae 019, 023
Cordyceps 263, 343
Cordyceps Sinensis 044, 051, 085, 160, 188, 232, 249, 292, 308, 311
Cornu Cervi 054
Cornu Cervi Degelatinatum 187
Cornu Cervi Pantotrichum 319
Cornu Cervi Slice 055, 366
Cornu Naemorhedis 202
Cortex Acanthopanacis 026, 104

Cortex Cinnamomi 024, 032, 054, 063, 102, 118, 121, 153, 187, 231
Cortex Eucommiae 194, 231, 319
Cortex Fraxini 161, 163, 318, 328
Cortex Lycii 087, 098, 118
Cortex Magnoliae 120, 186, 351
Cortex Magnoliae Officinalis 022, 052, 087, 105, 274, 303
Cortex Magnoliae Praeparata 091
Cortex Mori 021, 051, 080, 100, 152, 193, 255, 349
Cortex Mori Praeparata 090
Cortex Moutan 022, 232
Cortex Phellodendri 260
Cortex Radix Gossypii 368
Coulis Phragmitis 019, 188, 312
Cù zhì yuán huā 068
ròu cōng róng 260

D

Dà Bǔ Yuán Jiān 133
dà fù pí 120
dà huáng 023, 114, 161, 173, 225
Daige Powder 114, 116
Dài Gé Sǎn 058, 187, 290
dài gé sǎn 114, 116

Dài Mài Yǎng Fèi Zhǐ Ké Tāng 058
dài zhě shí 153
dà jǐ 119
dàn dòu chǐ 103, 289, 290
dàn gān jiāng 115, 344
dāng guī 032, 060, 115, 163, 250, 318
Dāng Guī Shēng Jiāng Yáng Ròu Tāng 250
Dǎng shēn 029
dǎng shēn 022, 068, 084, 091, 133, 188, 193, 202, 262, 267, 268, 310, 341, 350
dǎn nán xīng 023, 060, 078, 103, 114, 139, 256
dān pí 184, 232, 342
dān shēn 021, 091, 188, 350
Dān Shēn Zhù Shè Yè 167, 173
Dān Zhī Xiāo Yiáo Sǎn 117
Dǎo Tán Tāng 301
Dà Qīng Lóng Tāng 284
dà qīng yè 099
dì biē chóng 239, 344, 358
dì fū zǐ 344
dì gǔ pí 087, 098, 118
Dìng Chuǎn Fāng 360
Dìng Chuǎn Tāng 106, 266, 301, 373
Dí Tán Tāng 343
dì yú 083
dōng chóng xià cǎo 044,

051, 085, 160, 188, 232, 249, 250, 263, 292, 308, 311, 343
dōng guā pí 101, 107
dōng guā zǐ 114
dōng huā 103
duàn lóng gǔ 026
duàn mǔ lì 026, 029, 267
dú huó 199
Dú Shēn Tāng 162
dù zhòng 194, 231, 319

E

é guǎn shí 048, 302, 366
ěi shā shēn 091
ē jiāo 077, 118, 133
ē jiāo zhū 281, 283
Epicarpium Benincasae 101, 107
Èr Chén Tāng 076, 121, 130, 150, 282
Èr Mǔ Níng Sòu Wán 282
èr yá 056
Euphorbiae seu Knoxiae Radix 119
Eupolyphaga seu steleophaga 239, 344, 358
Exocarpium Citri Grandis 093, 114
Exocarpium Citri Rubrum 053, 081, 223
Exocarpium Citri Rubrum Praeparata 050, 084
Exremitas Gecko 286
Exremitas Gecko Pulveratum 102

é zhú 052, 359

F

fǎ bàn xià 021, 087, 101, 137, 190, 256, 257, 270, 301, 310
Fǎ Bàn Xià Hòu Pò Tāng 283
fáng fēng 017, 199, 227, 278, 279, 280, 312, 317, 323, 341, 345, 346, 347, 350, 352, 357
fáng jǐ 173
Fǎ xià 068
fǎ xià 017, 018, 060, 093
Fèi Fù Kāng Hé Jì 039
Fèi Kāng Chōng Jì 190
Fèi Kāng Fāng 187
Fèi Kāng Fāng Jiān Jì 205
Fèi Níng Hé Jì 155, 156
Fèi Qì Zhǒng Yàn Fāng 051
fěi zǐ 288
fēng mì 038, 045
Flos Carthami 024, 039, 186, 271, 344
Flos Carthami Tinctorii 270
Flos Caryophylli 044, 249, 318, 329
Flos Chrysanthemi 081, 083, 158, 346
Flos Daturae 244, 329
Flos Farfarae 087, 103, 193, 222, 272, 280, 354, 364

Flos Farfarae Praeparata 029, 050, 091, 149, 344
Flos Genkwa Praeparata 068
Flos Inulae 049, 099, 143, 153, 346
Flos Lonicerae 060, 069, 090, 098, 112, 317
Flos Lonicerae Japonicae 245, 345, 365
Flos Magnoliae 247, 365
Flos Tussilaginis Farfarae 287
Fluoritum 055, 263
fó ěr cǎo 040, 049, 192
Folium Artemisiae 199, 327
Folium Camelliae Sinensis 098
Folium Eriobotryae 047, 064, 077, 078, 079, 081, 084, 090, 150, 156, 191, 230, 275, 276, 328
Folium Eriobotryae Praeparata 075, 279
Folium Eriobotryae Tostum 091
Folium Ginkgo 192, 368
Folium Ilex 066, 262
Folium Isatidis 099
Folium Microcotis 049
Folium Mori 080, 112, 158, 275, 317, 346
Folium Nelumbinis Nuciferae 076
Folium Perillae 017, 051,

150, 199, 249, 256, 306, 317, 345
Folium Pyrrosiae 368
fó shǒu 044, 190, 322, 328
Fructrus Evodiae 328, 329, 330
Fructus Alpiniae Oxyphyllae 231
Fructus Amomi 056, 231
Fructus Arctii 020, 245
Fructus Arctii Tostum 259
Fructus Aristolochiae 060, 082, 118, 142
Fructus Aurantii 066, 087, 182, 225
Fructus Aurantii Immaturus 023, 137
Fructus Aurantii Tostum 082, 092
Fructus Canarii 118, 141
Fructus Cannabis 075, 082, 175
Fructus Chebulae 098, 140
Fructus Citri Sarcodactylis 044, 190, 249, 322, 328
Fructus Citri Tostum 134
Fructus Cnidii 344
Fructus Corni 026, 056, 102, 188, 231
Fructus Corni Officinalis 281, 311
Fructus Crataegi 068, 190, 263
Fructus Eriobotryae 249
Fructus Forsythiae 053, 112, 191, 202, 243, 259
Fructus Gardeniae 099, 117, 290
Fructus Gleditsiae 056
Fructus Gleditsiae Abnormalis 288, 303, 304
Fructus Gleditsiae Sinensis 055, 246
Fructus Hordei Germinatus 056, 068, 162
Fructus Hordei Vulgaris Germinatus 263
Fructus Jujubae 018, 121, 246, 351
Fructus Kochiae 344
Fructus Ligustri Lucidi 263, 308
Fructus Lycii 044, 134, 164, 194, 304
Fructus Momordicae 044, 249, 252
Fructus Mori 088
Fructus Mume 101, 140, 314
Fructus Nandinae Domesticae 040, 137, 260, 314
Fructus Perillae 021, 121, 171, 301
Fructus Perillae Tostum 052, 093, 143
Fructus Persicae Viride 049
Fructus Piperis Nigri 249
Fructus Mume 137
Fructus Psoraleae 108, 160, 256, 311
Fructus Rosae Laevigatae 231
Fructus Schisandrae Chinensis 018, 100, 183, 281, 308
Fructus Setariae Germinatus 056, 101
Fructus Sophorae Japonicae 082
Fructus Terminaliae 140
Fructus Terminaliae Chebulae 137, 315
Fructus Terminaliae Immaturus 140
Fructus Tribuli 081
Fructus Trichosanthis 019, 051, 118, 263, 365
Fructus Tritici Levis 029
Fructus Viticis 039
Fructus Viticis Negundo 127
Fructus Xanthii 064, 259, 353
Fructus Ziziphi Jujubae 189, 300
Fù Fāng Dān Shēn Zhù Shè Yè 203
Fù Fāng Xiè Bái Jiāo Náng 201
Fù Guì Bā Wèi Wán 105
fú líng 018, 048, 101
Fú Líng Gān Cǎo Tāng 128
fú xiǎo mài 029
fù zǐ 104, 189, 232
Fù Zǐ Lǐ Zhōng Tāng 117

fù zǐ piàn 067

G

Gamoderma Lucidim 164
gān dì lóng 038, 142, 344
gān jiāng 017, 071, 098, 238, 349
gān sōng 328
gān suí 119, 357
gān zhī 038
gǎo běn 327, 329
gāo liáng jiāng 328, 329, 330
gāo lì shēn 171
Gardeniae Praeparatus 063
Gecko 032, 108, 160
gé jiè 044, 250
Gé Jiè Dìng Chuǎn Jiāo Náng 369, 374
Gé Jiè Dìng Chuǎn Wán 233, 354
Glehniae 101, 151
Gnaphalium Affine D.Don 049, 192
gōng láo yè 066, 067, 262
gǒu qǐ 194
gōu téng 024, 328, 329
guā lóu 051, 082
guā lóu pí 063, 107, 156
guā lóu rén 103, 180
guǎng dì lóng 190, 244
Gù Běn Shí Wèi Sǎn 352, 370
Guì Fù Bā Wèi Wán 143
Guì Fù Dì Huáng Tāng 286

Guì Líng Wǔ Wèi Gān Cǎo Tāng 070
Guì Lóng Ké Chuān Níng Jiāo Náng 340
Guì Lóng Níng Jiāo Náng 355
guì zhī 017, 052
Guì Zhī Fú Líng Wán 021, 170
Guì Zhī Jiā Hòu Pò Xìng Rén Tāng 137
Guì Zhī Jiā Hòu Pò Xìng Zǐ Tāng 120, 351, 370
Guì Zhī Tāng 287
gǔ yá 101
Gypsum Fibrosum 019, 038, 283

H

Haematitum 099, 153, 171
hǎi fú shí 262, 289, 291, 314
hǎi gé fěn 103
hǎi mǎ 292, 315
hǎi shí 184
Hǎi Shí Hé Jì 369, 374
hàn fáng jǐ 167, 192
háng sháo 117
Hán Xiào Píng Kǒu Fú Yè 339
Hé Chē Dà Zào Wán 233, 261
hēi fù kuài 115
hēi shān zhī 289
Hēi Xī Dān 304
Heleocharis dulcis 082

Herba Agastachis 094, 327
Herba Agrimoniae 263
Herba Ajugae 329
Herba Aloes 329
Herba Ardisiae Japonicae 038, 328
Herba Artemisiae Annuae 060
Herba Cistanches 056, 231, 260, 366
Herba Cynomorii 231
Herba Elsholtziae Seu Moslae 317
Herba Ephedrae 017, 113, 247, 369
Herba Ephedrae 071
Herba Ephedrae Praeparata 019, 254, 354
Herba Ephedrae Recens 259
Herba Epimedii 054, 291
Herba Eupatorii 231
Herba Euphorbiae Helioscopiae 056, 065
Herba Geranii 049
Herba Gnaphalii 040
Herba Hedyotidis 064
Herba Houttuyniae 019, 064, 194
Herba Houttuyniae Cordatae 112
Herba Inulae 098, 289
Herba Leonuri 025
Herba Lobeliae Chinensis 328
Herba Lycopi 025, 026, 197

Herba Menthae 098, 120, 317
Herba Menthae Haplocalycis 225
Herba Patriniae 318
Herba Plantaginis 090, 192
Herba Sargassi 180
Herba Schizonepetae 051, 158, 278
Herba Scutellariae Barbatae 328
Herba Siegesbeckiae 242, 360
Herba Stemonae 053
Herba Taraxaci 087, 112, 136, 312, 318, 323
Herba Tetrastigmatis Hypoglauci 048
hé táo 044, 249, 286
hē zǐ 098, 137, 180
Hē Zǐ Qīng Dài Wán 184
Hirudo 187, 190
hóng huā 024, 185, 271, 344
hóng shēn 026, 139
hóng zǎo 134, 243, 304
hòu pò 022, 151
Hòu Pò Má Huáng Tāng 283
Hòu Pò Shēng Jiāng Bàn Xià Gān Cǎo Rén Shēn Tāng 122
Hóu Zǎo Sǎn 034
huái jiǎo 082
huái niú xī 285
huái shān 171
huái shān yào 046
huà jú hóng 093, 114
huáng bǎi 260
huáng jīng 163, 190, 318
huáng jiǔ 052
huáng lián 114
Huáng Lóng Shū Chuǎn Tāng 264
huáng qí 022, 091, 304
huáng qín 019, 087, 114, 292, 364
Huáng Qín Jiā Bàn Xià Shēng Jiāng Tāng 128
Huáng Qí Zhù Shè Yè 196, 355, 371
huà shān shēn 036
Huà Shān Shēn Jìn Gāo 036
huá shí 077
Huí Yáng Dìng Chuǎn Tāng 321, 330
Huí Yáng Jiù Jí Tāng 320
hú jiāo 249, 328
hú lú bā 294
huǒ má rén 082, 175
huò xiāng 094, 327
Huó Xuè Huà Yū Fāng 185
Huó Xuè Huà Yū Tāng 343
hú táo 038
hǔ zhàng 021, 023
Hylocereus undatus 251

I

Indigo Naturalis 059, 180

J

Jiā Jiǎn Zé Qī Tāng 065
Jiā Jiǎn Zhǐ Sòu Sǎn 150
jiān bàn xià 049, 348
jiāng cán 060, 307, 353
Jiàng Qì Dìng Chuǎn Kē Lì Chōng Jì 254
Jiàng Qì Dìng Chuǎn Tāng 367, 374
jiàn huā 251
Jiàn Pí Bú Fèi Chōng Jì 172
Jiàn Pí Yì Fèi Chōng Jì 193
jiāo liù qū 259
jiāo mù 249, 314
jiāo sān xiān 101, 263
jiāo shān zhī 063
jiāo shén qū 102
Jiā Wèi Mài Wèi Dì Huáng Tāng 057
Jiā Wèi Xìng Rén Tāng 347, 370
Jiā Wèi Yòu Guī Wán 194, 207
Jié Chuǎn Tāng 049, 260
jié gěng 038, 087, 257
Jié Gěng Tāng 128
Jié Láo Tāng 133
Jǐ Jiāo Lì Huáng Tāng 192, 206
jí lín shēn 244, 250
jīn fèi cǎo 098, 099, 142, 190, 289, 290, 302
Jīng Fáng Bài Dú Sǎn 161
jīng jiè 051, 104, 135, 278, 346

jīng mǐ 046
Jīn Guì Shèn Qì Tāng 148
Jīn Guì Shèn Qì Wán 108, 294, 322
Jīn qiáo mài 039
jīn qiáo mài 064, 090
Jīn Shuǐ Bǎo 034
Jīn Shuǐ Liù Jūn Jiān 061, 131, 146, 343
jīn yīng zǐ 231
jīn yín huā 060, 112, 191, 275
jì yú 044
Jú hóng 053, 064
jú hóng 056, 099, 114, 223
Jú Hóng Tán Ké Gāo 033
jú huā 081, 158, 346
jú luò 049, 259

K

Ké Chuǎn Gù Běn Tāng 350, 370
Ké Chuǎn Hé Jì 039
Ké Chuǎn Kāng Fù Jiāo Náng 094, 095
Ké Chuǎn Kāng Fù Wán 095
Ké Chuǎn Líng 348
Ké Chuǎn Níng Fěn Jì 368
kuǎn dōng huā 087, 159
Kuǎn Xìng Èr Chén Tāng 151
kǔ shēn 328
kǔ xìng rén 045, 155

L

lái fú zǐ 021, 099, 256, 346

Lái Fú Zǐ Sǎn 245, 350, 370
lǎo guàn cǎo 049
Lasiosphaerae seu Calvatia 136, 260
léi gōng téng 363
Lěng Xiào Wán 103, 288
lián mǐ 046, 253
lián qiào 053, 317
lián zǐ 044, 249
Lignum Aquilariae Resinatum 056, 267
Lignum Aquilariae Resinatumare 108
Lignum Santali Albi 291
Líng Guì Zhú Gān Tāng 146
Líng Guì Zhū Gān Tāng 078, 301
líng zhī 164
Liù Ān Jiān 129
liú huáng 237, 359
Liù Jūn Zǐ Tāng 030, 067, 107, 115, 131, 146
Liù Jūn Zǐ Wán 139, 286
Liù Wèi Dì Huáng Tāng 282, 298, 366
Liù Wèi Dì Huáng Wán 057, 133, 164, 322, 348
Liù Wèi Huí Yáng Yǐn 133
Liù Wèi Wán 183
Lǐ Yīn Jiān 131
Lǐ Zhōng Tāng 131, 133
lì zǐ 194
lóng dǎn cǎo 117
lóng gǔ 122, 171
lú gēn 112, 225

lú huì 329
lù jiǎo jiāo 032, 054, 187
lù jiǎo piàn 054, 366
lú jīng 188
Lumbricus 038, 202, 306
luó hàn guǒ 249
lù róng 319

M

Má Bái Hé Jì 246
mǎ bó 136, 139, 260
mǎ dōu líng 060, 082, 368
Magnetitum 032, 102
Má Huáng 330
Má huáng 055, 069
má huáng 017, 100, 245, 350
Má Huáng Fù Zǐ Xì Xīn Tāng 128
má huáng gēn 228, 230
Má Huáng Tāng 122
Má Huáng Yuè Bì Jiā Bàn Xià Tāng 183
mài dōng 044, 151, 186
Mài Luò Níng Zhù Shè Yè 203
mài mén dōng 052, 281, 348, 350
Mài Wèi Dì Huáng Tāng 107, 118, 122, 145
Mài Wèi Dì Huáng Wán 153
mài yá 068, 162
máng guǒ hé 049
Mangifera indicae 049
máng xiāo 175, 246, 348,

354
màn jīng zǐ 039
máo dōng qīng 173
máo gēn 053, 189, 329
mǎ qián zǐ 239
má rén 103
Massa Fermentata 263
Massa Fermentata
　Praeparatus 102
Massa Medicata
　Fermentata 259
Má Xìng Bǔ Fèi Tāng 100
Má Xìng Dū Qì Tāng 102
Má Xìng Èr Sān Tāng 099,
　100
Má Xìng Liù Jūn Zǐ Tāng
　101
Má Xìng Lóu Shí Tāng
　098
Má Xìng Shè Dǎn Tāng
　257
Má Xìng Shí Gān Tāng
　019, 087, 112, 272
Má Xìng Sū Chá Tāng 098
Má Xìng Zhǐ Xiào Sǎn
　358, 372
Mel 038
Měng Shí Gǔn Tán Wán
　175
mián gēn pí 368
mì zhì má huáng 259
mò yú gú fěn 368
mǔ dān pí 102, 159, 232
mǔ jīng zǐ 127
mǔ lì 122, 171, 268
mù xiāng 318, 328

N

nán shā shēn 085, 186, 190
nán tiān zhú zǐ 260
Nǎo Fèi Kāng 201, 208
Natrii Sulfas 175, 246, 348,
　354
Nervilia Fordii 225, 312
niú bàng zǐ 020, 087, 099,
　112, 245
Niú Xī 363
Nodus Nelumbinis
　Rhizomatis 118
nuò dào gēn 228
nǚ zhēn zǐ 263, 308, 318

O

Olumula Cinnamomi 294
Oryza Sativa 046
Os Costaziae 142, 184,
　262, 289, 290, 291, 314
Os Draconis 122, 171
ǒu jié 118

P

pàng dà hǎi 060
pào jiāng 187
pèi lán 231
Pericarpium Arecae 120
Pericarpium Citri Reticulatae
　017, 044, 137, 349
Pericarpium Citri
　Reticulatae Viride 249,
　291, 314
Pericarpium Papaveris
　119, 140

Pericarpium Trichosanthis
　063, 107, 155
Pericarpium Zanthoxyli
　103, 253
Pericarpium Zanthoxyli
　Bungeani 288
Periostracum Cicadae
　136, 158, 258, 307, 353
Phragmites 190
Pí Gōng Fāng 066
Píng Chuǎn Fāng 261
Píng Chuǎn Gù Běn Tāng
　031
Píng Chuǎn Hé Jì 369, 374
Píng Chuǎn Jiàng Qì Tāng
　360
Píng Chuǎn Tāng 346, 370
píng dì mù 340
Píng Gān Xiào Chuǎn
　Tāng 353, 371
Píng Wèi Èr Chén Tāng
　105
Píng Wèi Sǎn 107, 288
pí pa guǒ 249
pí pa yè 047, 079, 230, 275,
　328
pī shí 103, 363
Placenta Hominis 108,
　139, 249, 315
Placenta Hominis
　Pulveratum 115
Placenta Pill 322
Polyporus 079, 093
Poria 018, 073, 131
Pò Xìng Èr Chén Tān 151
Pseudosciaena crocea 252,

311
pú gōng yīng 087, 112, 136, 312, 318, 323
Puilvis Os Sepiella seu Sepiae 368
Pulvis Concha Meretricis seu Cyclinae 059, 139
Pulvis Fellis Suis 202
Pulvis Massa Medicata Fermentata 103
Pulvis Meretricis seu Cyclinae 103

Q

qiāng huó 199, 223
qián hú 053, 106, 155, 328
Qián Hú Tāng 275, 276
Qiān Jīn Mài Mén Dōng Tāng 066
Qiān Mín Tāng 303
qiàn shí 044, 108, 171, 249, 253
Qián Shì Yì Gōng Sǎn 128
Qián Xìng Èr Chén Tāng 151
qīng bàn xià 050, 081, 142
qīng chén pí 127
qīng dài 180
Qīng É Wán 134
Qīng Fèi Dìng Chuǎn Tāng 063
qīng guǒ 141
qīng hāo 060
Qīng Huà Wán 184
Qīng Lóng Tiē 238
qīng pí 249, 291, 314

Qīng Qì Huà Tán Tāng 019
qīng tiān kuí 312, 323
Qīng Yuán Huà Tán Kē Lì 193, 206
Qīng Zào Jiù Fèi Tāng 124, 161
qín jiāo 319
qín pí 161, 318
Qín Yí Hé Jì 365, 373
Qī Wèi Dū Qì Wán 105, 302
Qī Wèi Qīng Fèi Yǐn 114
Qì Zhǒng Fāng 048
quán guā lóu 019, 023, 049, 081, 190, 262
quán xiē 188, 266, 291, 314, 344
Quán Zhēn Yī Qì Tāng 285
Qū Fēng Jiě Jìng Píng Chuǎn Tāng 306
Qū Tán Zhǐ Ké Chōng Jì 033, 068

R

Radix Aucklandiae 318
Radix Achyranthis Bidentatae 285
Radix Aconiti 103, 288
Radix Aconiti Carmichaeli 238
Radix Aconiti Lateralis 104
Radix Adenophorae 085, 186, 190

Radix Angelicae 115, 310
Radix Angelicae Pubescentis 199
Radix Angelicae Sinensis 032, 131, 286, 347
Radix Asparagi 088, 115, 318, 350
Radix Astragali 022, 153, 249, 347
Radix Aucklandiae Lappae 328
Radix Bupleuri 117, 130, 365
Radix Campylotropis Harmsii 038
Radix Codonopsis 022
Radix Codonopsis Lanceolatae 192
Radix Curcumae 021, 051, 118, 150, 322
Radix et Rhizoma Asari 017, 118
Radix et Rhizoma Asteris 032, 127, 274, 301
Radix et Rhizoma Clematidis 223
Radix et Rhizoma Cynanchi Paniculati 346
Radix et Rhizoma Cynanchi Stauntonii 053, 136, 187, 278
Radix et Rhizoma Cynanchi Stauntonii Praeparata 084
Radix et Rhizoma Ephedrae 228, 230

Radix et Rhizoma
    Fagopyri Cyrosi 346
Radix et Rhizoma
    Gentianae 117
Radix et Rhizoma Ginseng
    Rubra 026, 051
Radix et Rhizoma
    Nardostachyos 328
Radix et Rhizoma
    Notoginseng 194
Radix et Rhizoma
    Polygoni Cuspidati 021
Radix et Rhizoma Rhei
    021, 161, 348
Radix et Rhizoma Rhei
    Praeparata 186, 202
Radix et Rhizoma Salviae
    Miltiorrhizae 021, 090,
    162, 246
Radix et Rhizoma
    Sophorae Tonkinensis
    192, 328, 329
Radix Gentianae
    Macrophyllae 319
Radix Ginseng 038, 190,
    352
Radix Ginseng Alba 109,
    260
Radix Ginseng Indici 244
Radix Glehniae 084, 262
Radix Glehniae seu
    Adenophorae 044, 197,
    263
Radix Ilicis Pubescentis
    173
Radix Isatidis 060, 136,
    191, 343
Radix Isatidis seu
    Baphicacanthi 139
Radix Kansui 119, 164,
    198, 237, 357
Radix Morindae
    Officinalis 231
Radix Ophiopogonis 044,
    088, 183, 346
Radix Oryza Sativa 228
Radix Paeoniae 071, 162
Radix Paeoniae Alba 018,
    137, 222
Radix Paeoniae Rubra
    025, 173, 329
Radix Panacis
    Quinquefolii 028, 078
Radix Peucedani 053, 106,
    112, 120, 121, 124, 246,
    328
Radix Physochlainae 036
Radix Platycodonis 038,
    098, 228
Radix Polygalae 138, 189
Radix Polygalae Tostum
    085
Radix Pseudostellariae
    048, 088, 189
Radix Pulsatillae 163
Radix Rehmanniae
    Glutinosae 062, 175,
    197, 342
Radix Rehmanniae
    Glutinosae Praeparata
    054, 187, 194
Radix Rehmanniae
    Praeparata 100, 263
Radix Rehmanniae Recens
    160, 260
Radix Sanguisorbae 082
Radix Saposhnikoviae
    017, 060, 278, 341
Radix Scrophulariae 020,
    078, 151, 175, 260
Radix Scutellariae 031,
    117, 194, 260, 300, 365
Radix Scutellariae
    Baicalensis 304
Radix Sophorae
    Flavescentis 328, 344
Radix Stemonae 039, 134
Radix Stemonae
    Praeparata 084, 348
Radix Stephaniae
    Tetrandrae 167, 173,
    192
Radix Trichosanthis 020,
    088, 276
Radix Tripterygii Wilfordi
    363
Ramulus Cinnamomi 017,
    071, 101, 106, 238, 351
Ramulus Cinnamomi
    Cassiae 071, 173, 223
Ramulus Uncaria 329
Ramulus Uncariae cum
    Uncis 024, 328
rén shēn 038, 059, 229,
    249, 304
Rén Shēn Dìng Chuǎn
    Tāng 285
Rén Shēn Gé Jiè Sǎn 153,

250
Rén Shēn Má Huáng Tāng 285
Retinervs Citri Reticulatae Fructus 049, 259
Rè Xiào Píng Kǒu Fú Yè 340
Rhioma Polygonati 085
Rhioma Polygonati Odorati 262, 345
Rhizhoma Paridis 357
Rhizoma Acori Tatarinowii 023, 264, 329
Rhizoma Alismatis 026, 077, 101
Rhizoma Alismatis Orientalis 298
Rhizoma Alpiniae Officinarum 329
Rhizoma Anemarrhenae 020, 099, 118, 132, 137, 151, 258, 260, 275, 281, 282
Rhizoma Arisaematis Praeparata 143, 197, 223
Rhizoma Atractylodis 022, 067, 105
Rhizoma Atractylodis Macrocephalae 017, 104, 172, 188, 310, 352
Rhizoma Atractylodis Macrocephalae Tostum 091, 344
Rhizoma Belamcandae 020, 161, 222, 365
Rhizoma Bistortae 065

Rhizoma Bletillae 118
Rhizoma Chuanxiong 039, 167, 185, 365
Rhizoma Cimicifugae 317
Rhizoma Coptidis 114
Rhizoma Corydalis 094, 164, 237, 357
Rhizoma Curculiginis 291, 315
Rhizoma Curcumae 052, 237, 359
Rhizoma Cyperi 117, 152
Rhizoma Dioscoreae 030, 102
Rhizoma et Radix Ligustici 327
Rhizoma et Radix Notopterygii 199, 223
Rhizoma Fagopyri Dibotryis 019, 090, 186
Rhizoma Gastrodiae 024
Rhizoma Imperatae 328
Rhizoma Imperatae Cylindricae 053, 189
Rhizoma Metaplexis 064
Rhizoma Metaplexis Japonicae 137, 260
Rhizoma Paridis 065
Rhizoma Phragmitis 112
Rhizoma Phragmitis Communis 225
Rhizoma Phragmitis Communis Recens 090
Rhizoma Pinelliae 029, 071, 106, 142, 238, 367
Rhizoma Pinelliae cum

Succus Bambusae 090
Rhizoma Pinelliae Fermentata 085, 288,103,
Rhizoma Pinelliae Praeparata 050, 081, 093, 142
Rhizoma Pinelliae Praeparatum 021, 269, 292, 301, 353
Rhizoma Pinelliae Preparata 049, 259, 348
Rhizoma Pinelliae Ternatae Praeparata 017, 060, 068
Rhizoma Polygonati 163, 190, 318, 345
Rhizoma Polygonati Odorati 264
Rhizoma Zingiberis 017, 068, 135, 238
Rhizoma Zingiberis Officinalis 032, 256, 284, 300
Rhizoma Zingiberis Praeparatum 187
Rhizoma Zingiberis Recens 038, 052, 066, 283, 312
Rhizoma Zingiberis Tostum 131, 310
Rhododendron Hance 328
Rhododendron Mariae Hance 068
ròu cōng róng 056, 231, 366

ròu guì 024, 054, 063, 153, 231
ròu guì xīn 294

S

Saccharum Granorum 253
sāng bái pí 021, 051, 159
Sāng Bái Pí Tāng 105, 296
Sāng Jú Yǐn 124, 150
sāng shèn zǐ 088
sāng yè 080, 112, 158, 275, 317, 346
Sān Jīn Gāo 289
Sān Niù Tāng 050, 106, 120, 152, 284, 296, 343
sān qī 194
Sān Qī Zhù Shè Yè 167
sān yè qīng 344
Sān Zǐ Yǎng Qīn Tāng 021, 061, 148, 280, 296, 301
Scorpio 188, 266, 291, 314
Secretio Moschi 237, 292, 316, 359
Semen Arecae 098, 350
Semen Benincasae 114
Semen Bilobae 247
Semen Cannabis Sativae 103
Semen Cassiae 329
Semen Coicis 078, 186
Semen Cuscutae 066, 134, 194, 294, 311
Semen Euryales 044, 108, 171, 249, 253
Semen Ginkgo 043, 252, 307
Semen Ginkgo Bilobae 352
Semen Juglandis 044, 249
Semen Juglandis Regiae 032, 108, 122, 353
Semen Lablab Album Tostum 115
Semen Lepidii 254, 262
Semen Lepidii seu Descurainiae 018, 151, 226, 238, 354
Semen Lepidii seu Descurainiae Tostum 142
Semen Nelumbinis 249
Semen Persicae 021, 173, 339, 350
Semen Phaseoli 279
Semen Plantaginis 025, 039, 077
Semen Platycladi 046, 175
Semen Pruni 082, 175
Semen Pruni Armeniacae 369
Semen Raphani 021, 048, 051, 062, 112, 188, 194, 245, 278, 367
SemenRaphani Sativi 350
Semen Raphani Tostum 093, 121, 159
Semen Sinapis Albae 021, 032, 050, 236, 239, 303
Semen Sinapis Albae Tostum 121
Semen Sojae Praeparatum 103, 289
Semen Sterculiae Lychnophorae 060
Semen Strychni 239, 358
Semen Torreyae 288
Semen Trichosanthis 103, 137, 180
Semen Trigonellae 294
Semen Vaccariae 240
Semen Zanthoxyli Bungeani 192, 249, 291, 314
Semen Ziziphi Spinosae 347
shān dòu gēn 192, 328, 329
Shān Ěr Hé Jì 191, 206
sháng yáng jiáo 202
shān hǎi luó 192
shān yào 030, 088, 102, 231
shān yú ròu 153, 232
shān zhū yú 026, 160
sháo yào 162, 351
Sháo Yào Gān Cǎo Tāng 128
shā rén 056, 231
shā shēn 044, 101, 151
shé chuáng zǐ 344
Shé Dǎn Chuān Bèi Yè 034
shè gān 020, 348, 365, 367
Shè Gān Má Huáng Tāng 066, 113, 121, 142, 145, 303, 340
Shēn Bèi Liù Xián Sǎn 078
Shēn Fù Lóng Mǔ Tāng 026

Shēn Fù Tāng 138, 320
shēng bái fán 103
shēng bái guǒ 244
shēng dà huáng 021, 099, 107
shēng dì 062, 067, 197
shēng dì huáng 160, 175, 260, 353
shēng dì yú 082
Shēng Dì Zhù Shè Yè 203, 209
Shēn Gé Sǎn 105, 121
shēn gé sǎn 269
shēng fǎ bàn xià 315
shēng gé qiào 262
shēng huáng qí 187
shēng lí 039
shēng má 317
shēng má huáng 127, 259, 330, 358
Shēng Mài Jiāo Náng 034
Shēng Mài Sǎn 058, 076, 088, 122, 153, 170
Shēng Má Tāng 128
shēng mǔ lì 081, 228
shēng shài shēn 186
shēng shí gāo 019, 098, 264, 291, 344
shēng shú dì huáng 263, 342
shēng zhě shí 099
Shēn Mài Sǎn 026
Shēn Mài Zhù Shè Yè 162, 172
Shèn Qì Wán 078, 122, 164, 231, 286, 301

shén qū mò 103
Shēn Zhě Zhèn Qì Tāng 153, 171
Shé shé cǎo 064
shè xiāng 237, 292, 316, 359
shí chāng pú 023, 186, 264, 329
shí gāo 038, 069, 137
shí hú 088
Shiraia Bambusicola 137, 161
shí wěi 368
Shí Zǎo Tāng 119
Shuāng Huáng Lián Zhēn Fěn Jì 162
shú dì 054, 100, 131, 187, 194
shú fù piàn 192
shú fù zǐ 024, 118, 294
shuǐ zhì 187, 190
shuǐ zhì má huáng 259
shǔ jiāo 288
Sì Chóng Qū Fēng Gù Běn Tāng 344, 370
Sì Jūn Zǐ Tāng 085, 160, 229, 282
Sì Nì Sǎn 124, 152, 343
Sì Nì Tāng 171
Sī Qí Kāng Zhù Shè Yè 196
Sì Wù Tāng 182
Sì Zǐ Píng Chuǎn Tāng 061
Spina Gleditsiae Abnormalis 245, 350

Stalactitum Calcinatun 138
Stamen Nelumbinis 044, 046
Stamen Nelumbinis Nuciferae 253
suān zǎo rén 347
Succus Bambusae 019, 063, 139, 182
Sū Chén Jiǔ Bǎo Tāng 120, 124
sū gěng 263
Sulphur 237, 359
suǒ yáng 231
sū yè 017, 052, 199, 264, 345
sū zǐ 098, 100, 142
Sū Zǐ Jiàng Qì Tāng 061, 089, 121, 324

T

tāi pán 292, 315
Tāi Pán Wán 143, 322
tài zǐ shēn 048, 088, 189
Talcum 077, 079
Tán Ké Jìng 233
Tán Rè Qīng Zhù Shè Yè 202, 208
tán xiāng 291, 314
Táo Hóng Sì Wù Tāng 343
táo rén 021, 039, 069, 184, 339, 350
Tetrastlgma hemsleyanum 344
tiān dōng 088, 115
tiān huā fěn 020, 088, 276

tiān jiāng ké 137, 260
tiān má 024
tiān mén dōng 318, 350
tián xìng rén 044
tiān zhú huáng 019, 023
Tiáo Bǔ Fèi Shèn Jiāo
  Náng 194, 207
Tiáo Wèi Chéng Qì Tāng
  261
Tíng Bèi Jiāo Náng 202
Tíng Lì Dà Zǎo Xiè Fèi
  Tāng 021, 282
Tíng Lì Píng Chuǎn Shuān
  246, 354, 371
tíng lì zǐ 021, 106, 226,
  323, 368
Tōng Sè Kē Lì 186, 201
Tremela 044
tù sī zǐ 066, 134, 194, 294,
  311

V

Venenum Bufonis 329

W

wáng bù liú xíng zǐ 240
wěi jīng 019, 031, 088, 190,
  312, 323
Wěi Jīng Tāng 019, 170
wēi líng xiān 223
Wēn Dǎn Tāng 147, 349,
  370
Wēn Fèi Dìng Chuǎn Tāng
  255
Wēn Fèi Tāng 296
Wǔ Hǔ Tāng 296

wǔ jiā pí 026, 104
Wǔ Líng Sǎn 078
wū méi 101, 141, 291, 314
Wū Méi Wán 128
Wǔ Wèi Yì Gōng Sǎn 286
wǔ wèi zǐ 018, 121, 189,
  274, 367
wǔ zhuǎ lóng 048
wú zhū yú 328, 329, 330
Wǔ Zǐ Dìng Chuǎn Tāng
  278, 280
Wǔ Zǐ Píng Chuǎn Tāng
  170

X

xiān dì sù 082
Xiān Fāng Huó Mìng Yín
  161
xiāng fù 117, 152, 180, 184
xiāng rú 317
Xiāng Shā Liù Jūn Zǐ Tāng
  066, 122, 162, 324
Xiāng Sū Yǐn 124
xiān hè cǎo 263
xiān líng pí 066, 067
xiān lú gēn 090
xiān máo 291, 315, 319
xiān zhú lì 116
Xiān Zhú Lì Kǒu Fú Yè
  033
xiān zhú xīn 044
Xiǎo Chái Hú Tāng 128
Xiǎo Luó Zào Wán 103
Xiǎo Qīng Lóng Jiā Shí
  Gāo Tāng 132, 184
Xiǎo Qīng Lóng Tāng 018,

070, 106, 113, 121, 130,
145, 222, 284, 298, 300,
330, 342
xiǎo yá zào 303
xiè bái 329, 365
Xiè Bái Sǎn 087, 106, 124,
  152
Xiè Tíng Hé Jì 200, 201,
  208
Xìng Bèi Chōng Jì 245
xìng rén 019, 120, 256,
  291, 351, 365
Xìng Rén Hú Táo Sǎn 038
Xìng Rén Tāng 347
Xìng Sū Èr Chén Tāng
  106, 107
Xīn Jiā Xiāng Rú Yǐn 124
Xīn Jiè Gāo 236
xīn yí 247, 327
xióng dǎn fěn 202
Xī qīng guǒ 141
xī qīng guǒ 140, 141
xī xiān cǎo 242, 360
xì xīn 017, 018, 022, 060, 071,
  106, 118, 127, 130, 135, 164,
  198, 283, 310, 369
xī yáng shēn 028, 078, 308
xuán fù huā 049, 050, 079,
  099, 143, 153, 328, 344,
  346
Xuán Mài Gān Jié Jiāo
  Náng 033
xuán shēn 020, 078, 079,
  099, 115, 118, 151, 175,
  260
xú cháng qīng 346

xuě ěr 044
Xuè Fǔ Zhú Yū Tāng 147

Y

Yáng Hé Píng Chuǎn Tāng 054
Yáng Hé Tāng 187, 205, 288
yáng jīn huā 244, 329, 339, 354
yáng ròu 250
Yǎng Yīn Qīng Fèi Zhú Yū Tāng Jiāng 191
yán hú suǒ 164, 237, 239, 357, 358, 359
Yán Nián Zǐ Wǎn Sǎn 085
yá zào 288, 303, 304
yě qiáo mài gēn 346, 348
yě rén shēn 270
Yì Fèi Jiàn Pí Fāng 193, 206
yì mǔ cǎo 025
yīng sù ké 119, 140
yín huā 090
Yín Huáng Hé Jì 069
Yín Qiào Sǎn 112, 150, 161
yín xìng 143
yín yáng huò 054, 308, 315
Yì Qì Fú Zhèng Tāng 195, 207
Yī Yīn Jiān 133
yì yǐ rén 078, 186
yì zhì rén 231
Yòu Guī Wán 133, 261
Yòu Guī Yǐn 133

yuán hú 094
yuán huā 119
yuǎn zhì 138, 143, 189, 302
yú biāo jiāo 252, 311
Yuè Bì Jiā Bàn Xià Tāng 121, 123, 179, 184
Yuè Bì Jiā Fǎ Bàn Xià Tāng 296
Yuè Bì Zhú Xià Tāng 283
yù jīn 021, 051, 118, 150
yù lǐ rén 175
Yú Mián Píng Chuǎn Fāng 368, 374
yún líng 189, 190, 232
Yù Píng Fēng 228
Yù Píng Fēng Sǎn 028, 030, 066, 109, 145, 164, 226, 312, 319, 324
yú xīng cǎo 019, 069
Yú Xīng Cǎo Zhù Shè Yè 162, 196, 203, 204, 209, 355, 371
yù zhú 262, 345

Z

zàng hóng huā 270
zào jiá 103, 246, 354
zào jiǎo 055, 103
Zào Jiá Wán 243, 303
zào jiá zǐ 114
zǎo xiū 065
zé lán 025, 197
zé qī 056, 065
Zé Qī Tāng 065
zé xiè 026, 077, 079, 094, 101, 102, 189, 232, 294,

298, 342
zhè bèi mǔ 019, 051, 081, 107, 119, 136, 150, 188, 190, 258, 348
Zhēn Wǔ Tāng 025, 122, 146
Zhēn Yuán Yǐn 286
zhēn zhū mǔ 094
zhě shí 171
zhì bǎi bù 084, 348
zhì bái qián 084
zhì bàn xià 349
zhì chuān hòu pò 091
zhì dà huáng 186, 192, 202
zhì dōng huā 029
zhì fǎ bàn xià 259
zhì fù zǐ 194, 197, 360
zhì jú hóng 050, 084, 149
Zhǐ Ké Dìng Chuǎn Tāng 050, 149
Zhǐ Ké Píng Chuǎn Gāo 197, 207
Zhǐ Ké Qīng Fèi Kǒu Fú Yè 191, 206
zhì kuǎn dōng 050, 149, 152
zhì má huáng 019, 031, 050, 087, 106, 186, 194, 254, 264, 310
zhī mǔ 118, 132, 137, 151, 260, 275, 281
zhì nán xīng 143, 197, 223
zhì pa yè 075, 279
zhǐ qiào 066, 087, 182, 225, 263, 347, 365
zhì sāng bái pí 090

zhǐ shí 023, 175, 247, 349
Zhǐ Sòu Sǎn 124, 135, 150
zhì sū zǐ 278, 344
Zhǐ Xiào Píng Chuǎn Fāng 373
Zhǐ Xiào Píng Chuǎn Tāng 364
zhì zào jiá 243
zhī zǐ 099
Zhì zǐ wǎn 029
zhì zǐ wǎn 084, 092, 278, 279
Zhū Bèi Dìng Chuǎn Wán 033
zhú huáng 099, 137, 161
zhú lì 019, 063, 099, 137, 139, 182, 259, 340
zhū líng 079, 093
Zhū Líng Tāng 077, 079
zhú lì shuǐ 023
Zhū Pāo Tāng 128
zhú rú 081, 083, 104, 137, 349
zhū shā 036
zhū yá zào jiǎo 245, 350
zǐ hé chē 108, 115, 139, 249, 297, 318, 319, 352
zǐ huā dù juān 038, 068, 328
Zǐ Jīn Dān 103
zǐ jīn niú 328
zǐ quán 065
Zī Shèn Yǎng Fèi Yǐn 115
zǐ shí yīng 055, 263
zǐ sū 158, 249, 256, 257, 317, 327
zǐ sū yè 051, 150
zǐ sū zǐ 051, 151, 186
zǐ wǎn 049, 222, 272, 301
Zuǒ Guī Wán 133, 261

General Index

A

abdominal distention 117, 169, 170, 174, 175, 259, 269
Accumulation of Cold Phlegm 049
accumulation of cold-phlegm in the Lung 055
accumulation of Lung heat 123
accumulation of phlegm-fire 276
Accumulation of Phlegm-Heat 019, 271
Accumulation of Phlegm-Heat 069
Accumulation of Phlegm-Heat Mixed with Stasis 089
Accumulation of phlegm-heat mixed with stasis 090
Accumulation of Phlegm-Stasis 021
Accumulation of Turbid-Phlegm 277

acid regurgitation 251
acral coldness 169
ACTH 366, 373
acute bronchitis 156
Acute respiratory failure 168
adverse rising of Lung qi 219
agitation 019, 147, 171, 178, 184
ǎi dì chá 038
ài yè 199, 327
Alimentary tract hemorrhage 168
allergic asthma 312, 325
Allergic Bronchial Asthma 265
allergic reaction 249
allergic rhinitis 353
Alumen 068, 103, 288, 292, 315
AMP 368, 369
Ān Dá Píng Kǒu Fú Yè 033
anasarca 016
anorexia 138
anoxemic PAH 200
anoxia 144, 187, 195, 320
Anoxic Pulmonary Hypertension 208
anxiety 047
apathy 147
Ardisia Japonica 328
Arisaema cum Bile 023, 060, 078, 103, 114, 136, 256, 288, 294, 311
Armeniacae Semen Amarum 032, 038, 039, 043, 053, 062, 069, 071, 073, 077, 083, 098, 120, 124, 130, 134, 137, 142, 149, 150, 159, 180, 188, 198, 222, 225, 239, 245, 252, 256, 257, 266, 274, 278, 288, 291, 293, 301, 310, 311, 314, 321, 327, 334, 339, 341, 347, 351, 358, 364
Armeniacae Semen Amarum Tostum 084
Armenicae Semen Amarum 019, 021, 030
Arsenicum 103, 363, 364
Asarum and Brassicae Albae Semen Plaster 236
ascites 016

asthmatic bronchitis 060, 100, 254, 297, 298
asthmatic prostration 220
aversion to cold 017, 051, 120, 144, 221, 325
aversion to wind 029, 086

B

bā jǐ tiān 231, 232, 260, 322, 353, 366
Bá Wèi Dì Huáng Wán 133
Bā Wèi Wán 131
bǎi bù 039, 049, 060, 134, 150, 159, 202, 318, 327
bǎi bù cǎo 053
bái dòu kòu 068, 328
bái fán 068, 103, 288, 292, 315
bái guǒ 043, 121, 247, 249, 264, 292, 307, 311, 328, 352, 364
Bái Guǒ Dìng Chuǎn Tāng 284
bái guǒ rén 291, 314, 315
Bái Guǒ Tāng 296
bǎi hé 043, 116, 189, 249, 328
Bǎi Hé Gù Jīn Tāng 147
bái jí 118
bái jiāng cán 112, 258, 339
bài jiàng cǎo 318
bái jiāng chán 259
Bái jiè zǐ 055, 062, 256
Bǎi Lìng Jiāo Náng 033, 190

bái máo xià kū cǎo 329
bái qián 053, 065, 136, 187, 278
bái sháo 024, 133, 264, 307, 313, 318, 327, 341, 365
bái shēn 109, 260
bái tóu wēng 163
bái zǎo xiū 357
bái zhǐ 310, 318, 327, 329, 353
Bái zhú 032, 227
bǎi zǐ rén 046, 175
Balanophyllia 048, 302, 366
BALF 363
Bambusae Succus 023
bàn biān lián 328, 330
bǎn lán gēn 060, 136, 191, 342
bàn xià 029, 114, 123, 149, 180, 193, 225, 340
Bàn xià 062, 065, 071
bàn xià qū 085, 103
bàn zhī lián 328
Bǎo Fèi Dìng Chuǎn Chōng Jì 192, 206
Bǎo Fèi Tāng 133
Bǎo Hé Wán 124
bèi mǔ 114, 186, 190
Běi Qí Zhù Shè Yè 162
běi shā shēn 084, 262, 348
běi xìng 310
belching 117, 251
bì táo gān 049
biē jiǎ 060

bīng láng 098, 350
bīng piàn 237, 359
bitter taste 082, 223
blockage of cold phlegm 032
blockage of damp-phlegm 034
blockage of phlegm-qi 339
blood deficiency 060
bò hé 098, 120, 225, 317
Bombyx Batryticatus 060, 112, 258, 307, 339
Borneolum Syntheticum 237, 359
breathlessness 028, 097
bronchial asthma 050, 322
bronchial spasms 329
bronchiectasis 065
bronchitis 064, 154, 176
Bǔ Fèi Shèn Fāng 308
Bǔ Fèi Tāng 145, 202, 208
Bǔ Fèi Yì Shèn Gāo 046
Bǔ Fèi Yì Shèn Kē Lì 188, 205
bǔ gǔ zhī 108, 311
Bǔ Shèn Dìng Chuǎn Piān 095
Bǔ Shèn Dìng Chuǎn Tāng 366, 373
Bǔ Shèn Yáng Fāng 366
Bǔ Zhōng Yì Qì Tāng 160, 162, 164, 170, 171
Bǔ Zhōng Yì Qì Wán 139
bù zhā yè 049
Bulbus Allii 120

Bulbus Allii Macrostemi 329
Bulbus Fritillariae 053, 114, 186, 190, 348
Bulbus Fritillariae Cirrhosae 032, 044, 078
Bulbus Fritillariae Powder 310
Bulbus Fritillariae Thunbergii 019, 051, 150
Bulbus Lilii 043, 116, 189, 190, 249, 328, 329

C

Cacumen Platycladi 328, 348
cAMP 329, 369, 374
Cāng ěr zǐ 064
cāng ěr zǐ 259, 353
cāng zhú 022, 067, 105
cǎo hé chē 065
cǎo jué míng 329
Carapax Trionycis 060
cardiac arrhythmia 012
cardiac dullness 009
cardiac insufficiency 093
Caulis Bambusae in Taeniis 081, 083, 104, 137, 349
Caulis Dendrobii 088
Caulis Perillae 263
CD3 196
CD4 196, 203
CD4/CD8 196, 203
CD8 196, 203
cè bǎi yè 328, 348

cementation of the blood stasis 343
Chá yè 098
Chái Chén Jiān 130
chái hú 117, 130, 365
chán sū 329
Chán yī 307
Chāng Pú Yù Jīn Tāng 023
chǎo bái jiè zǐ 121
chǎo bái zhú 091, 344
chǎo biǎn dòu 115
chǎo chén pí 090
chǎo dāng guī 091
chǎo dǎng shēn 344
chǎo dì lóng 354
chǎo ěr yá 190
chǎo gān jiāng 131
chǎo lái fú zǐ 093, 121
chǎo niú bàng zǐ 259
chǎo pí pā yè 090, 091
chǎo sū zǐ 052, 093
chǎo tíng lì zǐ 142
chǎo xìng rén 084
chǎo yuǎn zhì 085
chǎo zhǐ qiào 082, 092
Charcot-Leyden crystals 218
chē qián cǎo 090, 192
chē qián zǐ 025, 026, 039, 077, 078
chén dǎn xīng 288
Chén Xià Liù Jūn Zǐ Tāng 312, 324
chén xiāng 056, 108
chest fullness 096
chest hyperinflation 296

chest oppression 009, 051
chest pain 269
chest qi 314
chest stuffiness 096
Chest vexation 082
chì sháo 025, 032, 039, 159, 167, 173, 184, 202, 329
Chì Sháo Zhù Shè Yè 167
Chì Shí 128
chì xiǎo dòu 279
chief herb 227, 229
childhood asthma 288
chills 130, 223, 256
chronic bronchitis 048, 104, 195
Chronic cough 125
chronic cough 125, 158
chronic larygopharyngitis 058
Chronic Obstructive Pulmonary Disease 127, 204
chronic respiratory failure 158
Chú Yún Zhǐ Ké Tāng 052, 053
chuǎn 313
chuān bèi 032, 270, 288
chuān bèi mò 310
chuān bèi mǔ 044, 078, 084, 134, 186, 246
Chuǎn Hǔ Níng Zhù Shè Yè 196
chuān jiāo 103
chuān jiāo mù 192

chuǎn tuō 168, 171, 220
chuān wū 103, 288
chuān xiōng 039, 167, 247
Chuān Xiōng Qín Zhù Shè Yè 167
chuǎn zhèng 012
cì jí lì 081
cí shí 032, 102
Cinnabaris 036
clear qi 169, 173
coagulation and stagnation of phlegm and stasis 054
coarse breathing 096, 098
cold 028, 064
Cold Asthma 221, 255, 256
cold enveloping fire 284
cold evil lying deep in the Lung 342
cold extremities 063
cold fluid retention 071, 125
Cold Fluids Transforming to Heat 125
Cold in the Exterior and Fluid Retention in the Interior 017
Cold in the Lung and Heat in the Diaphragm 265
cold limbs 032, 067, 074, 091, 122, 168, 258, 320, 334
cold panting 045, 066
cold sweats 024
cold-and-heat mixed asthma 313, 326
Cold-excess 097
Cold-Phlegm Obstructing the Lung 268
cold-phlegm trasforming into heat 056
Colla Corii Asini 077, 118, 133, 281
Colla Cornus Cervi 032, 054, 055, 187, 194
coma 016, 147
Concha Margaritifera 094
Concha Meretricis seu Cyclinae 020, 078, 087, 262, 302, 315
Concha Ostreae 081, 122, 171, 228, 268
Concha Ostreae Calcinatun 026, 267
Concretio Silicea Bambusae 019, 023
Concurrent deficiency and excess 263
congested throat 259
constipation 021, 056, 082, 083, 099, 107, 174, 198, 223, 281
Contraction of Wind-Heat 086
COPD 009, 014, 016
cor pulmonale 010
Cordyceps 263, 343
Cordyceps Sinensis 044, 051, 085, 160, 188, 232, 249, 292, 308, 311
Cornu Cervi 054
Cornu Cervi Degelatinatum 187
Cornu Cervi Pantotrichum 319
Cornu Cervi Slice 055, 366
Cornu Naemorhedis 202
Cortex Acanthopanacis 026, 104
Cortex Cinnamomi 024, 032, 054, 063, 102, 118, 121, 153, 187, 231
Cortex Eucommiae 194, 231, 319
Cortex Fraxini 161, 163, 318, 328
Cortex Lycii 087, 098, 118
Cortex Magnoliae 120, 186, 351
Cortex Magnoliae Officinalis 022, 052, 087, 105, 274, 303
Cortex Magnoliae Praeparata 091
Cortex Mori 021, 051, 080, 100, 152, 193, 255, 349
Cortex Mori Praeparata 090
Cortex Moutan 022, 232
Cortex Phellodendri 260
Cortex Radix Gossypii 368
cough-variant asthma 351
Cough-Variant Asthma 370
Coulis Phragmitis 019, 188, 312

counterflow of qi 223, 259
critical asthma 320, 321, 324, 330, 331
Cù zhì yuán huā 068
Cushing's disease 321, 333
cyanosis 013, 017, 021, 024, 147, 165, 170
cyanotic lips 138, 320, 334

D

dōng chóng xià cǎo 044, 051, 085, 160, 188, 232, 249, 250, 263, 292, 308, 311, 343
dōng guā pí 101, 107
dōng guā zǐ 114
dōng huā 103
Dà Bǔ Yuán Jiān 133
dà fù pí 120
dà huáng 023, 114, 161, 173, 225
dà jǐ 119
Dà Qīng Lóng Tāng 284
dà qīng yè 099
Dài Gé Sǎn 058, 187, 290
dài gé sǎn 114, 116
Dài Mài Yǎng Fèi Zhǐ Ké Tāng 058
dài zhě shí 153
Daige Powder 114, 116
dàn dòu chǐ 103, 289, 290
dàn gān jiāng 115, 344
dǎn nán xīng 023, 060, 078, 103, 114, 139, 256
dān pí 184, 232, 342
dān shēn 021, 091, 188, 350
Dān Shēn Zhù Shè Yè 167, 173
Dān Zǐ Xiāo Yiáo Sǎn 117
dāng guī 032, 060, 115, 163, 250, 318
Dāng Guī Shēng Jiāng Yáng Ròu Tāng 250
dǎng shēn 022, 068, 084, 091, 133, 188, 193, 202, 262, 267, 268, 310, 341, 350
Dǎng shēn 029
Dǎo Tán Tāng 301
debilitation 138
debility 152, 153
deficienct asthma 360
deficiency asthma 126, 233, 282, 286
deficiency cold 133, 134
deficiency fullness 177
deficiency of both Kidney yin and Kidney yang 294
Deficiency of Both Qi and Yin 058
deficiency of both the Lung and Kidney 057, 144, 199, 326, 341, 342, 343
deficiency of both the Lung and Spleen 038, 107, 326
Deficiency of both the Lung and Spleen 048
deficiency of both the Spleen and Kidney 326
deficiency of both the Spleen and Stomach 107
Deficiency of Both Yin and Yang 171
deficiency of Kidney qi 044
Deficiency of Kidney yang 263
Deficiency of Kidney yin 263
Deficiency of Lung Qi 028, 226
Deficiency of Spleen Qi 228
deficiency of the Lung 188, 271
Deficiency of the Lung and excess of the Stomach 263
deficiency of the Lung, Spleen and Kidney 185
deficiency of the Spleen and Lung 085
Deficiency of the Spleen and Stomach 013
deficiency panting 034, 036, 168, 177
delirious speech 147, 180
delirium 023
depletion of Kidney essence 296
depletion of Kidney yang 032
depletion of Kidney yin and yang 322

dì biē chóng 239, 344, 358
dì fū zǐ 344
dì gǔ pí 087, 098, 118
Dí Tán Tāng 343
dì yú 083
diarrhea 066, 075, 128, 133, 184, 272
DIC 174
difficult breath 223
difficulty in laying flat 257, 265
Dìng Chuǎn Fāng 360
Dìng Chuǎn Tāng 106, 266, 301, 373
dizziness 074, 076, 081, 083, 094, 197, 297
drowsiness 131
dry cough 064, 154, 183
Dry heat in the Lung 262
dry mouth 017, 020, 027, 077, 082, 088, 105, 122, 146, 147, 150, 170, 223, 249, 251
dry stools 069, 075, 080
dry throat 197, 262
dry tongue 262
dryness of the Lung and Stomach 130
dú huó 199
Dú Shēn Tāng 162
dù zhòng 194, 231, 319
Dual deficiency of both the Lung and Spleen 084
dual deficiency of Lung and Kidney 194

Dual Deficiency of Qi and Yin 074
Dual Deficiency of the Lung and Kidney 031, 057, 145
Dual Deficiency of the Lung and Spleen 029, 084, 146
dual deficiency of the Spleen and Kidney 094, 095, 164
dual infection 332
duàn lóng gǔ 026
duàn mǔ lì 026, 029, 267
dull pain in the epigastrium 251
dyspnea 009, 101, 254, 309

E

é guǎn shí 048, 302, 366
ē jiāo 077, 118, 133
ē jiāo zhū 281, 283
é zhú 052, 359
Earth 228
ECG 089
edema 009, 014, 073, 091, 101, 220, 332
EF-1 368
ěi shā shēn 091
emaciation 044, 147, 168, 169, 228, 263, 281
emphysema 048, 049, 050, 070, 109, 133, 144, 149, 247
endogenous asthma 316
enuresis 128

envoy herb 230
Epicarpium Benincasae 101, 107
èr Chén Tāng 076, 121, 130, 150, 282
èr Mǔ Níng Sòu Wán 282
èr yá 056
Euphorbiae seu Knoxiae Radix 119
Eupolyphaga seu steleophaga 239, 344, 358
excess asthma 360
Excess Heat with Symptoms of Cold 126
excess in the Lung and deficiency in the Kidney 063
excess-heat 134
exhaustion of both qi and yin 028
Exocarpium Citri Grandis 093, 114
Exocarpium Citri Rubrum 053, 081, 223
Exocarpium Citri Rubrum Praeparata 050, 084
exogenous asthma 316
exogenous cold and internal fluid retention 120
expiratory dyspnea 217
Exremitas Gecko 286
Exremitas Gecko Pulveratum 102
exterior cold and interior fluid retention 340

exterior cold and interior heat 034, 299
exterior cold with interior fluids 284
exterior constrainr of wind-cold 280
exterior deficiency 227, 230
exterior heat 098
exteriorly constraint of cold evil 311
external cold and internal heat 312, 325
extrinsic asthma 217

F

fǎ bàn xià 021, 087, 101, 137, 190, 256, 257, 270, 301, 310
Fǎ Bàn Xià Hòu Pò Tāng 283
fā wù 249
fǎ xià 017, 018, 060, 093
Fǎ xià 068
facial edema 128
failure of the clear yang to rise 076
failure of the defensive exterior to consolidate 109
failure of the Kidney to receive qi 109, 281, 294, 304
failure of the Lung qi to diffuse 258
Failure of the Lung to Clear and Depurate 080
failure of the Lung to clear and depurate 080
fáng fēng 017, 199, 227, 278, 279, 280, 312, 317, 323, 341, 345, 346, 347, 350, 352, 357
fáng jǐ 173
fatigue 170
Fèi Fù Kāng Hé Jì 039
Fèi Kāng Chōng Jì 190
Fèi Kāng Fāng 187, 205
Fèi Níng Hé Jì 155, 156
Fèi Qì Zhǒng Yàn Fāng 051
fèi zhàng 012, 039, 220
fěi zǐ 288
fen 237, 241, 298
fēng mì 038, 045
fēng wēn 112
feverish sensation in the chest 263
five emotions 276
flaring nose 179
Flos Carthami 024, 039, 186, 271, 344
Flos Carthami Tinctorii 270
Flos Caryophylli 044, 249, 318, 329
Flos Chrysanthemi 081, 083, 158, 346
Flos Daturae 244, 329
Flos Farfarae 087, 103, 193, 222, 272, 280, 354, 364
Flos Farfarae Praeparata 029, 050, 091, 149, 344
Flos Genkwa Praeparata 068
Flos Inulae 049, 099, 143, 153, 346
Flos Lonicerae 060, 069, 090, 098, 112, 317
Flos Lonicerae Japonicae 245, 345, 365
Flos Magnoliae 247, 353, 365
Flos Tussilaginis Farfarae 287
fluid retention 017, 119, 123, 124, 293, 300
Fluoritum 055, 263
flushed cheeks 027
fó ěr cǎo 040, 049, 192
fó shǒu 044, 190, 322, 328
Folium Artemisiae 199, 327
Folium Camelliae Sinensis 098
Folium Eriobotryae 047, 064, 077, 078, 079, 081, 084, 090, 150, 156, 191, 230, 275, 276, 328
Folium Eriobotryae Praeparata 075, 279
Folium Eriobotryae Tostum 091
Folium Ginkgo 192, 368
Folium Ilex 066, 262
Folium Isatidis 099

Folium Microcotis 049
Folium Mori 080, 112, 158, 275, 317, 346
Folium Nelumbinis Nuciferae 076
Folium Perillae 017, 051, 150, 199, 249, 256, 306, 317, 345
Folium Pyrrosiae 368
food retention 123, 124
forehead sweats 026
frequent urination 077
Fructrus Evodiae 328, 329, 330
Fructus Alpiniae Oxyphyllae 231
Fructus Amomi 056, 231
Fructus Arctii 020, 245
Fructus Arctii Tostum 259
Fructus Aristolochiae 060, 082, 118, 142
Fructus Aurantii 066, 087, 182, 225
Fructus Aurantii Immaturus 023, 137
Fructus Aurantii Tostum 082, 092
Fructus Canarii 118, 141
Fructus Cannabis 075, 082, 175
Fructus Chebulae 098, 140
Fructus Citri Sarcodactylis 044, 190, 249, 322, 328
Fructus Citri Tostum 134
Fructus Cnidii 344
Fructus Corni 026, 056, 102, 188, 231
Fructus Corni Officinalis 281, 311
Fructus Crataegi 068, 190, 263
Fructus Eriobotryae 249
Fructus Forsythiae 053, 112, 191, 202, 243, 259
Fructus Gardeniae 099, 117, 290
Fructus Gleditsiae 056
Fructus Gleditsiae Abnormalis 288, 303, 304
Fructus Gleditsiae Sinensis 055, 246
Fructus Hordei Germinatus 056, 068, 162
Fructus Hordei Vulgaris Germinatus 263
Fructus Jujubae 018, 121, 246, 351
Fructus Kochiae 344
Fructus Ligustri Lucidi 263, 308
Fructus Lycii 044, 134, 164, 194, 304
Fructus Momordicae 044, 249, 252
Fructus Mori 088
Fructus Mume 101, 140, 314
Fructus Mume 137
Fructus Nandinae Domesticae 040, 137, 260, 314
Fructus Perillae 021, 121, 171, 301
Fructus Perillae Tostum 052, 093, 143
Fructus Persicae Viride 049
Fructus Piperis Nigri 249
Fructus Psoraleae 108, 160, 256, 311
Fructus Rosae Laevigatae 231
Fructus Schisandrae Chinensis 018, 100, 183, 281, 308
Fructus Setariae Germinatus 056, 101
Fructus Sophorae Japonicae 082
Fructus Terminaliae 140
Fructus Terminaliae Chebulae 137, 315
Fructus Terminaliae Immaturus 140
Fructus Tribuli 081
Fructus Trichosanthis 019, 051, 118, 263, 365
Fructus Tritici Levis 029
Fructus Viticis 039
Fructus Viticis Negundo 127
Fructus Xanthii 064, 259, 353
Fructus Ziziphi Jujubae 189, 300
Fù Fāng Dān Shēn Zhù Shè Yè 203
Fù Fāng Xiè Bái Jiāo Náng

201
Fù Guì Bā Wèi Wán 105
fú líng 018, 048, 101
Fú Líng Gān Cǎo Tāng 128
fu organs 085, 116, 123, 128, 161, 198, 225, 282
fu qi 174
fú xiǎo mài 029
fù zǐ 104, 189, 232,
Fù Zǐ Lǐ Zhōng Tāng 117
fù zǐ piàn 067
fullness 336
FVC 010, 189

G

gōng láo yè 066, 067, 262
gōu téng 024, 328, 329
Gallbladder cough 128
Gamoderma Lucidim 164
gān dì lóng 038, 142, 344
gān jiāng 017, 071, 098, 238, 349
gān sōng 328
gān suí 119, 357
gān zhī 038
gǎo běn 327, 329
gāo lì shēn 171
gāo liáng jiāng 328, 329, 330
Gardeniae Praeparatus 063
gasping 265, 296, 321, 323, 335
gastric and duodenal ulcer 332
gastric distention 263

gastrointestinal congestion 174
gastrointestinal excess 261
gathering qi 169, 236, 250
gé jiè 044, 250
Gé Jiè Dìng Chuǎn Jiāo Náng 369, 374
Gé Jiè Dìng Chuǎn Wán 233, 354
Gecko 032, 108, 160
general arthralgia 223
general debility 227
general edema 119
general pain 017, 145
general weakness 038
Glehniae 101, 151
GMP 368, 369
Gnaphalium Affine D.Don 049, 192
gǒu qǐ 194
Gù Bén Shí Wèi Sǎn 352, 370
gǔ yá 101
guā lóu 051, 082
guā lóu pí 063, 107, 156
guā lóu rén 103, 180
guǎng dì lóng 190, 244
Guì Fù Bā Wèi Wán 143
Guì Fù Dì Huáng Tāng 286
Guì Líng Wǔ Wèi Gān Cǎo Tāng 070
Guì Lóng Ké Chuān Níng Jiāo Náng 340
Guì Lóng Níng Jiāo Náng

355
guì zhī 017, 052
Guì Zhī Fú Líng Wán 021, 170
Guì Zhī Jiā Hòu Pò Xìng Rén Tāng 137
Guì Zhī Jiā Hòu Pò Xìng Zǐ Tāng 120, 351, 370
Guì Zhī Tāng 287
Gypsum Fibrosum 019, 038, 283

H

hacking cough 262
Haematitum 099, 153, 171
hǎi fú shí 262, 289, 291, 314
hǎi gé fěn 103
hǎi mǎ 292, 315
hǎi shí 184
Hǎi Shí Hé Jì 369, 374
half deficiency and half excess 285
halitosis 019, 099
hàn fáng jǐ 167, 192
Hán Xiào Píng Kǒu Fú Yè 339
háng sháo 117
Hé Chē Dà Zào Wán 233, 261
hé táo 044, 249, 286
hē zǐ 098, 137, 180
Hē Zǐ Qīng Dài Wán 184
headache 073, 081, 221, 255, 271
Heart cough 128

heart failure 009, 012, 157, 174, 331
heat asthma 234, 295, 302, 307, 340
heat damaging the Lung yin 088
heat evil attacking the Lung 312
heat in the Large Intestine causing fluid exhaustion 082
heat panting 260, 264
heat phlegm 315
Heat-excess 098
heavy sweating on the head 303
hēi fù kuài 115
hēi shān zhī 289
Hēi Xī Dān 304
Heleocharis dulcis 082
hemoptysis 198
hemorrhoids 082
hepatomegaly 009
Herba Agastachis 094, 327
Herba Agrimoniae 263
Herba Ajugae 329
Herba Aloes 329
Herba Ardisiae Japonicae 038, 328
Herba Artemisiae Annuae 060
Herba Cistanches 056, 231, 260, 366
Herba Cynomorii 231
Herba Elsholtziae Seu Moslae 317
Herba Ephedrae 017, 113, 247, 369
Herba Ephedrae 071
Herba Ephedrae Praeparata 019, 254, 354
Herba Ephedrae Recens 259
Herba Epimedii 054, 291
Herba Eupatorii 231
Herba Euphorbiae Helioscopiae 056, 065
Herba Geranii 049
Herba Gnaphalii 040
Herba Hedyotidis 064
Herba Houttuyniae 019, 064, 194
Herba Houttuyniae Cordatae 112
Herba Inulae 098, 289
Herba Leonuri 025
Herba Lobeliae Chinensis 328
Herba Lycopi 025, 026, 197
Herba Menthae 098, 120, 317
Herba Menthae Haplocalycis 225
Herba Patriniae 318
Herba Plantaginis 090, 192
Herba Sargassi 180
Herba Schizonepetae 051, 158, 278
Herba Scutellariae Barbatae 328
Herba Siegesbeckiae 242, 360
Herba Stemonae 053
Herba Taraxaci 087, 112, 136, 312, 318, 323
Herba Tetrastigmatis Hypoglauci 048
hiccup 145
Hirudo 187, 190
hoarse breathing 296
hóng huā 024, 185, 271, 344
hóng shēn 026, 139
hóng zǎo 134, 243, 304
hormone-dependent asthma 321
hòu pò 022, 151
Hòu Pò Má Huáng Tāng 283
Hòu Pò Shēng Jiāng Bàn Xià Gān Cǎo Rén Shēn Tāng 122
Hóu Zǎo Sǎn 034
HPA axis 366
hú jiāo 249, 328
hú lú bā 294
hú táo 038
hǔ zhàng 021, 023
huà jú hóng 093, 114
huà shān shēn 036
Huà Shān Shēn Jìn Gāo 036
huá shí 077
huái jiǎo 082
huái niú xī 285
huái shān 171
huái shān yào 046

huáng bǎi 260
huáng jīng 163, 190, 318
huáng jiǔ 052
huáng lián 114
Huáng Lóng Shū Chuǎn Tāng 264
huáng qí 022, 091, 304
Huáng Qí Zhù Shè Yè 196, 355, 371
huáng qín 019, 087, 114, 292, 364
Huáng Qín Jiā Bàn Xià Shēng Jiāng Tāng 128
Huí Yáng Dìng Chuǎn Tāng 321, 330
Huí Yáng Jiù Jí Tāng 320
huǒ má rén 082, 175
huò xiāng 094, 327
Huó Xuè Huà Yū Fāng 185
Huó Xuè Huà Yū Tāng 343
Hylocereus undatus 251
hyperactivity of Liver-yang 081, 083
hypercapnia 010, 157
hyperhidrosis 266
hyperinflation of the chest 323
hypochondriac pain 117, 259
hypoxemia 009, 010, 157
hypoxia 165, 174, 204, 334

I

IgE 218, 367, 374

IL-12 367
IL-2 374
IL-4 367
IL-6 364
Indigo Naturalis 059, 180
infectious asthma 312, 325
Insecurity of the lower origin 281
insomnia 036, 077, 093, 147, 171
insufficiency of both the Lung and Kidney 269
interior obstruction of turbid phlegm 258
Interior retention of cold fluids 262
Internal accumulation of phlegm-heat 261
internal fluid retention 287
internal heat with yin deficiency 067
Internal Obstruction of Turbid Phlegm 144
internal obstruction of turbid phlegm 144
internal retention of latent phlegm 219
intolerance of cold 032, 063, 138, 168, 169, 231, 263, 271, 273
intolerance of wind 153, 226
intrinsic asthma 217
Invasion of Wind-Cold 050

itching 059, 127, 136, 154, 252
itching and stridor in the throat 258
itching throat 053, 147

J

Jǐ Jiāo Lì Huáng Tāng 192, 206
jí lín shēn 244, 250
jì yú 044
Jiā Jiǎn Zé Qī Tāng 065
Jiā Jiǎn Zhǐ Sòu Sǎn 150
Jiā Wèi Mài Wèi Dì Huáng Tāng 057
Jiā Wèi Xìng Rén Tāng 347, 370
Jiā Wèi Yòu Guī Wán 194, 207
jiāng bàn xià 049, 348
jiàn huā 251
Jiàn Pí Bú Fèi Chōng Jì 172
Jiàn Pí Yì Fèi Chōng Jì 193
jiāng cán 060, 307, 353
Jiàng Qì Dìng Chuǎn Kē Lì Chōng Jì 254
Jiàng Qì Dìng Chuǎn Tāng 367, 374
jiāo liù qū 259
jiāo mù 249, 314
jiāo sān xiān 101, 263
jiāo shān zhī 063
jiāo shén qū 102
Jié Chuǎn Tāng 049, 260
jié gěng 038, 087, 257

Jié Gěng Tāng 128
Jié Láo Tāng 133
jīn fèi cǎo 098, 099, 142, 190, 289, 290, 302
Jīn Guì Shèn Qì Tāng 148
Jīn Guì Shèn Qì Wán 108, 294, 322
Jīn qiáo mài 039
jīn qiáo mài 064, 090
Jīn Shuǐ Bǎo 034
Jīn Shuǐ Liù Jūn Jiān 061, 131, 146, 343
jīn yín huā 060, 112, 191, 275
jīn yīng zǐ 231
Jīng Fáng Bài Dú Sǎn 161
jīng jiè 051, 104, 135, 278, 346
jīng mǐ 046
Jú hóng 053, 064
jú hóng 056, 099, 114, 223
Jú Hóng Tán Ké Gāo 033
jú huā 081, 158, 346
jú luò 049, 259

K

Ké Chuǎn Gù Běn Tāng 350, 370
Ké Chuǎn Hé Jì 039
Ké Chuǎn Kāng Fù Jiāo Náng 094, 095
Ké Chuǎn Kāng Fù Wán 095
Ké Chuǎn Líng 348
Ké Chuǎn Níng Fěn Jì 368
Kidney asthma 296

Kidney cough 128
Kidney deficiency and exterior excess 263
Kidney deficiency and fluid exhaustion 183
Kidney Deficiency Failing to Receive Qi 061
Kidney essence depletion 219
Kidney qi deficiency 122, 169, 299
Kidney yang deficiency 153, 189
Kidney yin deficiency 118, 153
knee weakness 297
kǔ shēn 328
kǔ xìng rén 045, 155
kuǎn dōng huā 087, 159
Kuǎn Xìng èr Chén Tāng 151

L

lái fú zǐ 021, 099, 256, 346
Lái Fú Zǐ Sǎn 245, 350, 370
lǎo guàn cǎo 049
laryngeal edema 114
Lasiosphaerae seu Calvatia 136, 260
lassitude 107, 151, 231
Latent cold fluids upwardly invading the Lung 070
léi gōng téng 363
Lěng Xiào Wán 103, 288
lethargy 016
leukocytosis 274

Lǐ Yīn Jiān 131
Lǐ Zhōng Tāng 131, 133
lì zǐ 194
lián mǐ 046, 253
lián qiào 053, 317
lián zǐ 044, 249
Lignum Aquilariae Resinatum 056, 267
Lignum Aquilariae Resinatumare 108
Lignum Santali Albi 291
Líng Guì Zhū Gān Tāng 078, 301
Líng Guì Zhú Gān Tāng 146
líng zhī 164
lip cyanosis 052
listlessness 107
Liù Ān Jiān 129
liú huáng 237, 359
Liù Jūn Zǐ Tāng 030, 067, 107, 115, 131, 146
Liù Jūn Zǐ Wán 139, 286
Liù Wèi Dì Huáng Tāng 282, 298, 366
Liù Wèi Dì Huáng Wán 057, 133, 164, 322, 348
Liù Wèi Huí Yáng Yǐn 133
Liù Wèi Wán 183
Liver cough 128
Liver qi depression and binding constraint 322
Liver-wind internally stirring 024
lóng dǎn cǎo 117
lóng gǔ 122, 171

loose stools 029, 068, 084, 107, 115, 138, 146, 175, 228, 231, 272
low fever 060, 271
lú gēn 112, 225
lú huì 329
lù jiǎo jiāo 032, 054, 187
lù jiǎo piàn 054, 366
lú jīng 188
lù róng 319
lumbago 094
lumbar pain 101
lumbar soreness 118, 168, 169, 231, 269, 297
Lumbricus 038, 202, 306
Lung Abscess 338
Lung affected by Liver fire 198
Lung and Kidney qi deficiency 188
Lung and Spleen qi deficiency 193, 263
Lung cough 128
Lung deficiency 100, 109, 118, 141, 153
Lung Deficiency and Phlegm-Damp 086
Lung deficiency cold 178
Lung distention 012, 039, 144, 177, 220
Lung excess with heat and panting 178
Lung exhaustion 180
Lung heat depression and blockage 121
Lung qi deficiency 045, 169, 173, 189, 197, 202
Lung Qi Deficiency 144
Lung qi obstruction and counterflow 296
Lung Wilting 338
Lung yang deficiency 125, 126
Lung yin deficiency 250
Lung, Spleen and Kidney all deficiencies 313
Lung-cold 353
Lung-dryness 263
Lung-heat 263, 353
luó hàn guǒ 249

M

Má Bái Hé Jì 246
mǎ bó 136, 139, 260
mǎ dōu líng 060, 082, 368
má huáng 017, 100, 245, 350
Má huáng 055, 069
Má Huáng 330
Má Huáng Fù Zǐ Xì Xīn Tāng 128
má huáng gēn 228, 230
Má Huáng Tāng 122
Má Huáng Yuè Bì Jiā Bàn Xià Tāng 183
mǎ qián zǐ 239
má rén 103
Má Xìng Bǔ Fèi Tāng 100
Má Xìng Dū Qì Tāng 102
Má Xìng Èr Sān Tāng 099, 100
Má Xìng Liù Jūn Zǐ Tāng 101
Má Xìng Lóu Shí Tāng 098
Má Xìng Shè Dǎn Tāng 257
Má Xìng Shí Gān Tāng 019, 087, 112, 272
Má Xìng Sū Chá Tāng 098
Má Xìng Zhǐ Xiào Sǎn 358, 372
Magnetitum 032, 102
mài dōng 044, 151, 186
Mài Luò Níng Zhù Shè Yè 203
mài mén dōng 052, 281, 348, 350
Mài Wèi Dì Huáng Tāng 107, 118, 122, 145
Mài Wèi Dì Huáng Wán 153
mài yá 068, 162
màn jīng zǐ 039
máng guǒ hé 049
máng xiāo 175, 246, 348, 354
Mangifera indicae 049
máo dōng qīng 173
máo gēn 053, 189, 329
masses 050
Massa Fermentata 263
Massa Fermentata Praeparatus 102
Massa Medicata Fermentata 259
measles 290, 314
Mel 038
melancholy 047

Měng Shí Gǔn Tán Wán 175
mì zhì má huáng 259
mián gēn pí 368
middle jiao 020, 064, 133, 135, 146, 230, 283, 324
middle qi 117, 325
middle-cold failing to warm Lung qi 130
mixed asthma 313, 325
mò yú gú fěn 368
mǔ dān pí 102, 159, 232
mǔ jīng zǐ 127
mǔ lì 122, 171, 268
mù xiāng 318, 328
muscle soreness 271, 273

N

nán shā shēn 085, 186, 190
nán tiān zhú zǐ 260
Nǎo Fèi Kāng 201, 208
nasal discharge 128, 149, 259, 325
nasal obstruction 051, 149, 280
Natrii Sulfas 175, 246, 348, 354
nausea 093, 131, 330
Nervilia Fordii 225, 312
night sweats 231, 250
niú bàng zǐ 020, 087, 099, 112, 245
Niú Xī 363
nocturia 168, 322
Nodus Nelumbinis Rhizomatis 118
non-consolidation of the exterior 228
nǚ zhēn zǐ 263, 308, 318
nuò dāo gēn 228

O

obstruction of mixed phlegm and stasis 325
obstruction of the Lung by heat-phlegm 342, 343
oliguria 077, 078
Olumula Cinnamomi 294
oppression in the chest 258, 276
original essence 132
original qi 054
Original Yang about to Expire 026
orthopnea 323
Oryza Sativa 046
Os Costaziae 142, 184, 262, 289, 290, 291, 314
Os Draconis 122, 171
osteoporosis 321, 332
ǒu jié 118

P

pain 263
pain and distention of the head 259
pain in the throat 252
palpitation 147, 148, 171, 262, 297
pàng dà hǎi 060
panting 013, 016, 020, 070, 074, 092, 099, 144, 170
Panting 029, 057, 061, 069, 096, 179, 221, 309, 338, 369
panting 266
panting collapse 168, 171
pào jiāng 187
paroxysmal choking cough 127
pèi lán 231
peptic ulcers 321
Pericarpium Arecae 120
Pericarpium Citri Reticulatae 017, 044, 137, 349
Pericarpium Citri Reticulatae Viride 249, 291, 314
Pericarpium Papaveris 119, 140
Pericarpium Trichosanthis 063, 107, 155
Pericarpium Zanthoxyli 103, 253
Pericarpium Zanthoxyli Bungeani 288
Periostracum Cicadae 136, 158, 258, 307, 353
perspiration 227, 326, 331
pertusis 060
pharyngeal congestion 060
pharyngodynia 086
pharyngolaryngitis 141
phlegm and fluid retention 284
Phlegm and Fluids

Lodged in the Lung 061
phlegm and stasis in the Lung 056
phlegm and stasis obstruction 312
phlegm asthma 295
Phlegm Clouding the Spirit-orifice 023
phlegm-heat obstruction in the Lung 204
Phlegm Obstructing the Lung Collaterals 261
phlegm obstruction 118, 149, 172, 190, 196, 219
phlegm stasis and qi obstruction 342, 343
Phlegm Turbidity Assailing the Lung 151
phlegm wheezing 221, 223
Phlegm-Damp Cough 068
phlegm-damp internally flourishing 105
phlegm-damp internally smoldering 107
Phlegm-Damp Obstructing 084
phlegm-damp obstruction in the middle jiao 084
Phlegm-Drool Congestion 260
Phlegm-excess 099
Phlegm-Fire Assailing the Lung 274
Phlegm-fire assailing the Lung 275
Phlegm-Fluid Retention 013
phlegm-fluid retention 016, 066, 074, 080, 104, 119, 144, 301
phlegm-fluid retetion 072
phlegm-heat 017, 034, 064, 066, 081, 083, 088, 099, 105, 106, 120, 161, 197
phlegm-heat accumulated in the Lung 193
phlegm-heat blocking the Lung 150
phlegm-heat cough 117
Phlegm-Heat Internally Accumulating 080
Phlegm-heat internally accumulating 080
phlegm-heat obstructing the Lung 082, 083, 175
phlegm panting 295
phlegm-stasis in the Lung 125, 126
Phlegm-Stasis Obstruction in the Lung 170
phlegm-stasis stagnating in the Lung 125, 126
phlegm-turbidity obstruction 296
Phragmites 190
physical fatigue 094
Pí Gōng Fāng 066
pí pa guǒ 249
pí pa yè 047, 079, 230, 275, 328
pī shí 103, 363
Píng Chuǎn Fāng 261
Píng Chuǎn Gù Běn Tāng 031
Píng Chuǎn Hé Jì 369, 374
Píng Chuǎn Jiàng Qì Tāng 360
Píng Chuǎn Tāng 346, 370
píng dì mù 340
Píng Gān Xiào Chuǎn Tāng 353, 371
Píng Wèi Er Chén Tāng 105
Píng Wèi Sǎn 107, 288
Placenta Hominis 108, 139, 249, 315
Placenta Hominis Pulveratum 115
Placenta Pill 322
pneumonia 123
Pneumoniae gravis 168
Pò Xìng èr Chén Tān 151
polydipsia 020
Polyporus 079, 093
poor appetite 009, 029, 060, 074, 076, 101, 105, 146, 151, 162, 168, 169, 170, 198, 251, 259
poor digestion 169
Poria 018, 073, 131
postcapillary pulmonary hypertension 166
potential collapse due to qi deficiency 026
pre-capillary pulmonary

artery hypertension 165
preference for hot drinks 255, 257
primary pulmonary hypertension 166
productive cough 036
profuse perspiration 335
prolonged expiration 217
Pseudosciaena crocea 252, 311
pú gōng yīng 087, 112, 136, 312, 318, 323
puffy limbs 122
Puilvis Os Sepiella seu Sepiae 368
Pulmonary Artery Hypertension 165, 209
pulmonary emphysema 074, 077, 089, 092
pulmonary heart disease 092, 138, 164
Pulmonary Hypertension 205, 206
pulmonary tuberculosis 138
Pulvis Concha Meretricis seu Cyclinae 059, 139
Pulvis Fellis Suis 202
Pulvis Massa Medicata Fermentata 103
Pulvis Meretricis seu Cyclinae 103

Q

qi counterflow 099, 130, 149, 151, 178, 180, 183, 228
qi deficiency 066, 080, 091, 162, 173, 190, 260, 286, 338
qi deficiency and blood stasis 039
qi deficiency of both the Lung and Kidney 144
qi deficiency of both the Lung and Spleen 169, 341
qi deficiency of the Lung and Kidney 038
qi deficiency of the Lung and Spleen 188, 263
qi deficiency of the Lung, Spleen and Kidney 168, 170
Qi Depression 152
qi depression and phlegm obstruction 342
qi stagnation 123, 253
Qī Wèi Dū Qì Wán 105, 302
Qī Wèi Qīng Fèi Yǐn 114
Qì Zhǒng Fāng 048
qián hú 053, 106, 155, 328
Qián Hú Tāng 275, 276
Qiān Jīn Mài Mén Dōng Tāng 066
Qiān Mín Tāng 303
qiàn shí 044, 108, 171, 249, 253
Qián Shì Yì Gōng Sǎn 128
Qián Xìng èr Chén Tāng 151
qiāng huó 199, 223
qín jiāo 319
qín pí 161, 318
Qín Yí Hé Jì 365, 373
qīng bàn xià 050, 081, 142
qīng chén pí 127
qīng dài 180
Qīng E Wán 134
Qīng Fèi Dìng Chuǎn Tāng 063
qīng guǒ 141
qīng hāo 060
Qīng Huà Wán 184
Qīng Lóng Tiē 238
qīng pí 249, 291, 314
Qīng Qì Huà Tán Tāng 019
qīng tiān kuí 312, 323
Qīng Yuán Huà Tán Kē Lì 193, 206
Qīng Zào Jiù Fèi Tāng 124, 161
Qū Fēng Jiě Jìng Píng Chuǎn Tāng 306
Qū Tán Zhǐ Ké Chōng Jì 033, 068
quán guā lóu 019, 023, 049, 081, 190, 262
quán xiē 188, 266, 291, 314, 344
Quán Zhēn Yī Qì Tāng 285

R

Radix Aucklandiae 318

General Index

Radix Achyranthis Bidentatae 285
Radix Aconiti 103, 288
Radix Aconiti Carmichaeli 238
Radix Aconiti Lateralis 104
Radix Adenophorae 085, 186, 190
Radix Angelicae 115, 310
Radix Angelicae Pubescentis 199
Radix Angelicae Sinensis 032, 131, 286, 347
Radix Asparagi 088, 115, 318, 350
Radix Astragali 022, 153, 249, 347
Radix Aucklandiae Lappae 328
Radix Bupleuri 117, 130, 365
Radix Campylotropis Harmsii 038
Radix Codonopsis 022
Radix Codonopsis Lanceolatae 192
Radix Curcumae 021, 051, 118, 150, 322
Radix et Rhizoma Asari 017, 118
Radix et Rhizoma Asteris 032, 127, 274, 301
Radix et Rhizoma Clematidis 223
Radix et Rhizoma Cynanchi Paniculati 346
Radix et Rhizoma Cynanchi Stauntonii 053, 136, 187, 278
Radix et Rhizoma Cynanchi Stauntonii Praeparata 084
Radix et Rhizoma Ephedrae 228, 230
Radix et Rhizoma Fagopyri Cyrosi 346
Radix et Rhizoma Gentianae 117
Radix et Rhizoma Ginseng Rubra 026, 051
Radix et Rhizoma Nardostachyos 328
Radix et Rhizoma Notoginseng 194
Radix et Rhizoma Polygoni Cuspidati 021
Radix et Rhizoma Rhei 021, 161, 348
Radix et Rhizoma Rhei Praeparata 186, 202
Radix et Rhizoma Salviae Miltiorrhizae 021, 090, 162, 246
Radix et Rhizoma Sophorae Tonkinensis 192, 328, 329
Radix Gentianae Macrophyllae 319
Radix Ginseng 038, 190, 352
Radix Ginseng Alba 109, 260
Radix Ginseng Indici 244
Radix Glehniae 084, 262
Radix Glehniae seu Adenophorae 044, 197, 263
Radix Ilicis Pubescentis 173
Radix Isatidis 060, 136, 191, 343
Radix Isatidis seu Baphicacanthi 139
Radix Kansui 119, 164, 198, 237, 357
Radix Morindae Officinalis 231
Radix Ophiopogonis 044, 088, 183, 346
Radix Oryza Sativa 228
Radix Paeoniae 071, 162
Radix Paeoniae Alba 018, 137, 222
Radix Paeoniae Rubra 025, 173, 329
Radix Panacis Quinquefolii 028, 078
Radix Peucedani 053, 106, 112, 120, 121, 124, 246, 328
Radix Physochlainae 036
Radix Platycodonis 038, 098, 228
Radix Polygalae 138, 189
Radix Polygalae Tostum 085
Radix Pseudostellariae

048, 088, 189
Radix Pulsatillae 163
Radix Rehmanniae
    Glutinosae 062, 175,
    197, 342
Radix Rehmanniae
    Glutinosae Praeparata
    054, 187, 194
Radix Rehmanniae
    Praeparata 100, 263
Radix Rehmanniae Recens
    160, 260
Radix Sanguisorbae 082
Radix Saposhnikoviae
    017, 060, 278, 341
Radix Scrophulariae 020,
    078, 151, 175, 260
Radix Scutellariae 031,
    117, 194, 260, 300, 365
Radix Scutellariae
    Baicalensis 304
Radix Sophorae Flavescentis
    328, 344
Radix Stemonae 039, 134
Radix Stemonae Praeparata
    084, 348
Radix Stephaniae
    Tetrandrae 167, 173, 192
Radix Trichosanthis 020,
    088, 276
Radix Tripterygii Wilfordi
    363
Ramulus Cinnamomi 017,
    071, 238, 351
Ramulus Cinnamomi 101,
    106

Ramulus Cinnamomi
    Cassiae 071, 173, 223
Ramulus Uncaria 329
Ramulus Uncariae cum
    Uncis 024, 328
rapid breathing 269
Rè Xiào Píng Kǒu Fú Yè
    340
reluctance to talk 251, 262
rén shēn 038, 059, 229,
    249, 304
Rén Shēn Dìng Chuān
    Tāng 285
Rén Shēn Gé Jiè Sǎn 153,
    250
Rén Shēn Má Huáng Tāng
    285
respiratory failure 011,
    040, 157
respiratory muscle fatigue
    160, 193, 219
Respiratory Muscle
    Fatigue 206
respiratory tract infection
    274
restlessness 023, 102, 121,
    183, 258, 276, 336
retention of damp-heat in
    the interior of the Lung
    282
retention of phlegm and
    fluids in the Lung 280
Retention of Water due to
    Yang Deficiency 024
Retinervs Citri Reticulatae
    Fructus 049, 259

Rhioma Polygonati 085
Rhioma Polygonati
    Odorati 262, 345
Rhizhoma Paridis 357
Rhizoma Acori Tatarinowii
    023, 264, 329
Rhizoma Alismatis 026,
    077, 101
Rhizoma Alismatis
    Orientalis 298
Rhizoma Alpiniae
    Officinarum 329
Rhizoma Anemarrhenae
    020, 099, 118, 132, 137,
    151, 258, 260, 275, 281,
    282
Rhizoma Arisaematis
    Praeparata 143, 197,
    223
Rhizoma Atractylodis
    022, 067, 105
Rhizoma Atractylodis
    Macrocephalae 017,
    104, 172, 188, 310, 352
Rhizoma Atractylodis
    Macrocephalae Tostum
    091, 344
Rhizoma Belamcandae
    020, 161, 222, 365
Rhizoma Bistortae 065
Rhizoma Bletillae 118
Rhizoma Chuanxiong
    039, 167, 185, 365
Rhizoma Cimicifugae 317
Rhizoma Coptidis 114
Rhizoma Corydalis 094,

164, 237, 357
Rhizoma Curculiginis 291, 315
Rhizoma Curcumae 052, 237, 359
Rhizoma Cyperi 117, 152
Rhizoma Dioscoreae 030, 102
Rhizoma et Radix Ligustici 327
Rhizoma et Radix Notopterygii 199, 223
Rhizoma Fagopyri Dibotryis 019, 090, 186
Rhizoma Gastrodiae 024
Rhizoma Imperatae 328
Rhizoma Imperatae Cylindricae 053, 189
Rhizoma Metaplexis 064
Rhizoma Metaplexis Japonicae 137, 260
Rhizoma Paridis 065
Rhizoma Phragmitis 112
Rhizoma Phragmitis Communis 225
Rhizoma Phragmitis Communis Recens 090
Rhizoma Pinelliae 029, 071, 106, 142, 238, 367
Rhizoma Pinelliae cum Succus Bambusae 090
Rhizoma Pinelliae Fermentata 085, 288
Rhizoma Pinelliae Fermentata 103
Rhizoma Pinelliae Praeparata 050, 081, 093, 142
Rhizoma Pinelliae Praeparatum 021, 269, 292, 301, 353
Rhizoma Pinelliae Preparata 049, 259, 348
Rhizoma Pinelliae Ternatae Praeparata 017, 060, 068
Rhizoma Polygonati 163, 190, 318, 345
Rhizoma Polygonati Odorati 264
Rhizoma Zingiberis 017, 068, 135, 238
Rhizoma Zingiberis Officinalis 032, 256, 284, 300
Rhizoma Zingiberis Praeparatum 187
Rhizoma Zingiberis Recens 038, 052, 066, 283, 312
Rhizoma Zingiberis Tostum 131, 310
Rhododendron Hance 328
Rhododendron Mariae Hance 068
right cardiomegaly 010
right qi 016, 029, 043, 070
right qi deficiency 145
right-sided heart failure 040, 166
ròu cōng róng 056, 231, 260, 366
ròu guì 024, 054, 063, 153, 231
ròu guì xīn 294
runny nose 277, 280

S

Saccharum Granorum 253
Sān Jīn Gāo 289
Sān Niù Tāng 050, 106, 120, 152, 284, 296, 343
sān qī 194
Sān Qī Zhù Shè Yè 167
sān yè qīng 344
Sān Zǐ Yǎng Qīn Tāng 021, 061, 148, 280, 296, 301
sāng bái pí 021, 051, 159
Sāng Bái Pí Tāng 105, 296
Sāng Jú Yǐn 124, 150
sāng shèn zǐ 088
sāng yè 080, 112, 158, 275, 317, 346
Scorpio 188, 266, 291, 314
Secretio Moschi 237, 292, 316, 359
seeking yang from yin 309
seeking yin from yang 309
Semen Arecae 098, 350
Semen Benincasae 114
Semen Bilobae 247
Semen Cannabis Sativae 103
Semen Cassiae 329

Semen Coicis 078, 186
Semen Cuscutae 066, 134, 194, 294, 311
Semen Euryales 044, 108, 171, 249, 253
Semen Ginkgo 043, 252, 307
Semen Ginkgo Bilobae 352
Semen Juglandis 044, 249
Semen Juglandis Regiae 032, 108, 122, 353
Semen Lablab Album Tostum 115
Semen Lepidii 254, 262
Semen Lepidii seu Descurainiae 018, 151, 226, 238, 354
Semen Lepidii seu Descurainiae Tostum 142
Semen Nelumbinis 249
Semen Persicae 021, 173, 339, 350
Semen Phaseoli 279
Semen Plantaginis 025, 039, 077
Semen Platycladi 046, 175
Semen Pruni 082, 175
Semen Pruni Armeniacae 369
Semen Raphani 021, 048, 051, 062, 112, 188, 194, 245, 278, 367
Semen Raphani Tostum 093, 121, 159
Semen Sinapis Albae 021, 032, 050, 236
Semen Sinapis Albae 239, 303
Semen Sinapis Albae Tostum 121
Semen Sojae Praeparatum 103, 289
Semen Sterculiae Lychnophorae 060
Semen Strychni 239, 358
Semen Torreyae 288
Semen Trichosanthis 103, 137, 180
Semen Trigonellae 294
Semen Vaccariae 240
Semen Zanthoxyli Bungeani 192, 249, 291, 314
Semen Ziziphi Spinosae 347
SemenRaphani Sativi 350
Senile Asthma 295
shā rén 056, 231
shā shēn 044, 101, 151
shān dòu gēn 192, 328, 329
Shān ěr Hé Jì 191, 206
shān hǎi luó 192
shān yào 030, 088, 102, 231
shān yú ròu 153, 232
shān zhū yú 026, 160
sháng yáng jiáo 202
sháo yào 162, 351
Sháo Yào Gān Cǎo Tāng 128
shé chuáng zǐ 344
Shé Dǎn Chuān Bèi Yè 034
shè gān 020, 348, 365, 367
Shè Gān Má Huáng Tāng 066, 113, 121, 142, 145, 303, 340
Shé shé cǎo 064
shè xiāng 237, 292, 316, 359
Shēn Bèi Liù Xián Sǎn 078
Shēn Fù Lóng Mǔ Tāng 026
Shēn Fù Tāng 138, 320
Shēn Gé Sǎn 105, 121
shēn gé sǎn 269
Shēn Mài Sǎn 026
Shēn Mài Zhù Shè Yè 162, 172
Shèn Qì Wán 078, 122, 164, 231, 286, 301
shén qū mò 103
Shēn Zhě Zhèn Qì Tāng 153, 171
shēng bái fán 103
shēng bái guǒ 244
shēng dà huáng 021, 099, 107
shēng dì 062, 067, 197
shēng dì huáng 160, 175, 260, 353
shēng dì yú 082
Shēng Dī Zhù Shè Yè 203, 209
shēng fǎ bàn xià 315
shēng gé qiào 262
shēng huáng qí 187

shēng lí 039
shēng má 317
shēng má huáng 127, 259, 330, 358
Shēng Má Tāng 128
Shēng Mài Jiāo Náng 034
Shēng Mài Sǎn 058, 076, 088, 122, 153, 170
shēng mǔ lì 081, 228
shēng shài shēn 186
shēng shí gāo 019, 098, 264, 291, 344
shēng shú dì huáng 263, 342
shēng zhě shí 099
shí chāng pú 023, 186, 264, 329
shí gāo 038, 069, 137
shí hú 088
shí wěi 368
Shí Zǎo Tāng 119
Shiraia Bambusicola 137, 161
shortness of breath 009, 014, 022, 029, 046, 061, 076, 086, 093, 094, 100, 101, 107, 121, 145, 153, 177, 194, 226, 228, 250, 258, 281, 297, 323
shú dì 054, 100, 131, 187, 194
shú fù piàn 192
shú fù zǐ 024, 118, 294
shǔ jiāo 288
Shuāng Huáng Lián Zhēn Fēn Jì 162

shuǐ gǔ 016
shuǐ zhì 187, 190
shuǐ zhì má huáng 259
Sì Chóng Qū Fēng Gù Běn Tāng 344, 370
Sì Jūn Zǐ Tāng 085, 160, 229, 282
Sì Nì Sǎn 124, 152, 343
Sì Nì Tāng 171
Sī Qí Kāng Zhù Shè Yè 196
Sì Wù Tāng 182
Sì Zǐ Píng Chuǎn Tāng 061
Sinking of the Gathering Qi 170
slurred speech 023
sneezing 277, 278, 280, 325
SOD 202
soluble intercellular adhesion molecule 187
sore throat 300
spasm 268, 291, 314, 331
spasmodic cough 295
Spina Gleditsiae Abnormalis 245, 350
Spleen and Kidney dual deficiency 313
Spleen and Lung qi deficiency 195
Spleen and Stomach qi deficiency 322
Spleen cough 128
Spleen deficiency 101, 131, 132, 138

Spleen qi deficiency 162, 169
Spleen yang deficiency 189, 197
spontaneous cold sweats 026
spontaneous perspiration 226, 231, 250, 296
spontaneous sweating 028, 029, 060, 089, 091, 170, 197
St. George's respiratory questionaire 189
stagnated cold transforming into heat 125
stagnated heat in the Lung 064
stagnation and obstruction of the Lung collaterals 271
Stagnation of Phlegm and Stasis 054
stagnation of wind-phlegm 154
Stalactitum Calcinatun 138
Stamen Nelumbinis 044, 046
Stamen Nelumbinis Nuciferae 253
Status asthmaticus 247
steaming bones 118
Stomach affecting the Lung 128
Stomach qi deficiency 251, 330

stridor 021, 077, 145, 151, 255, 280, 298, 336
stuffy nose 259
Sū Chén Jiǔ Bǎo Tāng 120, 124
sū gěng 263
sū yè 017, 052, 199, 264, 345
sū zǐ 098, 100, 142
Sū Zǐ Jiàng Qì Tāng 061, 089, 121, 324
suān zǎo rén 347
Succus Bambusae 019, 063, 139, 182
sudden collapse of yang qi 325, 334
sudden desertion of yang qi 312, 320, 326
Sulphur 237, 359
suǒ yáng 231
sweating 017, 019, 022, 029, 102, 111, 120, 131, 142, 145, 153, 168, 171, 178, 181, 182, 228, 258, 266, 320, 330, 334
sweats 230
swelling 110, 258, 259

T

Tōng Sè Kē Lì 186, 201
tachypnea 009, 056, 093, 112, 148
tāi pán 292, 315
Tāi Pán Wán 143, 322
tài zǐ shēn 048, 088, 189
Taiji 041
taiyang wind stroke 120
Talcum 077, 079
Tán Ké Jìng 233
Tán Rè Qīng Zhù Shè Yè 202, 208
tán xiāng 291, 314
tán yǐn 016
Táo Hóng Sì Wù Tāng 343
táo rén 021, 039, 069, 184, 339, 350
taxation fatigue 219
Tetrastlgma hemsleyanum 344
thirst 069, 077, 098, 121, 221, 255, 275, 296, 325
thoracic fluid retention 071
thoracic hyperinflation 217
tiān dōng 088, 115
tiān huā fěn 020, 088, 276
tiān jiāng ké 137, 260
tiān má 024
tiān mén dōng 318, 350
tián xìng rén 044
tiān zhú huáng 019, 023
Tiáo Bǔ Fèi Shèn Jiāo Náng 194, 207
Tiáo Wèi Chéng Qì Tāng 261
tidal fever 118, 171
Tíng Bèi Jiāo Náng 202
Tíng Lì Dà Zǎo Xiè Fèi Tāng 021, 282
Tíng Lì Píng Chuǎn Shuān 246, 354, 371
tíng lì zǐ 021, 106, 226, 323, 368
tinnitus 094, 118, 197
tonsillitis 258, 259
trachitis 058
Tremela 044
tù sī zǐ 066, 134, 194, 294, 311
tuberculosis 084
turbid phlegm retention 146
turbid phlegm smoldering in the Lung 087
TXB_2 201

U

ulcer 174
unconsciousness 012, 016
unsmooth breathing 219
unsmooth defecation 263, 277
upper respiratory infection 156

V

vacuity obesity 322, 326
Venenum Bufonis 329
vertigo 146
vexation 019, 020, 027, 059, 077, 122, 131, 147, 171, 184, 275, 284
vexing heat 150
vexing oppression 296
vexing thirst 225
viscous sweats 027
vomiting 093, 131, 145,

183, 336
vomiting phlegm 330

W

wáng bù liú xíng zǐ 240
Warm evil transforming into heat, contending with cold fluids 076
Water Flooding into the Flesh and Skin 147
water overflowing to form phlegm 131
weakness 170
wěi jīng 019, 031, 088, 190, 312, 323
Wěi Jīng Tāng 019, 170
wēi líng xiān 223
weight loss 009
Wēn Dǎn Tāng 147, 349, 370
Wēn Fèi Dìng Chuǎn Tāng 255
Wēn Fèi Tāng 296
wheezing 009, 086, 099, 103, 114, 149, 181, 217, 274, 290, 295, 296, 335
whooping cough 295
wind evils invading the Lung 156
wind-cold 017, 097, 106, 120, 142, 150, 154, 182, 220, 223, 225, 273, 278, 296, 299, 313, 330, 345, 361
wind-cold fettering the exterior 150, 296

Wind-Cold Fettering the Lung 257
wind-cold settling in the Lung 258
wind-cold tightening the Lung 317
wind-cold to transform into heat 156
wind-heat 017, 086, 150, 161, 273, 300, 345, 346
wind-heat attacking the Lung 317
wind-warm 112
Wood and Fire Torturing Metal 147
Wǔ Hǔ Tāng 296
wǔ jiā pí 026, 104
Wǔ Líng Sǎn 078
wū méi 101, 141, 291, 314
Wū méi 141
Wū Méi Wán 128
Wǔ Wèi Yì Gōng Sǎn 286
wǔ wèi zǐ 018, 121, 189, 274, 367
wú zhū yú 328, 329, 330
wǔ zhuǎ lóng 048
Wǔ Zǐ Dìng Chuǎn Tāng 278, 280
Wǔ Zǐ Píng Chuǎn Tāng 170

X

xī qīng guǒ 140, 141
Xī qīng guǒ 141
xī xiān cǎo 242, 360
xì xīn 017, 018, 022, 060,

071, 106, 118, 127, 130, 135, 164, 198, 283, 310, 369
xī yáng shēn 028, 078, 308
xiān dì sù 082
Xiān Fāng Huó Mìng Yǐn 161
xiān hè cǎo 263
xiān líng pí 066, 067
xiān lú gēn 090
xiān máo 291, 315, 319
xiān zhú lì 116
Xiān Zhú Lì Kǒu Fú Yè 033
xiān zhū xīn 044
xiāng fù 117, 152, 180, 184
xiāng rú 317
Xiāng Shā Liù Jūn Zǐ Tāng 066, 122, 162, 324
Xiāng Sū Yǐn 124
xiào 313
xiào bìng 335
Xiǎo Chái Hú Tāng 128
xiào chuǎn 276, 280, 290, 297, 338
xiào chuǎn bìng 314
Xiǎo Luó Zào Wán 103
Xiǎo Qīng Lóng Jiā Shí Gāo Tāng 132, 184
Xiǎo Qīng Lóng Tāng 018, 070, 106, 113, 121, 130, 145, 222, 284, 298, 300, 330, 342
xiǎo yá zào 303
xiào zhèng 219
xiè bái 329, 365
Xiè Bái Sǎn 087, 106, 124,

152
Xiè Tíng Hé Jì 200, 201, 208
Xīn Jiā Xiāng Rú Yǐn 124
Xīn Jiè Gāo 236
xīn yí 247, 327
Xìng Bèi Chōng Jì 245
xìng rén 019, 120, 256, 291, 351, 365
Xìng Rén Hú Táo Sǎn 038
Xìng Rén Tāng 347
Xìng Sū Er Chén Tāng 106, 107
xióng dǎn fěn 202
xú cháng qīng 346
xū chuǎn 168
xuán fù huā 049, 050, 079, 099, 143, 153, 328, 344, 346
Xuán Mài Gān Jié Jiāo Náng 033
xuán shēn 020, 078, 079, 099, 115, 118, 151, 175, 260
xuán yǐn 016, 119
xuě ěr 044
Xuè Fǔ Zhú Yū Tāng 147

Y

yá zào 288, 303, 304
yán hú suǒ 164, 237, 239, 357, 358, 359
Yán Nián Zī Wǎn Sǎn 085
yang deficiency 072, 126, 162, 173, 288, 338
yang deficiency affecting yin 056
Yang Deficiency and Phlegm-Stasis Turning to Heat 126
yang deficiency and water counterflow 122
yang deficiency and water overflowing 138
yang deficiency of the Kidney 353
Yang deficiency of the Spleen and Kidney 173
Yang Deficiency with Water Flooding 092
Yang deficiency with water flooding 093
Yáng Hé Píng Chuǎn Tāng 054
Yáng Hé Tāng 187, 205, 288
yáng jīn huā 244, 329, 339, 354
Yang qi deficiency 126
yáng ròu 250
Yǎng Yīn Qīng Fèi Zhú Yū Tāng Jiāng 191
yang-collapse 326
yě qiáo mài gēn 346, 348
yě rén shēn 270
Yì Fèi Jiàn Pí Fāng 193, 206
yì mǔ cǎo 025
Yì Qì Fú Zhèng Tāng 195, 207
yì yǐ rén 078, 186
Yī Yīn Jiān 133
yì yǐn 016
yì zhì rén 231
yin and yang deficiency 322
yin cold internally blocking 187
yin deficiency 059, 122, 175, 301, 338, 346
yin deficiency and insufficient blood 131
yin deficiency and phlegm-heat 289
yin deficiency of both the Lung and Kidney 039
yin deficiency of the Liver and Kidney 282
yin deficiency of the Lung 252
yin deficiency of the Lung and Kidney 241, 250, 345, 353
yin deficiency with heat 260
yin deficiency with hyperactivity of yang 330
yín huā 090
Yín Huáng Hé Jì 069
Yín Qiào Sǎn 112, 150, 161
yín xìng 143
yín yáng huò 054, 308, 315
yīng sù ké 119, 140
Yòu Guī Wán 133, 261
Yòu Guī Yǐn 133
yú biāo jiāo 252, 311
yù jīn 021, 023, 051, 118, 150
yù lǐ rén 175
Yú Mián Píng Chuǎn Fāng 368, 374

Yù Píng Fēng 228
Yù Píng Fēng Sǎn 028, 030, 066, 109, 145, 164, 226, 312, 319, 324
yú xīng cǎo 019, 069
Yú Xīng Cǎo Zhù Shè Yè 162, 196, 203, 204, 209, 355, 371
yù zhú 262, 345
yuán hú 094
yuán huā 119
yuǎn zhì 138, 143, 189, 302
Yuè Bì Jiā Bàn Xià Tāng 121, 123, 179, 184
Yuè Bì Jiā Fǎ Bàn Xià Tāng 296
Yuè Bì Zhú Xià Tāng 283
yún líng 189, 190, 232

Z

zàng hóng huā 270
zang organ 085, 115, 116, 123, 128, 148, 282
zào jiá 103, 246, 354
Zào Jiá Wán 243, 303
zào jiá zǐ 114
zào jiǎo 055, 103
zǎo xiū 065
zé lán 025, 197
zé qī 056, 065
Zé Qī Tāng 065
zé xiè 026, 077, 079, 094, 101, 102, 189, 232, 294, 298, 342
zhè bèi mǔ 019, 051, 081, 107, 119, 136, 150, 188,
190, 258, 348
zhě shí 171
Zhēn Wǔ Tāng 025, 122, 146
Zhēn Yuán Yǐn 286
zhēn zhū mǔ 094
zhì bǎi bù 084, 348
zhì bái qián 084
zhì bàn xià 349
zhì chuān hòu pò 091
zhì dōng huā 029
zhì dà huáng 186, 192, 202
zhì fǎ bàn xià 259
zhì fù zǐ 194, 197, 360
zhì jú hóng 050, 084, 149
Zhǐ Ké Dìng Chuǎn Tāng 050, 149
Zhǐ Ké Píng Chuǎn Gāo 197, 207
Zhǐ Ké Qīng Fèi Kǒu Fú Yè 191, 206
zhì kuǎn dōng 050, 149, 152
zhì má huáng 019, 031, 050, 087, 106, 186, 194, 254, 264, 310
zhī mǔ 118, 132, 137, 151, 260, 275, 281
zhì nán xīng 143, 197, 223
zhì pa ye 075, 279
zhǐ qiào 066, 087, 182, 225, 263, 347, 365
zhì sāng bái pí 090
zhǐ shí 023, 175, 247, 349
Zhǐ Sòu Sǎn 124, 135, 150
zhì sū zǐ 278, 344

Zhǐ Xiào Píng Chuǎn Fāng 373
Zhǐ Xiào Píng Chuǎn Tāng 365
zhì zào jiá 243
zhī zǐ 099
Zhì zǐ wǎn 029
zhì zǐ wǎn 084, 092, 278, 279
Zhū Bèi Dìng Chuǎn Wán 033
zhú huáng 099, 137, 161
zhú lì 019, 063, 099, 137, 139, 182, 259, 340
zhú lì shuǐ 023
zhū líng 079, 093
Zhū Líng Tāng 077, 079
Zhū Pāo Tāng 128
zhú rú 081, 083, 104, 137, 349
zhū shā 036
zhū yá zào jiǎo 245, 350
zǐ hé chē 108, 115, 139, 249, 297, 318, 319, 352
zǐ huā dù juān 038, 068, 328
Zǐ Jīn Dān 103
zǐ jīn niú 328
zǐ quán 065
Zī Shèn Yǎng Fèi Yīn 115
zǐ shí yīng 055, 263
zǐ sū 158, 249, 256, 257, 317, 327
zǐ sū yè 051, 150
zǐ sū zǐ 051, 151, 186
zǐ wǎn 049, 222, 272, 301
Zuǒ Guī Wán 133, 261

Notes

Notes

图书在版编目（CIP）数据

中医临床实用系列：慢性阻塞性肺疾病与哮喘（英文）/刘伟胜等主编；—北京：人民卫生出版社，2007.10
ISBN 978-7-117-09112-1

Ⅰ.中… Ⅱ.刘… Ⅲ.①哮喘—中医治疗法—英文 ②慢性病：肺栓塞—中医治疗法—英文 Ⅳ.R256.1

中国版本图书馆CIP数据核字（2007）第122392号

中医临床实用系列：慢性阻塞性肺疾病与哮喘（英文）

主　　编：刘伟胜　林　琳
出版发行：人民卫生出版社（中继线 +8610-6761-6688）
地　　址：中国北京市丰台区方庄芳群园三区3号楼
邮　　编：100078
网　　址：http://www.pmph.com
E - mail：pmph @ pmph.com
发　　行：zzg@pmph.com.cn
购书热线：+8610-6769-1034（电话及传真）
开　　本：787×1092　1/16
版　　次：2007年10月第1版　2007年10月第1版第1次印刷
标准书号：ISBN 978-7-117-09112-1/R · 9113

版权所有，侵权必究，打击盗版举报电话：+8610-8761-3394
（凡属印装质量问题请与本社销售部联系退换）